Vitamin K and Vitamin K-Dependent Proteins in Relation to Human Health

Special Issue Editors

Martin J. Shearer
Leon J. Schurgers

MDPI • Basel • Beijing • Wuhan • Barcelona • Belgrade

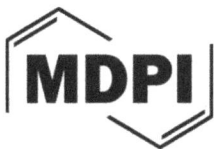

MDPI

Special Issue Editors
Martin J. Shearer
St. Thomas' Hospital
UK

Leon J. Schurgers
University of Maastricht
The Netherlands

Editorial Office
MDPI AG
St. Alban-Anlage 66
Basel, Switzerland

This edition is a reprint of the Special Issue published online in the open access journal
Nutrients (ISSN 2072-6643) from 205–2016 (available at:
http://www.mdpi.com/journal/nutrients/special_issues/vitamin-k-dependent-proteins).

For citation purposes, cite each article independently as indicated on the article
page online and as indicated below:

Lastname, F.M.; Lastname, F.M. Article title. *Journal Name.* **Year** *Article number,*
page range.

First Edition 2018

ISBN 978-3-03842-831-2 (Pbk)
ISBN 978-3-03842-832-9 (PDF)

Table of Contents

About the Special Issue Editors

Martin J. Shearer is a biochemist who worked in Guy's and St Thomas' NHS Foundation Trust as a Consultant Clinical Scientist (now emeritus). He is internationally recognized in the field of vitamin K research, in which his main research interests have been the role of vitamin K nutrition/metabolism and Gla proteins in health and disease, and the development of analytical methods for the evaluation of vitamin K status. This work was supported by prestigious academic or government institutions including the UK Medical Research Council, Department of Health and Food Standards Agency, collaborations with the US FDA and NIH, as well as industry. Martin is author or co-author of over 150 peer-reviewed scientific articles, book chapters, or symposium proceedings and has edited a book on vitamin K. Since 1988 he has served on several national or international expert committees and working groups including those convened by the WHO, FAO UN, UK Department of Health, and UK MHRA.

Leon J. Schurgers did his PhD on the role of vitamin K in bone and vasculature health in Maastricht and is now working as professor of vascular calcification in the Department of Biochemistry, which is part of the Cardiovascular Research Institute of the University of Maastricht. His project line aims to elucidate the molecular mechanisms of vitamin-K-dependent proteins (VKDP) by which (vascular) calcification is initiated and propagated: key cellular events include the activation and apoptosis of vascular smooth muscle cells (VSMC), fibroblasts and chondrocytes and extracellular vesicles containing VKDP. The regulation of VKDP biosynthesis, its sites of action, and the paradoxical observation that patients with low vitamin K status during oral anticoagulant treatment develop massive ectopic calcification is insufficient to understand the pathogenesis of calcification at a level that allows the development of novel diagnostic tools and therapeutic strategies for VKDP.

Preface to "Vitamin K and Vitamin K-Dependent Proteins in Relation to Human Health"

Vitamin K comprises a family of highly lipophilic molecules that possess a common 2-methyl-1, 4-naphthoquinone nucleus and a variable polyisoprenoid side chain at the 3-position that can vary in both length and degree of saturation. In nature, these forms are found as a single plant form (phylloquinone or vitamin K1) and a series of bacterial forms (menaquinones or vitamin K2).

In the four decades since the discovery of the vitamin-K-dependent mechanism of the γ-glutamyl carboxylation of proteins, our perception of vitamin K has been transformed from a single-function 'haemostasis vitamin' to that of a 'multi-function vitamin' with roles in processes as diverse as bone and cardiovascular mineralization, vascular integrity, energy metabolism, immune response, and brain metabolism. At the cellular level, some of these effects appear to be mediated by pathways involving cellular growth, survival, and signalling. The transformational mechanistic discovery was made in 1974, namely that vitamin K acts as a cofactor for a microsomal enzyme, γ-carboxyglutamyl carboxylase, that catalyzes the conversion of specific peptide-bound glutamate residues found in certain specialized proteins to γ-carboxyglutamate (Gla). While attention initially focused on how this post-translational modification could explain the essentiality of vitamin K for the synthesis of the already-known vitamin-K-dependent blood coagulation proteins, a search for evidence of other non-haemostatic vitamin-K-dependent proteins (also known as Gla proteins) in other tissues quickly led to the discovery of osteocalcin and matrix Gla protein (MGP) and later to several other Gla-proteins that include Gas6, proline-rich Gla proteins, Gla-rich protein and periostin. Alongside these discoveries came the revelation that the process of γ-glutamyl carboxylation in the endoplasmic endothelium of cells was intimately linked to the production of the metabolite vitamin K epoxide and to an enzymatic pathway, whereby the epoxides of various molecular forms of vitamin K are reduced back to the substrate form and thereby retained for future cofactor functions in membrane γ-glutamyl carboxylation reactions. This salvage pathway is called the vitamin K (epoxide) cycle, of which a major feature is the reduction of vitamin K epoxide by the enzyme vitamin K epoxide reductase (VKOR). It is the inhibition of VKOR by vitamin K antagonists such as warfarin that forms the pharmacological basis of the anticoagulant therapy that has been a mainstay of the treatment and prevention of thrombotic disorders.

A major aim of this book was to compile a set of articles that reflect the diversity of modern research into vitamin K, which ranges from pure nutrition to the structural biology of key regulators of vitamin K function and metabolism. As with other vitamins, a central tenet is the occurrence of states of vitamin K deficiency and their prevention. It is also important to distinguish between overt and subclinical vitamin K deficiency. The classic symptoms of overt vitamin K deficiency is a reduction in the four vitamin-K-dependent procoagulant proteins (factors II, VII, IX and X) sufficient to cause bruising and/or bleeding. Although very rare in adults, except in malabsorption syndromes, vitamin K deficiency bleeding (VKDB) is less rare in newborns and early infancy. At this age VKDB has potentially devastating and fatal consequences because bleeding commonly occurs in the brain. In addition, bleeding in neonates can occur spontaneously so that with no available screening test, it is now common paediatric practice throughout the world to protect all newborn infants by giving them vitamin K prophylaxis as soon as they are born. However, in spite of prophylaxis, VKDB is still a significant cause of morbidity and mortality in early infancy, especially in developing countries. This volume includes two articles that address the topic of VKDB or vitamin K status in early infancy, one article focusses on the prevalence of vitamin K insufficiency in Uganda, and the other article focusses on the nutritional intakes and sources of phylloquinone in preterm infants in the UK.

Although oral vitamin K antagonists have been in clinical use as anticoagulants for some 60 years, the gene encoding VKOR was not discovered until the year 2004. This book contains three articles from the institute and authors credited with the co-discovery of the VKOR gene who have made prominent contributions to the current knowledge of the structure–function relationships of VKOR and its paralog VKORL1. These paralogous proteins possess similar or identical enzymatic functions and have persisted in vertebrates throughout approximately 400 million years of evolution. This book includes two articles that explore these evolutionary relationships in order to gain insights into the reasons for the ubiquitous presence of these enzymes in all taxa from the entire tree of life, with the exception of yeasts and fungi. The third article from this group addresses the structure–function relationships and molecular mechanisms of VKOR in humans. Such studies are clinically important due to there being two types of VKOR mutations with different phenotypes. Firstly, one class of several VKOR mutations confers a phenotype of 'warfarin resistance', for which much higher doses of VKA are required to achieve stable anticoagulation. Secondly, a single, rare autosomal recessive mutation of VKOR results in a bleeding disorder characterized by a combined deficiency of vitamin-K-dependent coagulation factors, which can be corrected by vitamin K supplementation. Also included in this book is a review article of the clinical and nutritional pros and cons of using traditional vitamin K antagonists as anticoagulants compared to the recently developed direct oral anticoagulants that do not depend for their effect on the inhibition of VKOR. This review reveals that a major downside of vitamin K antagonists such as warfarin is that they induce vascular calcification, probably by inhibiting MGP carboxylation (see also below). Due to their different mechanism of action, direct anticoagulants are not expected to cause vascular calcification, and importantly allow patients taking them to take vitamin K supplements for their putative health benefits without concern that they will disrupt anticoagulant efficacy.

An important modern area of vitamin K research comprises several topics that come under the umbrella of non-coagulation functions of vitamin K. Although many of these putative non-coagulation functions of vitamin K are thought to be mediated by the expression of different Gla proteins in target extrahepatic tissues, there is evidence that other cellular functions are driven by menaquinone-4. This vitamin K2 form is particularly abundant in endocrine and exocrine glands as well as in major organs such as the brain, bone and skin. Although some menaquinone-4 is present in the diet, most tissue menaquinone-4 derives from its synthesis within the body from dietary phylloquinone. These extrahepatic functions of vitamin K are covered in several articles. They include a study of human cognition based on longstanding evidence that vitamin K is implicated in the synthesis of brain sphingolipids. More recent evidence suggests that menaquinone-4 is concentrated in the brain and has unique cellular functions not shared by other forms of vitamin K. In this book, the relevance of menaquinone-4 synthesis from phylloquinone is addressed in an article describing a nutritional research study that investigated the tissue concentrations of these two vitamers in a lifetime study of rats.

Recently, an increasingly important research area is based on the knowledge that the Gla protein MGP is a major inhibitor of calcification. The obligatory requirement of a functional MGP throughout life was amply illustrated by findings in 1997 that MGP-knockout mice die within eight weeks of birth due to the rupture of severely calcified arteries. Many other studies have confirmed that only the γ-glutamyl carboxylated form of MGP is able to inhibit vascular calcification, and that vitamin K insufficiency is common among certain patient populations. The mechanism of arterial calcification is complex: it is not, as previously thought, a passive mineralization process, but an actively-regulated, cell-mediated interplay between promotors and inhibitors. Two patient populations in which cardiovascular calcification is associated with substantial morbidity and mortality, and in which vitamin K insufficiency is also common, are chronic kidney disease and diabetes mellitus. Because coronary artery calcification develops early in the pathogenesis of atherosclerosis, researchers have hypothesized that vitamin K supplementation aimed to maximize the γ-glutamyl carboxylation of MGP may have beneficial effects on the vasculature by ameliorating vascular calcification. This topic is covered in this book by two articles that explore the practical role of nutritional vitamin K supplementation in the reduction of cardiovascular calcification. One article reports data from a murine model and the other sets out the strategy and protocol of the first randomized trial of vitamin K supplementation using the vitamin K2 form, menaquinone-7, in patients with coronary artery disease.

Finally a timely review article addresses the importance of being able to accurately assess the nutritional status of vitamin K in humans. This review discusses the concepts and controversies in the evaluation of vitamin K status at both the individual and population level. This field is complicated because of the occurrence of multiple dietary forms of vitamin K, complex metabolism (which includes the conversion of phylloquinone to menaquinone-4), and the fact that the requirements for vitamin K appear to be tissue specific. This tissue specificity lies both with the variability of the efficiency of vitamin K transport mechanisms to different tissues and the wide heterogeneity of Gla proteins possessing different efficiencies for the γ-glutamyl carboxylation reaction. For such reasons, multiple biomarkers of vitamin K status are usually required that reflect both tissues stores and the function of the Gla protein(s) under study.

We believe this collection illustrates the variety of topics currently under study in the vitamin K field and is representative of the progress being made in our understanding of the structural biology, genetics, biochemistry, physiology and nutrition of vitamin K and/or vitamin-K-dependent proteins, particularly in relation to human health.

Martin J. Shearer and Leon J. Schurgers

Special Issue Editors

nutrients

MDPI

Article

Phylogeny of the Vitamin K 2,3-Epoxide Reductase (VKOR) Family and Evolutionary Relationship to the Disulfide Bond Formation Protein B (DsbB) Family

Carville G. Bevans [1], Christoph Krettler [2], Christoph Reinhart [2], Matthias Watzka [3] and Johannes Oldenburg [3,*]

[1] Im Hermeshain 6, 60388 Frankfurt am Main, Germany; E-Mail: bevans@jhu.edu
[2] Department of Molecular Membrane Biology, Max Planck Institute of Biophysics,
    60388 Frankfurt am Main, Germany; E-Mails: christoph.krettler@biophys.mpg.de (C.K.);
    christoph.reinhart@biophys.mpg.de (C.R.)
[3] Institute of Experimental Haematology and Transfusion Medicine, University Clinic Bonn,
    53105 Bonn, Germany; E-Mail: matthias.watzka@ukb.uni-bonn.de
*   Author to whom correspondence should be addressed; E-Mail: johannes.oldenburg@ukb.uni-bonn.de;
    Tel.: +49-228-287-15175; Fax: +49-228-287-14783.

Received: 18 May 2015 / Accepted: 9 July 2015 / Published: 29 July 2015

Abstract: In humans and other vertebrate animals, vitamin K 2,3-epoxide reductase (VKOR) family enzymes are the gatekeepers between nutritionally acquired K vitamins and the vitamin K cycle responsible for posttranslational modifications that confer biological activity upon vitamin K-dependent proteins with crucial roles in hemostasis, bone development and homeostasis, hormonal carbohydrate regulation and fertility. We report a phylogenetic analysis of the VKOR family that identifies five major clades. Combined phylogenetic and site-specific conservation analyses point to clade-specific similarities and differences in structure and function. We discovered a single-site determinant uniquely identifying VKOR homologs belonging to human pathogenic, obligate intracellular prokaryotes and protists. Building on previous work by Sevier *et al.* (*Protein Science* 14:1630), we analyzed structural data from both VKOR and prokaryotic disulfide bond formation protein B (DsbB) families and hypothesize an ancient evolutionary relationship between the two families where one family arose from the other through a gene duplication/deletion event. This has resulted in circular permutation of primary sequence threading through the four-helical bundle protein folds of both families. This is the first report of circular permutation relating distant α-helical membrane protein sequences and folds. In conclusion, we suggest a chronology for the evolution of the five extant VKOR clades.

Keywords: cyclic permutation; DsbB; homology modeling; phylogeny; sequence conservation; vitamin K; vitamin K 2,3-epoxide; VKOR; VKORC1; VKORC1L1

---

1. Introduction

In humans and other animals, vitamin K 2,3-epoxide complex subunit 1 (VKORC1) is the primary oxidoreductase enzyme that reduces vitamin K quinone (K), acquired in trace amounts by dietary uptake, to the hydroquinone (KH_2) form, functioning as the point of entry for vitamin K into the vitamin K cycle [1–3]. Subsequently, vitamin K hydroquinone is oxidized to vitamin K 2,3-epoxide (K>O) during the posttranslational activation of vitamin K-dependent (VKD) proteins involving enzymatic conversion of specific glutamate (Glu) residues to γ-carboxyglutamate (Gla) residues. To complete the cycle, VKORC1 sequentially reduces K>O to K and KH_2, ensuring that the limiting trace amounts of vitamin K are efficiently recycled to drive further rounds of γ-glutamyl carboxylation.

VKORC1 has been demonstrated to be essential to the production of VKD blood clotting factors which takes place in liver hepatocytes [4]. Suboptimal availability of K from dietary sources can eventually result in interruption of vitamin K cycle turnover and lead to pathophysiological anticoagulation and, in the extreme case, uncontrollable bleeding [3,5]. In the case of pathological hypercoagulative conditions such as thrombosis and embolism, 4-hydroxycoumarin based oral anticoagulants, including warfarin as a well-known example, are administered to block the enzymatic function of VKORC1, effectively diminishing turnover of the vitamin K cycle [6]. This results in induction of a controlled hypocoagulative state to counteract the tendency towards clot formation. Thus, the biological action of vitamin K on hemostasis, mediated by function of the VKORC1 enzyme, is entirely dependent on vitamin K nutritional status and, occasionally, on treatment with oral anticoagulant drugs. Very recently, evidence has been presented that a second VKOR enzyme, VKORC1-like 1 (VKORC1L1), is responsible for extrahepatic VKOR activity crucial to bone growth and homeostasis [7,8]. Interestingly, although VKORC1L1 carries out the same two enzymatic steps of the vitamin K cycle as does VKORC1, it appears to be far less sensitive to oral anticoagulant drugs, suggesting that its biological activity may not be substantially reduced when oral anticoagulants are administered at levels that effectively modulate hemostasis and reduce coagulation tendency [7,9].

To date, homologous VKOR enzymes have been detected in hundreds of prokaryotic and eukaryotic species through whole genome sequencing efforts. A number of representative VKOR enzymes from bacteria, plants and animals have been cloned and studied [7,9–16]. Surprisingly, bacterial and plant VKOR homologs studied so far have been shown to not possess K>O de-epoxidase (VKOR) activity and do not use K>O as a substrate. Alternatively, these enzymes possess only quinone reductase activity which reduces ubiquinone or K substrates to the respective hydroquinone forms. Thus, an updated analysis of VKOR oxidoreductase family phylogenetics and associated review of functional and structural similarities and differences is warranted.

Structural and functional similarities among prokaryotic periplasmic and eukaryotic ER-resident oxidoreductase families involved in oxidative protein folding have been previously suggested, although lack of significant sequence homology suggests these families arose independently during evolution [17]. Specifically, these include Endopasmic Reticulum Oxidoreductin 1 (ERO1, PFAM PF04137, common to all eukaryotes), Augmenter of Liver Regeneration (Erv1/Alr, PFAM PF04777, common to all eukaryotes, some proteobacteria, cyanobacteria and all known cytoplasmic DNA virus taxa), and Disulfide Bond-forming protein B (DsbB, PFAM PF02600, common only to prokaryotes) families that share similar pairs of redox-active disulfide motifs [18]. Recently, studies confirmed a direct role for VKORC1 in oxidative protein folding in addition to its classically reported role in the vitamin K cycle which enables post-translational γ-glutamyl carboxylation of vitamin K-dependent proteins including a number of blood clotting factors [19,20]. VKORC1 is a representative of the vitamin K epoxide reductase family (VKOR, PFAM PF07884), named for the enzymatic function first identified in humans and rodents, namely, vitamin K 2,3-epoxide reductase (VKOR) activity, which is potently inhibited by warfarin and other 4-hydroxycoumarin derivatives [10,11]. Since the 1950s, warfarin and homologous 4-hydroxycoumarins have been the most widely prescribed oral anticoagulants to treat thromboembolitic diseases in humans and, at much higher, lethal dosages as rodenticides [21]. VKOR family sequences also possess two redox-active cysteine pairs and have been detected in taxa from the entire Tree of Life except for yeasts and fungi [22,23]. In prokaryotes, either VKOR or DsbB homologs are required for oxidative protein folding (Figure 1) [24,25]. Both DsbB and VKOR enzymes receive reducing equivalents via thioredoxin-like (Trx-like) oxidoreductases from pairs of redox-active cysteines during oxidative protein folding, ultimately passing the reducing equivalents to diffusible quinone cofactors. DsbB cofactors include ubiquinones (UQ) principally for aerobically respiring taxa and menaquinones (MK, K_2 vitamins) for anaerobic respirants [26]. With the exception of only a very few obligate intracellular prokaryotic pathogens, all prokaryotic VKOR homologs apparently use UQ or MK, while plant VKORs use phylloquinone (PK, vitamin K_1) as the sole electron accepting cofactor. All other eukaryote genomes from single-celled protists through higher invertebrates and vertebrates, but not those of fungi, encode VKOR homologs that can use MK or PK as cofactors, while jawed vertebrates (gnathostomes) can additionally use the more highly oxidized 2,3-epoxides of K vitamins which are naturally produced only in taxa possessing genomically encoded-glutamyl carboxlase homologs. While menaquinone 2,3-epoxides have been found in vertebrates, they are not known to exist in any prokaryotes [27,28].

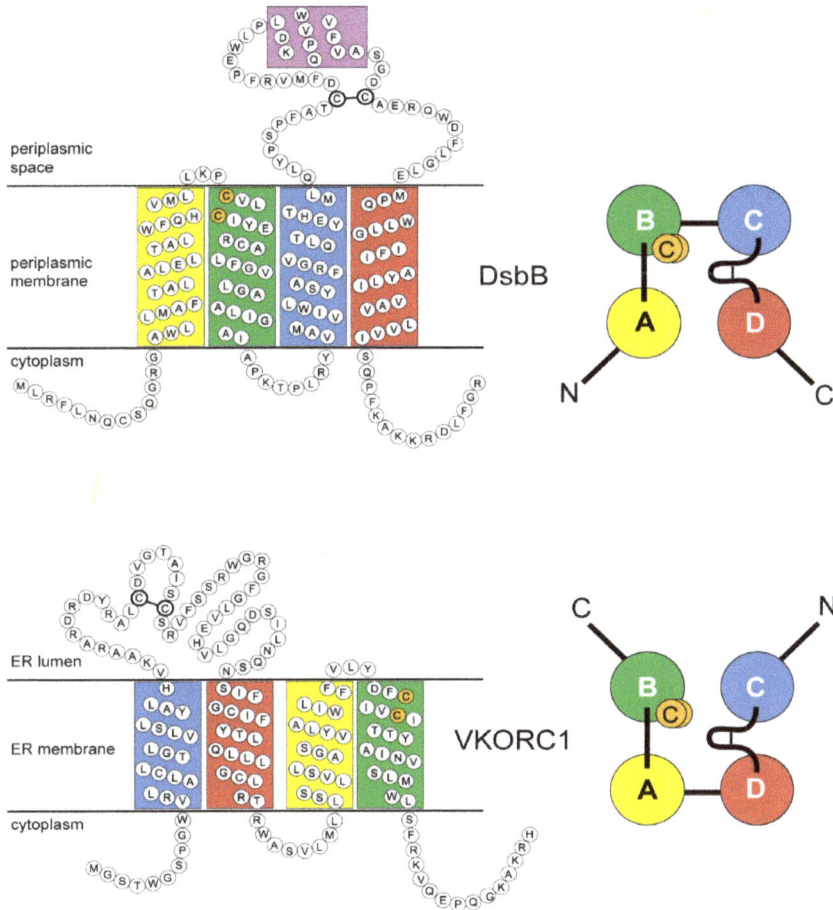

Figure 1. Relationship of structural elements for *E. coli* DsbB and human VKORC1. Single-letter amino acids (circles); transmembrane helices (four colored rectangles; coloring scheme according to [17]); two active site cysteines (orange circles); DsbB (top left) short helix (purple rectangle); two redox-active cysteines in DsbB large periplasmic loop (thick connected circles); Human VKORC1 (bottom left), transmembrane helix colors for homologous positions relative to DsbB. Transmembrane helical bundle organization and primary sequence threading (N, N-terminus; C, C-terminus) for DsbB (top right, view from periplasm) and VKORC1 (bottom right, view from ER lumen) are shown based on X-ray crystallographic structures. Letters A–D on the right side indicate helix designations used throughout the text. N- to C-terminus direction threading of the primary sequence through DsbB is "ABCD", but "CDAB" for VKORC1; thus, both threadings are related to each other by circular permutation (CP). Structural elements for DsbB from PDB entry 2HI7 [29], for VKORC1 from PDB entry 3KP9 [14].

Five studies have previously explored VKOR family phylogeny. Rost *et al.* (2004) reported cloning paralogous pairs of VKOR genes in human, rat, mouse and the fish Takifugu ruprides and identified VKOR homologs by gene annotations in the mosquito Anopheles gambiae, but not in the fruit fly Drosophila melangaster, suggesting that evolution of VKOR family proteins was later than the evolution of carboxylase enzymes for which *Drosophila* is known to possess a homologous gene [10]. They also noted the existence of two human VKORC1 retropseudogenes that arose independently. Goodstadt & Ponting (2004) presented a multiple sequence alignment analysis identifying VKOR homologs in 37 species of archaea, eubacteria, plants, invertebrates and vertebrates [22]. They further identified four conserved cysteines and a conserved serine/threonine as residues likely required for enzymatic function. Additionally, they noted that many plant and prokaryote VKOR homologs are multidomain proteins that often include a C-terminal thioredoxin-like domain in addition to the core VKOR domain. Using prediction algorithms, they also identified four putative transmembrane helices in the VKOR core domain. Indeed, a four-helical bundle organization of the VKOR domain was recently confirmed for a prokaryotic VKOR homolog by X-ray crystallographic analysis [14,30]. A study by Robertson (2004) confirmed that, while vertebrate genomes encode two VKOR paralogs, only single VKOR homologs are present in invertebrates, basal deuterostomes, protists and plants with no VKOR homologs detected in fungal taxa [23]. He also identified additional VKOR family retropseudogenes—three similar to human VKORC1L1, five similar to VKORC1L1 in mouse and three with VKORC1L1 similarity in rat. In contrast to the report by Rost *et al.*, Robertson was able to detect a VKOR homolog sequence in *Drosophila melanogaster* [10]. Robertson calculated an inferred phylogenetic tree with low bootstrap support using trypanosome protists as an outgroup, representing the most highly divergent homologs from higher animals. His results suggest that a gene duplication occurred resulting in VKORC1 and VKORC1L1 clades after vertebrates diverged from non-chordates. Schwarz *et al.* (2009) used profile hidden Markov models derived from multiple sequence alignments and correspondence analysis to distinguish between evolutionary and functional site-specific signals for VKORC1/VKORC1L1 paralog pairs of twelve vertebrate species [31]. Their analytical methods were able to distinguish functionally conserved and variable sites, detect clade-specific sequence clustering and revealed specific sites associated with clade splittings. Importantly, they identified the timing of the duplication event leading to VKORC1 and VKORC1L1 paralogs as occurring at the base of the vertebrate split from other metazoans. Finally, a recent study by Wan *et al.* (2014) that identified and characterized a VKOR family homolog in the tomato plant, presented evidence suggesting that all plant VKOR homologs possess an N-terminal signal peptide responsible for transit of the protein to inner thylakoid membranes and a C-terminal thioredoxin-like domain with four conserved cysteines [16]. They constructed a phylogenetic tree with 41 species that include plants, algae, photosynthetic bacteria and vertebrate animals. Vertebrates, monocot and dicot plants were segregated into three distinct clades, while conifers, mosses, cyanobacteria and green algae formed a weak clade with low branch support. Highest branch supports were for monocots and vertebrates.

In the present study, we reconstruct a comprehensive phylogeny for the VKOR family that includes 327 sequences from major representative phyla of the Kingdoms of Life and use the results to define major clades, explore clade-specific sequence differences that correlate with structural and functional differences of the clades, and propose an evolutionary scenario for the VKOR family that suggests an ancient common ancestor shared with the DsbB family.

2. Experimental Section

2.1. Protein Sequences and Multiple Sequence Alignments

Protein sequences were obtained from the NCBI Conserved Domain Database (http://www.ncbi.nlm.nih.gov/cdd/) and from the PFAM database (http://pfam.xfam.org) for VKOR (CDD: cl01729, VKOR Superfamily, 3748 raw sequences; PFAM: PF07884, VKOR family, 864 raw sequences) and DsbB (CDD: cl00649, DsbB Superfamily, 6673 raw sequences; PFAM:

PF02600, DsbB family, 2959 raw sequences) families [32,33]. For each family, sequences were initially aligned using the MAFFT fast algorithm (FFT-NS-1 option) implemented in JalView2.8 by masking non-core domain sequence segments (core domains defined as DsbB (*E. coli*): Trp15-Ile162 and VKOR (*Synechococcus* sp.): Ile22-Val148 including first residue of first transmembrane helix to last residue of fourth transmembrane helix based on X-ray crystallographic data from PDB entries 2HI7 and 3KP9, respectively) [34,35]. Identical sequences from redundant species, partial or unrelated sequences not fully encompassing the core domain lengths, and sequences lacking known conserved residues were manually culled. Further reduction of sequences in over-represented phyla and classes resulted in final data sets of 327 non-redundant VKOR and 514 non-redundant DsbB sequences for phylogenetic analysis. The DsbB family multiple sequence alignment (MSA) was not subjected to further phylogenetic analysis. For the full-length (multidomain) MSA for the VKOR family, N- and C-terminal non-core domains were aligned independently of the core domain. Core domain alignment was iteratively refined based on WSP and consistency scores using MAFFT (G-INS-i option) and manually adjusted to align any obvious positionally conserved residues while minimizing the number of gapped segments. Additional sequence-truncated versions of each MSA included either only the core domains (defined above) or a 44 residue subsequence comprising the large loop joining the 1st and 2nd transmembrane helices of the VKOR core domain ("VKORloop"—delimited by VKORC1(*H. sapiens*): Asp36-Ser79). All multiple sequence alignment and tree files are included with the online Supplementary Materials and Research Data.

2.2. Phylogenetic Analyses

Maximum Likelihood (ML) analyses were conducted using the TOPALi2 ver2.5 (http://www.topali.org/index.shtml) and IQ-TREE ver1.2.3 (http://www.cibiv.at/software/iqtree/) server-based phylogenetic packages [36,37]. Phylogenetic model testing and selection included 40 distinct models by TOPALi2 and 150 models by IQ-TREE. Model evaluation was based on standard Akaike infomation criterion (AIC), corrected AIC (cAIC) and Bayesian information criterion (BIC) scores, where best models correlate with minimized scores. Preliminary ML phylogenetic tree reconstructions were estimated using either PhyML3.0 [38] or RaxML8.0.0 [39] with branch supports for 1000 bootstrap replicates calculated by the rapid UFBoot method [40]. The final VKORloop consensus tree was constructed from 1000 bootstrap trees using the IQ-TREE1.0 tree search algorithm [37]. Branch lengths were optimized by maximum likelihood on original alignment and bootstrap branch support calculated. To simplify visual presentation, the consensus tree was further pruned to 310 sequences using IQ-TREE1.0 and graphically rendered using the Interactive Tree of Life (iTOL) server (http://itol.embl.de) [41].

2.3. Assessment of Residue-Specific Evolutionary Conservation and Structural Correlates

For determination of residue-specific sequence conservation from VKOR and DsbB family MSAs, we used the ConSurf server (http://consurf.tau.ac.il) [42,43]. Briefly, ConSurf computes position-specific evolutionary rate inferences as continuous-variable conservation scores using the empirical Bayesian algorithm. The server creates an output text file where the continuous conservation scores are binned into nine grades for visualization, from the most variable positions (grade 1, colored turquoise), through intermediately conserved positions (grade 5, colored white), to the most conserved positions (grade 9, colored maroon). We mapped these conservation grades onto MSAs using JalView2.8 for analysis and graphical rendering. We further explored structural features corresponding to the conservation data revealed by ConSurf analysis by using the TMPad server (http://bio-cluster.iis.sinica.edu.tw/TMPad/) to visualize and determine residues involved in direct interhelical contacts from the representative X-ray crystallographic structures (PDB entries 2HI7 and 3KP9) [44].

2.4. Homology Modeling of Human VKORC1 and VKORC1L1 Paralogs Using a Cyclic Permutation of E. coli DsbB as the Target Structure

Homology models of human VKORC1 and VKORC1L1 were created using template sequences from the NCBI Protein database (Accession: Q9BQB6.1 GI: 62511226 and Accession: Q8N0U8.2 GI: 62511214, respectively) and *E. coli* DsbB (PDB entry 2K74, model 1 [45]) as template structure. The nearly identical lengths of DsbB (176 aa), VKORC1 (163 aa) and VKORC1L1 (176 aa) suggested to us that indels would not be a major concern in modeling. Briefly, we swapped the first and second halves of the VKORC1 and VKORC1L1 primary sequences in order to create an optimized alignment to the DsbB sequence (see Figures S1–S4 and detailed methods in the online Supplementary Materials and Research Data) and generated initial models using MODELLER 9v7 [46]. In order to restore the native primary sequences and threading, the best quality initial models were edited to join the N- and C-termini and create new termini at the loop between the second and third transmembrane helices (TMHs) using Coot 0.6-pre-1 [47]. The 50 residue loops between the first and second TMHs of the edited models were replaced with same-sequence loops *de novo* modeled using the I-TASSER server [48]. Addition of hydrogen atoms and quality assessment of final models was performed using the MolProbity server [49]. Final models were submitted to the Protein Model DataBase (VKORC1: PMDB entry PM0075969, VKORC1L1: PM007970; both models deposited 21 September 2009, public release 1 September 2010).

3. Results

3.1. Multiple Sequence Alignments Reveal Greater Inhomogeneity in Indels for the VKOR Family Core Domain Relative to the DsbB Family

Initial inspection of high quality multiple sequence alignments for the core domains of the VKOR family (327 sequences, truncated to residues corresponding to human VKORC1: Leu13-Phe150 in order to remove highly variable N- and C-terminal sequences) and DsbB family (514 sequences, truncated to residues corresponding to *E. coli* DsbB: Gly13-Pro165 in order to remove highly variable N- and C-terminal sequences) revealed a larger heterogeneity in indel sizes and locations for the VKOR core domain (10 major indels for >1 sequences, ranging 2–27 residues in length) relative to the DsbB core domain (5 major indels for >1 sequences, ranging 2–11 residues in length) (see online Supplementary Materials Figures S5 and S6 and Research Data for FASTA-formatted MSA and graphical summary files; only non-terminal indels were counted in order to avoid possible incomplete sequencing reads in the original data; minor indels comprising single residues were not included.) Thus, the greater overall sequence diversity for the VKOR family core domain suggests greater overall evolutionary diversity, relative to the DsbB core domain. This is consistent with the evolutionary limitation of DsbB family taxa to prokaryotes *versus* the expansion of the VKOR family taxa into all major Kingdoms of Life.

3.2. VKOR Family Phylogeny is Organized into Five Principal Clades

Testing of standard phylogenetic amino acid substitution models using both TOPALi2 and IQ-TREE for the VKOR family MSA using 327 non-redundant full-length sequences resulted in the Whelan & Goldman rate heterogeneity model with invariant sites as the best model (see online Supplementary Materials and Research Data for sequences, MSAs and substitution model statistics). Subsequent phylogeny reconstruction using PhyML or RaxML revealed unrooted trees with five large cladistic groupings, although two clades included mixed prokaryotic, invertebrate and vertebrate VKOR homologs and animal sequences were found among the predominantly bacterial and plant clades. Similar results were obtained, with increased mingling of prokaryotic sequences among the predominantly invertebrate and vertebrate clades, when we truncated the MSA to include only the VKOR core domain (defined in Section 2.1). Previous reports have suggested that TMHs considerably contribute to phylogenetic noise, due to high frequency of occurrence and degeneracy among nonpolar residues in the hydrophobic membrane core and a relatively low selection pressure on residues that face into the lipid bilayer [50,51]. Also, a phylogenetic study of DsbB family homologs reported difficulties in automated sequence alignments due to amino acid compositional bias in the transmembrane region [52]. Accordingly, to enhance phylogenetic signal-to-noise levels for the VKOR family, we chose to further truncate the MSA to the large loop segment between the first two TMHs for two principal reasons: (1) the loop includes three out of five conserved residues known to be essential to VKOR enzymatic activity and other residues in this segment may also contribute to substrate specificity and/or catalysis; and (2) the loop is known to bind to and accept reducing equivalents from species-specific partner oxidoreductases essential for VKOR enzymatic function *in vivo* [53]. Thus, the loop-specific sequences (50 residues) encode a large amount of evolutionary information pertinent to enzyme function. Indeed, phylogeny reconstruction using the VKORloop sequences (corresponding to human VKORC1: Asp36-Ser79) and the best model (WAG + I + G) yielded a consensus tree with well-defined clades consistent with proposed versions of the Tree of Life based on, for example, ribosomal protein or tRNA synthase phylogeny (Figure 2) [54–57].

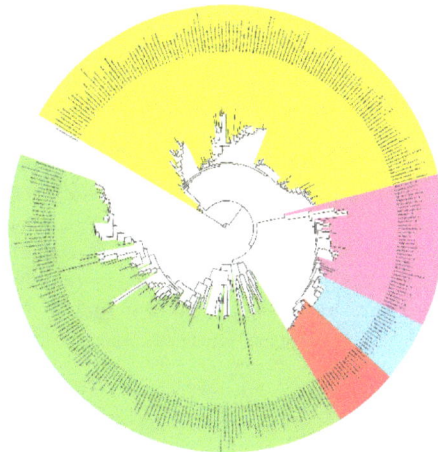

Figure 2. Maximum likelihood-estimated phylogeny for VKOR family based on VKORloop sequences for 327 non-redundant sequences (pruned to 310 sequences). Five major clades are shown in color (yellow, non-photosynthetic prokaryotes; green, photosynthetic prokaryotes and plants; magenta, primitive single-celled animals and invertebrates; blue, vertebrate VKORC1L1 homologs; red, vertebrate VKORC1 homologs. Tree is rooted using the archaeon *Caldivirga maquilingensis* as outgroup (single uncolored branch between yellow and green clades). Numbers at branches (see online Supplementary Materials and Research Data; visible when enlarged in PDF reader) indicate bootstrap supports (%). Accurate inclusion of all sequences in the VKORC1 and VKORC1L1 clades was manually verified despite incorrect annotations in some sequence database entries that led to false name assignments (e.g., where C1 and L1, representing VKORC1 and VKORC1L1, respectively, are indicated after the genus/species names). A PDF file of this figure is included with online supplementary data for enlarged viewing.

Figure 3 summarizes the major taxonomic classes and phyla comprising the five clades for the 327 non-redundant sequences. Clade 1 (Figure 2, colored yellow) is polyphyletic and includes non-photosynthetic archea and eubacteria. Actinobacteria, one of the three major Gram-positive phyla, comprise the major grouping along with acidobacteria, crenarchaeota (including species of the *Caldivirga*, *Pyrobaculum* and *Thermoproteus* genera grouped together in a discrete subclade), proteobacteria and spirochete representatives. All actinobacteria possess a predicted fifth transmembrane helix (TMH), but no C-terminal Trx-like domain, whereas proteobacteria and spirochetes possess both a fifth TMH and C-terminal Trx-like domain. Clades 2 and 3 (Figure 2, blue and red, respectively) are both individually and together monophyletic and include members of the vertebrate VKORC1 and VKORC1L1 paralogs, respectively, as single VKOR domains. Clade 4 (Figure 2, magenta) is paraphyletic and comprises single-domain VKOR homologs encoded in genomes of non-vertebrate animals including amoebazoans, choanoflagellates and lower metazoans through invertebrates. Clade 5 (Figure 2, green) is polyphyletic and comprises archaea, eubacteria and eukaryotes capable of various forms of photosynthesis from green sulfur-metabolizing hyperthermophilic prokaryotes through algae and higher plants. Bacteriodetes, Chloroflexus and Roseiflexus taxa all have additional N-terminal domains. Trx-like CXXC signature motifs are found in only the Chloroflexus and Roseiflexus N-terminal domains and these taxa lack C-terminal Trx-like domains. All other clade 5 taxa possess C-terminal Trx-like domains except for Archaea and Gemmatimonadetes. Interestingly, Clade 5 includes intermingled archaeal and eukaryotic taxa, suggesting horizontal gene transfer (HGT): a cluster of three archaeal *Pyrobaculum* species, all different from those in Clade 1, appear along with a single Verrucomicrobia representative (genus *Chthoniobacter*), the only non-photosynth grouping in Clade 5 (there are, however, other single Verrucomicrobia sequences intermingled among various Clade 5 branches, further suggesting HGT); a single Rhizaria eukaryote, *Paulinella chromatophora*, is found on a Clade 5 branch between branches bearing *Synechococcus* species. *P. chromatophora* is a freshwater amoeboid widely noted for its very recently acquired cyanobacterial symbiont previously believed to stem from an ancestor of either *Synechococcus* or *Prochlorococcus* genera [58]. Compared to free living *Synechococcus* species, the *P. chromatophora* plastid has retained ~26% of the original genome (*i.e.*, retained 867 protein-coding genes), although the VKOR family homolog (NCBI Protein: YP_002048937.1) was previously transferred, along with most of the plastid genes, to the *P. chromatophora* nuclear genome [59]. Thus, our reconstruction of the VKORloop phylogeny strongly suggests that the *P. chromatophora* chloroplast evolved from an acquired *Synechococcus* endosymbiont, further resolving the uncertainty of a phylogenetic reconstruction study by Marin *et al.*, based on analysis of concatenated rDNA operon or rRNA sequences, to determine if the ancestral endosymbiont was an ancestor of *Synechococcus* or *Prochlorococcus* [60].

3.3. Similarities and Differences among Sequence Position-Specific Substitutions Reveal VKOR Family Clade-Specific Structural and Functional Residues

In order to explore VKOR family clade-dependent and clade-independent sequence conservation, and to assess if conserved sites might have functional or structural correlates, we performed site-specific conservational analyses on the complete MSA as well as on the aligned sequences for each of the five identified VKOR family clades. Figure 4 graphically summarizes the conservation analysis results.

We identified 22 residue positions (Figure 4, bold black letters **s**, **f**, **x** below the Clade 1 line) that are highly conserved across all VKOR clades. We have assigned structural and functional roles to these positions as follows:

(1) The five fully conserved VKOR signature residue positions (Figure 4, marked **f**) are functional, playing direct roles in vitamin K 2,3-epoxide to vitamin K quinone and vitamin K quinone to vitamin K quinol reduction (Cys43, Cys51, Ser57, Cys132, Cys135 according to human VKORC1 numbering);

(2) Nine highly conserved positions (Figure 4, marked **s**) represent residues that form putative helix-helix structural contacts identified by visual inspection of the X-ray crystallographic structure for the prokaryotic VKOR homolog (PDB entry 3KP9, residue numbering corresponds to human VKORC1 sequence in Figure 4). On TMH1, Cys16, Gly19, Ser23 and Ala26 pack against TMH2, TMH2 and TMH4, TMH2, TMH2 and TMH3, respectively. On TMH2, Ser81 and Gly84 both pack against TMH1. On TMH3, Ser117 packs against TMH4, while Leu124 packs against only residues on the same helix (TMH3). On TMH4, Thr138 packs against TMH1;

(3) Eight highly conserved positions (Figure 4, marked **x**) may be putative functional residues either essential for quinone substrate reduction or involved in substrate binding and specificity (Asp44, Gly80, Gly84, Asn80, Tyr88, Gly95, Leu120, Leu128).

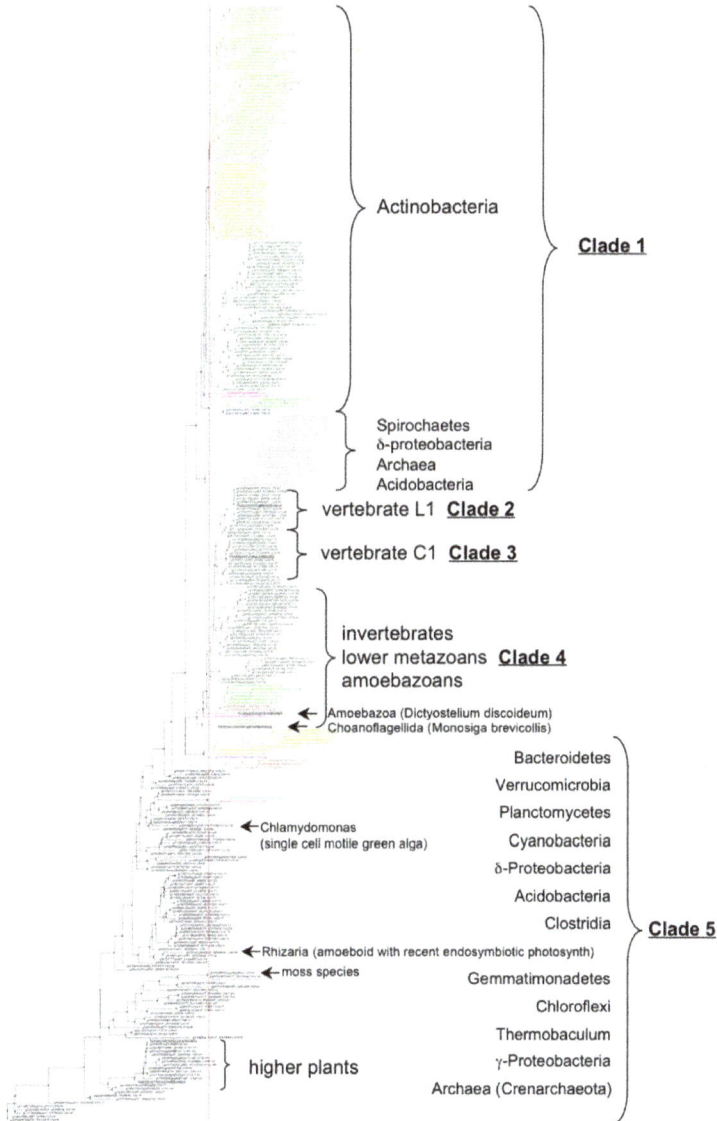

Figure 3. Cladogram (unrooted tree) of VKORloop sequences identifying groupings into highest common Linnaean taxonomic ranks. (See online supplemental data for a complete listing of protein identifiers in the FASTA-formatted MSA file; also, Figure S7 of the online Supplementary Materials and Research Data shows the full-length aligned sequences, including non-VKOR domains, corresponding to the cladogram in this figure).

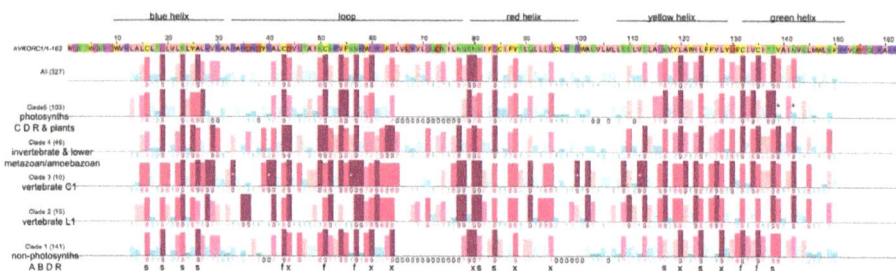

Figure 4. Comparison of Consurf conservational scoring for combined VKOR family sequences and the five individual VKOR clades. Human VKORC1 primary sequence is with relative postions of transmembrane helices (indicated using color scheme from [17]) and large loop as line segments (top); calculated Consurf conservation scores on lines below the sequence (six lines, top to bottom): All 327 VKOR sequences; Clade 5, 103 photosynthetic prokaryotes of the super-taxa C, D and R (prokaryotic super-taxa: A = Actinobacteria, B = Bacilli an related, C = Clostridia and related, D = double membrane Gram-negative bacteria, R = Archaea [56]); Clade 4, 46 invertebrates, lower metazoans, euglenozoans and mycetozoans; Clade 3, 10 vertebrate VKORC1 orthologs; Clade 2, 15 vertebrate VKORC1L1 orthologs; Clade 1, 141 non-photosynthetic prokaryotes of the super-taxa A, B, D and R. Darker red bars indicate greater positional conservation, darker blue bars indicate greater positional non-conservation (conservation scores below bars; lowest score 1 to highest score 9). Systematically absent from the prokaryotic sequences (clades 1 and 5) indicated with black zeros in place of Consurf scores. Fully conserved vertebrate VKORC1 residues (white asterisks superimposed upon dark red bars); Clade 5-specific absences of conserved Tyr139 and Asn142 (black asterisks above dark blue bars, human VKORC1 numbering). Letters and symbols (bottom) for positions highly conserved across all five major clades: s = structural residue contributing to helix-helix packing interactions; f = residues full conserved across all species and presumed to be catalytically active (Cys43, Cys51, Ser57, Cys132, Cys135); x = residues that are highly conserved, but presently lacking assignment as to structural or functional importance.

Notable differences in position-specific conservation between VKOR family clades include:

(1) Compared to non-animal VKOR homologs, there are conserved sequence insertions among animal VKOR homologs (clades 2–4; Figure 4, absence of animal-specific sequences indicated as conservation scores "0" for clades 1 and 5). A few of these insertions are individual or adjacent pairs of residues located in two groupings—one at the margin including the C-terminal portion of TMH1 and the large loop joining TMH1 and TMH2, and the other in the C-terminal margin of TMH2 and the variable-sized loop connecting TMH2 and TMH3. The largest insertion is a linear sequence of 13–14 residues that comprise and extension at the C-terminal end of the large loop which joins TMH1 and TMH2. Thus, these animal insertions positively correlate with the representative homologs possessing VKOR (*i.e.*, phyloquinone- and menaquinone-2,3-epoxidase) catalytic activity in addition to general quinone (*i.e.*, menaquinone, phyloquinone or ubiquinone) reductase activity common to all VKOR family members. To-date, with only the exception of demonstrated *in vitro* VKOR activity for two obligate intracellular bacteria that are pathogenic in eukaryotes (*M. tuberculosis*, *Corynebacterium jeikeium*) [13], all representative non-animal VKOR enzymes for which quinone substrate usage has been biochemically characterized were found to lack VKOR activity (eubacteria: *Synechococcus* species [14]; *Synechocystis* sp. PCC6803 [61]; *Roseiflexus* sp. RS-1, *Salinispora tropica* CNB-440 [13]; plants: *Arabidopsis thaliana* [15], *Solanum lycopersicum* [16]).

(2) A site-directed mutagenesis study by Matagrin *et al.* (2013) of rat VKORC1 revealed Tyr139 (homologous residue for human VKORC1 is also Tyr139) to be critical to VKOR catalysis in that removal of a 3-hydroxy group from vitamin K, once the epoxide oxirane ring has been opened, is apparently hindered by substitution of the tyrosine by cysteine, phenylalanine or serine as in naturally occurring

warfarin resistant VKORC1 variants in rats [62]. In agreement with their results, a previous study also reported the production of a proposed VKOR catalytic intermediate product, 3-hydroxyvitamin K, by liver microsomes from a homozygous warfarin-resistant HW Welsh rat strain later genotyped as VKORC1:Tyr139Ser [63,64]. We find that tyrosine is completely conserved at the primary sequence position homologous to human and rat Tyr139 among all metazoan VKOR family homologs belonging to Clades 2, 3 and 4. Alternative substitutions at this positions include chiefly tryptophan (infrequently, methionine or threonine) among Clade 1 homologs, while Clade 5 substitutions include chiefly residues with aliphatic side-chains (*i.e.*, Ala, Leu, Ile). Interestingly, the only Clade 1 or 5 homologs with Tyr at this position include prokaryotes of the genera *Leptospira* (spirochetes) and *Streptomyces* (filamentous soil bacteria), *Leishmania* (a genus of trypanosomatid protozoa) and *Trypanosoma* (a genus of kinetoplastid protozoa), all obligate intracellular pathogens in vertebrates, suggesting that these VKOR family homologs might catalyze VKOR activity. At least nine *Streptomyces* species have been reported to be pathogenic in humans (55) [65]. Also, *Leptospira interrogans* is known to possess a gene for a glutamyl carboxylase homolog presumed to have been obtained through HGT, lending support to the possibility that the genomically encoded VKOR family homolog enables production of vitamin K-dependent proteins involved in pathogenesis (56) [66]. For identification purposes, we name this the *LSLT* group of pathogenic organisms.

(3) We identified a covariant site for the *LSLT* pathogenic group at the residue homologous to human VKORC1: Ile136 immediately following the conserved active site CXXC motif. Species in the *LSLT* group possess a cysteine at this position homologous to the human sequence numbering VKORC1: Ile136Cys and include *T. brucei*, *L. major* strain Friedlin, *L. infantum*, and *Streptomyces* species (*coelicolor A3(2)*, *griseus* sub.sp. *griseus*, *sviceus*, sp. SPB74, and two distinctly non-identical VKOR family homologs for sp. Mg1) from our MSA data set. We could not identify any additional position-specific markers in the VKOR core domain for this group.

A notable, distinguishing feature of all vertebrate VKORC1 and VKORC1L1 sequences (clades 2 and 3) is the systematic absence of segments of the large loop region from the prokaryotic sequences (Figure 4; clades 1 and 5, indicated with black zeros among the Consurf scores). Thus, both prokaryotic clades are missing the equivalent of human VKORC1 sequence residues Leu65 through Asn77 that comprise the distal C-terminal residues of the large loops in clade 2, 3 and 4 sequences. Differential clade-specific absences of additional sequence segments occur in the N-terminal portion of the loop as well as in regions comprising portions of the red and yellow helices and adjoining small cytoplasmic loop for the prokaryotes (Figure 4; clades 1 and 5, indicated by black zeros). Vertebrate VKORC1 (clade 3-specific) full conservation is indicated in Figure 4 by white asterisks superimposed upon the highest conservation score bars (dark red) at Arg33, Arg40, Ser56, Arg100 and Val112 (human VKORC1 numbering). Interestingly, lack of clade 5-specific conservation at Tyr139 (human VKORC1 numbering), as well as at Asn142 (one helical turn away from Tyr139) indicates non-conservation at these positions, in striking contrast to conservation at these positions in the other four clades.

3.4. Evidence for an Evolutionary Relationship between VKOR and DsbB Families

In order to investigate our hypothesis that the VKOR and DsbB families may have evolved from a common ancestor, we explored sequence similarity and conservation by creating aligned Consurf profiles for homologous structural elements from each family based on the availability of high-resolution X-ray crystallographic structures for the representative *Synechococcus* sp. VKOR and *E. coli* DsbB homologs. Specifically, we aligned two different conservation profiles representing helix pair-loop modules. The first (AB) module encompasses the primary sequences including the first two TMHs of VKOR and the last two TMHs for DsbB and including the intervening large loops (Figure 5, upper half). Accordingly, the second (CD) module encompasses the last two TMHs of VKOR and the first two TMHs of DsbB, together with the respective short connecting loops (Figure 5, lower half). As individual sequences among the VKOR and DsbB families have variable lengths due to species-specific indels, we truncated the family MSAs to include only sites of the primary sequences of the human VKORC1 and VKORC1L1 paralogs and *E. coli* DsbB homolog. To align the VKOR and DsbB family conservation profiles for each module, the representative human and prokaryotic index sequences were translated relative to each other until the invariant CXXC motifs were aligned for the AB module; the CD module was aligned by assessing pairwise identity between the VKORC1 and DsbB index sequences and between the VKORC1L1 and DsbB index sequences (Figure 5, black bars). Altogether, the best AB module alignment resulted in a maximum of five identity sites among the three index sequences; the best CD module alignment resulted in a maximum of four identity sites among the three index sequences (Figure 5, for each upper and lower figure halves, compare black bars on both pairwise identity lines). Inspection of the aligned positional conservation scores representing 327 VKOR homologs and 514 DsbB homologs reveals a very strong correlation in position specific conservation (compare patterns of dark red bars representing high Consurf scores).

In addition to the interfamily conservation of the active site CXXC motifs in the AB module for both families, we could assign conserved interhelical contact residues for the DsbB family: five helix-helix contacts (HHCs) for the A helices, three HHCs for the B helices (by inspection of the best high-resolution NMR structure; PDB entry 2K74). Of these DsbB family AB module HHCs, there is a perfect match (Figure 5, top half, AB module alignment position 26) corresponding to an HHC with a Consurf score of 8 at the corresponding human VKORC1:S117 position in the A helix (see Figure 4) representing an HHC also common to all VKOR family members. Similarly, at AB module position 33, the DsbB family conserved HHC matches a VKOR family conserved HHC with a Consurf score of 9 at the corresponding human VKORC1: Leu124 position in the A helix. For the B helices of both families, a conserved HHC at VKORC1: Thr138 with Consurf score 9 matches a similar highly conserved HHC in the DsbB family (Figure 5, upper half, AB module position 47).

For the CD module, the C helix of the DsbB family has five conserved HHCs, of which four VKOR family conserved HHCs including VKORC1: Cys16 (CD module position 23), VKORC1: Gly19 (CD module position 26), VKORC1: Ser23 (CD module position 30) and VKORC1: Ala26 (CD module postion 33) are perfect matches. The DsbB family D helix has three conserved HHCs, for which one VKOR family conserved HHC (VKORC1: Ser81, CD module position 88) is a perfect match.

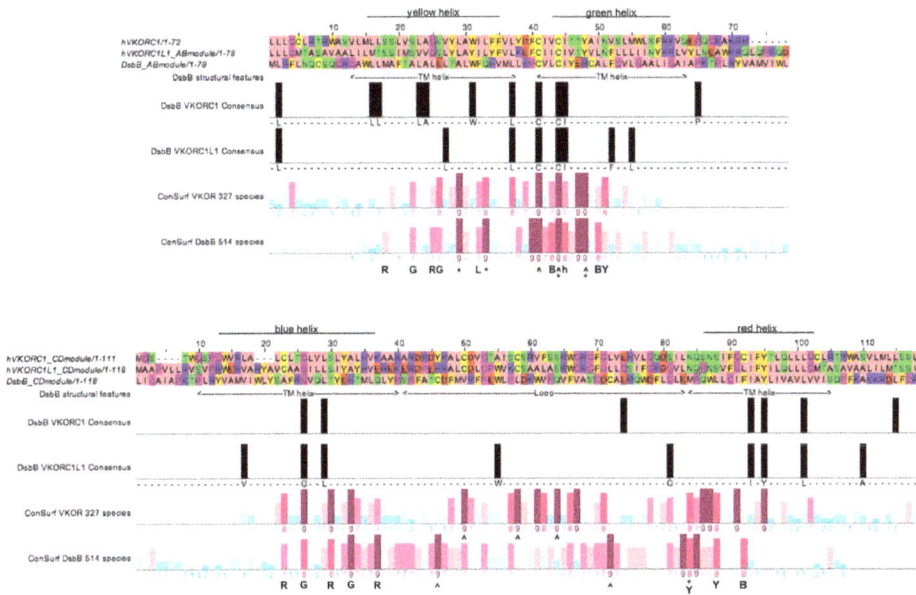

Figure 5. Alignment of helix pair-loop module sequences of VKORC1, VKORC1L1 and DsbB showing pairwise identity, Consurf conservational scoring and known DsbB secondary structure elements and interhelical packing residues (Note 1 [67]). ClustalW2 alignments for AB (top) and CD (bottom) modules. Positions of transmembrane helices for DsbB are indicated below alignment, helix color indicated above alignment. Vertical black bars, sequence identity between DsbB and VKOR proteins; bottom two lines, Consurf conservation scores for VKOR multiple sequence alignment (second from bottom line) and DsbB multiple sequence alignment (bottom line). Vertical colored bars, positional conservation as described in Figure 4—Letters and symbols below conservation score lines: R = interhelical contact to red helix, G = interhelical contact to green helix, B = interhelical contact to blue helix, Y = interhelical contact to yellow helix, * = residue making contact with quinone cofactor, L = residue mediating hydrophobic packing against a C-terminal segment of the large loop, ^ = residues completely conserved in all species, h = residue making hydrophobic contact with the small amphipathic helix of the large loop.

Thus, independent of different threading of primary sequences through the helical bundle for each family (*i.e.*, N- to C-terminus threading comprises helices ordered ABCD for the DsbB family, but CDAB for the VKOR family), a highly conserved network of altogether 8 interhelical structural contacts (3 AB module and 5 CD module HHCs) is shared by both VKOR and DsbB family protein folds.

Similarly, when we surveyed the available high-resolution structural data for position-specific matches between VKOR and DsbB residues interacting with bound ubiquinone substrates, out of a total of 9 DsbB residues contacting a bound ubiquinone-2 and 18 VKOR residues contacting a bound ubiquinone-4, we found conserved matches at AB module positions 25, 29, 33, 44 for both VKOR and DsbB families. The greater number of ubiquinone contacts for *Synechococcus* sp. VKOR compared to those for *E. coli* DsbB is primarily due to the longer isoprenoid chain length of ubiquinone-4 *versus* that of ubiquinone-2. Of the four positions common to ubiquinone binding for both representative high-resolution structures, position 44 represents one of the conserved active site cysteines in the CXXC motif (homologous to human VKORC1: Cys135) located on helix B, while positions 25 (Consurf scores 6 and 7), 29 (Consurf scores both 6) and 33 (Consurf scores 8 and 9) represent conserved residues on the adjacent helix A. We interpret these findings to be highly supportive for conservation of key homologous substrate binding site residues among VKOR and DsbB families. Taken together, we believe these results constitute substantial evidence for structural feature conservation for both VKOR and DsbB families in support of our hypothesis that both families share a common ancestor.

3.5. Identification of Transmembrane-Helical Bundle Protein Families Related by Cyclical Permuted Primary Sequences Can Extend Homology Modeling into the "Twilight Zone" (<30% Sequence Homology between Target and Template)

Figure 6 shows the human VKORC1 and VKORC1L1 models we produced along with the NMR structure of the DsbB template and the X-ray crystallographic structure of the prokaryotic VKOR family homolog (proVKOR) by Li *et al.* (2010) [14]. Stereochemical validation performed on both models indicated overall quality similar to that of the X-ray crystallographic and NMR structures (see online Supplementary Material & Experimental Data). Overall organization of the transmembrane helical bundles is quite similar between the DsbB and proVKOR experimentally determined structures, although the large loops (at the top of each structure) exhibit major structural differences. For DsbB, the loop extends across the bundle and is thought to be anchored in the lipid membrane by a short amphipathic helix (shown in purple). In contrast, for proVKOR, the loop is positioned entirely above the bundle (note that several short segments of the loop were not resolved in the crystallographic structure and are shown as dashed grey lines in Figure 6) with a short helix serving as a cap centered directly over the bundle (shown in magenta). The VKORC1 and VKORC1L1 models have transmembrane helical bundles organized very similarly to those of proVKOR and DsbB. Noticeably, the large loops of the models do not appear structurally homologous to that of DsbB because they were modeled separately using *de novo* modeling methods in order to avoid bias favoring structural features of the DsbB template loop region. The *de novo* modeling methods we used (see Section 2.4) identify pieces of structures from the PDB to use as templates for building up a realistic protein structure based on threading short segments of the target sequence. The resulting loop models were computationally annealed as small globular domains and could be easily fit to the respective helical bundles using standard X-ray crystallographic model building software. Interestingly, the *de novo* modeled loops for VKORC1 and VKORC1L1 prominently exhibit short helices located at nearly the same position in the final models as the short capping helix of the experimentally determined proVKOR structure (Figure 6, purple helix shown in the loop for VKORC1, for VKORC1L1 the helix is visible, but not colored, at the equivalent position). Taken together, the similarity between the experimental proVKOR loop and our modeled loops for VKORC1 and VKORC1L1 suggested to us that the large VKOR loops, in general, are likely to behave more like well-folded, small globular protein domains than the extended loop observed for the DsbB structure. Another potentially realistic feature of our modeled loops is that, for both VKORC1 and VKORC1L1, the loop cysteines appear to be within disulfide bonding distance from each other and, additionally, located at the very top periphery of the protein where they would theoretically be accessible for binding to, and for reduction by, ER lumenal partner oxidoreductases.

4. Discussion

Reconstruction of VKOR family phylogeny by standard ML methods revealed five distinct clades that follow a rationale consistent with evolution based on standard Tree of Life models. Analysis of overall VKOR family-specific and individual clade-specific sequence variability further revealed conserved sequence motifs and individual residue positions that suggest a possible evolutionary relationship with the DsbB family. Accordingly, results from our analysis of interhelical packing residues for representative experimentally determined structures from both families lends support to this hypothesis. Furthermore, differences in sequence conservation between VKOR clades have provided useful information for deducing a plausible evolutionary chronology for the VKOR family (Figure 7).

Of potentially broader implication to the structural biology of membrane proteins is the first discovery of cyclic permutation of sequence threading through seemingly unrelated protein folds for helical transmembrane proteins. In the case of the VKOR and DsbB families, there has been enough preservation of common structural elements for both protein fold and substrate binding, as well as preservation of enzymatic function, substrate class and functional partner proteins, to reveal a plausible underlying evolutionary relationship. Using phylogenetic conservation data from large multiple sequence alignments for both families, despite only 12.0%–13.6% shared primary sequence identity between the human VKOR paralogs and *E. coli* DsbB, we have presented the first evidence for evolutionary relatedness between these families.

Overall, polytopic membrane protein structures solved by X-ray and electron crystallographic and NMR methods account for <1% of Protein Data Bank entries [68], yet represent up to an estimated 30% of genomic proteins and include upwards of 70% of known or potential therapeutic drug targets [69, 70]. Identifying distant sequence homology targets for polytopic membrane protein templates with solved, high-resolution structures would prove beneficial to modeling efforts aimed at increasing structural coverage and would aid in defining functions for the rapidly growing number of new gene sequences from large-scale genomics efforts. Structural genomics aims to generate a minimum number of experimental structures to encompass all structural folds, including the subset of an estimated 550 (90% coverage) unique polytopic membrane protein folds [71]. Template-based models (TBMs) can be routinely constructed for target sequences sharing greater than 30% identity with an identified structural template [72] and used to guide hypothesis-driven experimentation [73] to study function [74] as well as to aid model building for crystallographic [75] and NMR data [76,77]. However, target sequences with less than 30% identity to any known template are considered to be in the "twilight zone" of template-based modeling [72,78], the case being exacerbated for membrane proteins where there are relatively few high-resolution structures [79].

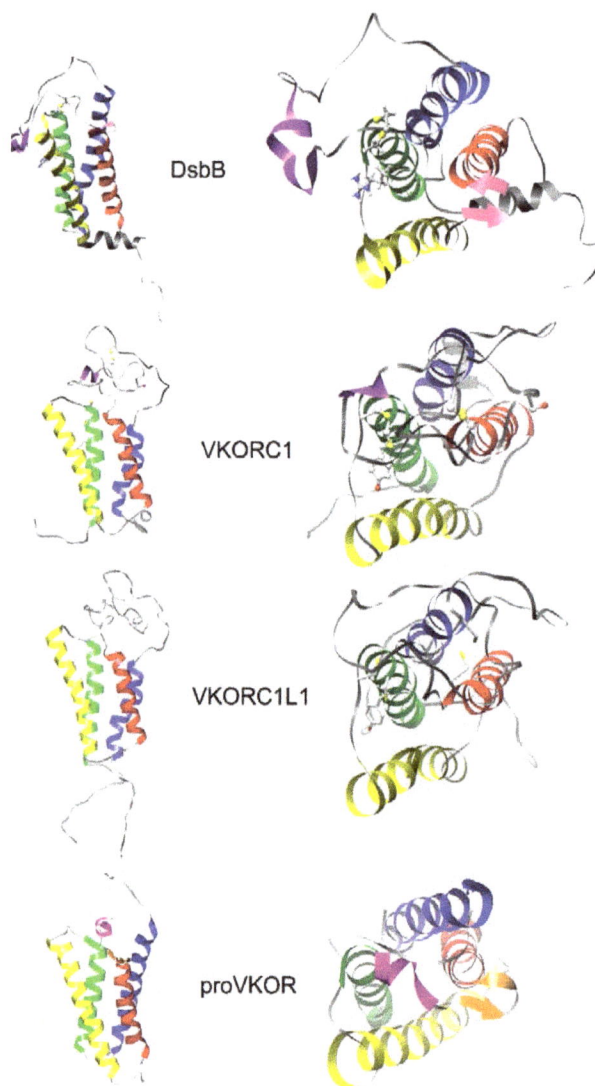

Figure 6. Backbone ribbon renderings of DsbB (PDB entry 2K74, model 1) [45], homology models of human VKORC1 and VKORC1L1 (Note 1 [67]), and Synechococcus sp. VKOR (proVKOR; PDB entry 3KP9) [14]. Views in the plane of the lipid bilayer (left) and normal (right) to the membrane plane from the ER lumenal (for VKORC1, VKORC1L1, proVKOR) or periplasmic (for DsbB) side. Transmembrane helices are colored (from N- to C-terminus) blue, red, yellow, green (designated as A, B, C and D, respectively, throughout the article text). Short loop helices for DsbB and VKORC1 (purple), for proVKOR (magenta); short β-sheet are regions (magenta or orange arrows); loop cysteines (ball and stick side-chains with yellow sulfur atoms).

E. coli DsbB and human VKORC1, for which experimental structures have been solved [14,29,30,45,80,81], share strikingly similar size, topology, two completely conserved functional cysteine pairs, lipidic quinone cofactors and oxidoreductase binding partners [19]. Moreover, primary sequence threading through the transmembrane α-helical secondary structural elements of both proteins is related by circular permutation (CP). Since 1979, there have been reports of CP relating the structural organization of naturally occurring soluble proteins (for a recent review see [82]) and underlying genetic principles leading to such permutations have been studied in the context of protein fold evolution [83]. We performed a literature-based survey of all published reports of CP in proteins and found examples for soluble protein domains, soluble domains of monotopic membrane proteins, sandwich transmembrane toxins, and a surprising number of engineered proteins including soluble domains as well as barrel transmembrane proteins occasionally genetically engineered to overcome crystallization problems for X-ray structural determinations. However, we could not identify any reports of CP for polytopic helical membrane proteins.

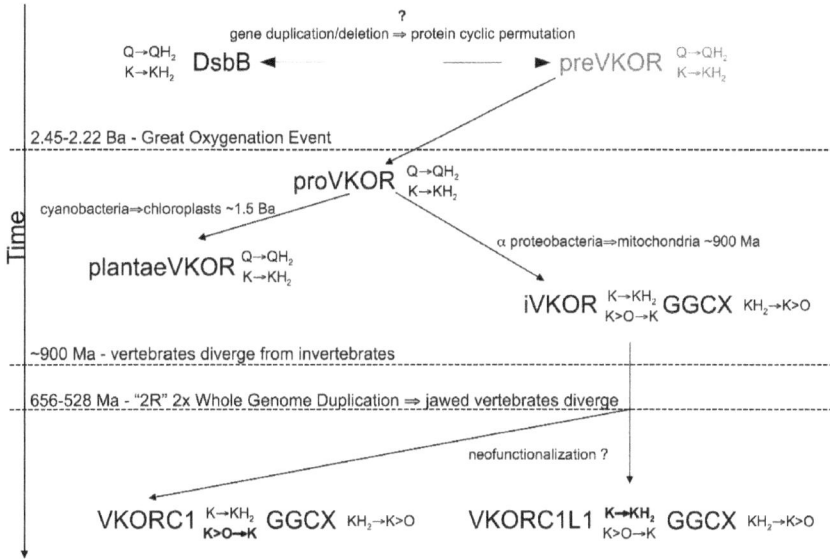

Figure 7. A comprehensive model for the evolution of the VKOR family and its hypothesized relationship to the DsbB family, suggested by the close relationship between the structure of the present reconstructed VKOR family phylogeny and that of the current consensus for the Tree of Life. Abbreviations and symbols (except if previously introduced): Ma, million years ago; Ba, billion years ago; Q, ubiquinone; QH$_2$, ubiquinol; K>O, vitamin K 2,3-epoxide; K, vitamin K quinone; KH$_2$, vitamin K hydroquinone; preVKOR, last universal common ancestral VKOR; proVKOR, prokaryotic VKOR; iVKOR, invertebrate VKOR; plantaeVKOR, plant VKOR; GGCX, γ-glutamyl carboxylase.

We advance the hypothesis and provide supporting evidence that both VKORC1 and DsbB families are evolutionarily divergent members of a single lipidic quinone:disulfide oxidoreductase superfamily (we suggest the nomenclature "LQOR superfamily") structurally related by CP threading homology that likely arose from an ancient gene duplication/deletion event. This event apparently occurred before eukaryotes evolved. It is likely that both families arose from a common ancestor in prokaryotes from a whole gene (ABCD) duplication that resulted in a concatenated linear tandem repeat (ABCDABCD), followed by deletions of the outer flanking helix pairs (A̶B̶CDABC̶D̶) to yield the CP-related secondary structure threading (CDAB). Unfortunately, this scenario confronts us with essentially another version of the "chicken or the egg" causality dilemma—we have no way of currently deducing which permutation, and hence which family, predates the CP event. However, considering cumulative results from genetic and biochemical studies to date, we may deduce that, whereas the enzymatic function of DsbB family members has remained rather constant over long evolutionary timescales and has remained exclusively restricted to prokaryotes, multiple *de novo* enzymatic functions have arisen for members of the VKOR family since the divergence of eukaryotes and prokaryotes (Figure 7). Furthermore, it seems reasonable that neofunctionalization of VKOR family enzymes to catalyze de-epoxidation likely did not first arise before the onset of the Great Oxygenation Event.

5. Conclusions

In the present report, we have updated the phylogenetic characterization of VKOR family proteins to include broader representative taxa from the entire Tree of Life than was possible only a few years ago. We hope these results will serve as a basis to further explore fundamental relationships between available genetic data and structure/function correlates for the VKOR family.

Moreover, our results suggest a generalized approach for detecting further distant protein homologs related by cyclic permutation of a primary sequence. Our results also suggest that pairs of transmembrane helices (TMHs) together with the connecting loop may form key minimal modular building blocks that enable such evolutionary fold changes for helical intrinsic membrane proteins.

We hope our results will encourage more researchers to strive to better understand the molecular-level function of the modern VKOR enzymes from each of the major clades and what roles they play in development, growth and homeostasis. Advances on these fronts will further help to understand the evolution of these only recently discovered enzymes.

Acknowledgments: This work was supported, in part, by funding from the Deutsche Forschungsgemeinschaft (DFG) grant Ol100 5-1 (to MW and JO), from DFG grant Mi236 6-1 (to Prof. Hartmut Michel, Director, Department of Molecular Membrane Biology, Max Planck Institute of Biophysics; support for CK), and from Baxter Germany GmbH (to JO).

Author Contributions: CGB and JO conceived and drafted the article and discussed and edited it with CK, CR and MW. CGB collected and analyzed data.

Conflicts of Interest: The authors declare no conflict of interest.

References

1. Oldenburg, J.; Bevans, C.G.; Müller, C.R.; Watzka, M. Vitamin K epoxide reductase complex subunit 1 (VKORC1): The key protein of the vitamin K cycle. *Antioxid. Redox Signal.* **2006**, *8*, 347–353. [CrossRef] [PubMed]
2. Shearer, M.J.; Fu, X.; Booth, S.L. Vitamin K nutrition, metabolism, and requirements: Current concepts and future research. *Adv. Nutr.* **2012**, *3*, 182–195. [CrossRef] [PubMed]
3. Shearer, M.J.; Newman, P. Recent trends in the metabolism and cell biology of vitamin K with special reference to vitamin K cycling and MK-4 biosynthesis. *J. Lipid Res.* **2014**, *55*, 345–362. [CrossRef] [PubMed]
4. Spohn, G.; Kleinridders, A.; Wunderlich, F.T.; Watzka, M.; Zaucke, F.; Blumbach, K.; Geisen, C.; Seifried, E.; Müller, C.; Paulsson, M.; *et al.* VKORC1 deficiency in mice causes early postnatal lethality due to severe bleeding. *Thromb. Haemost.* **2009**, *101*, 1044–1050. [CrossRef] [PubMed]
5. Dam, H. The antihaemorrhagic vitamin of the chick. *Biochem. J.* **1935**, *29*, 1273–1285. [PubMed]
6. Watzka, M.; Geisen, C.; Bevans, C.G.; Sittinger, K.; Spohn, G.; Rost, S.; Seifried, E.; Müller, C.R.; Oldenburg, J. Thirteen novel VKORC1 mutations associated with oral anticoagulant resistance: Insights into improved patient diagnosis and treatment. *J. Thromb. Haemost.* **2011**, *9*, 109–118. [CrossRef] [PubMed]
7. Hammed, A.; Matagrin, B.; Spohn, G.; Prouillac, C.; Benoit, E.; Lattard, V. VKORC1L1, an enzyme rescuing the vitamin K 2,3-epoxide reductase activity in some extrahepatic tissues during anticoagulation therapy. *J. Biol. Chem.* **2013**, *288*, 28733–28742. [CrossRef] [PubMed]
8. Caspers, M.; Czogalla, K.J.; Liphardt, K.; Müller, J.; Westhofen, P.; Watzka, M.; Oldenburg, J. Two enzymes catalyze vitamin K 2,3-epoxide reductase activity in mouse: VKORC1 is highly expressed in exocrine tissues while VKORC1L1 is highly expressed in brain. *Thromb. Res.* **2015**, *135*, 977–983. [CrossRef] [PubMed]
9. Westhofen, P.; Watzka, M.; Marinova, M.; Hass, M.; Kirfel, G.; Müller, J.; Bevans, C.G.; Müller, C.R.; Oldenburg, J. Human vitamin K 2,3-epoxide reductase complex subunit 1-like 1 (VKORC1L1) mediates vitamin K-dependent intracellular antioxidant function. *J. Biol. Chem.* **2011**, *286*, 15085–15094. [CrossRef] [PubMed]

10. Rost, S.; Fregin, A.; Ivaskevicius, V.; Conzelmann, E.; Hörtnagel, K.; Pelz, H.-J.; Lappegard, K.; Seifried, E.; Scharrer, I.; Tuddenham, E.G.D.; *et al.* Mutations in VKORC1 cause warfarin resistance and multiple coagulation factor deficiency type 2. *Nature* **2004**, *427*, 537–541. [CrossRef] [PubMed]

11. Li, T.; Chang, C.-Y.; Jin, D.-Y.; Lin, P.-J.; Khvorova, A.; Stafford, D.W. Identification of the gene for vitamin K epoxide reductase. *Nature* **2004**, *427*, 541–544. [CrossRef] [PubMed]

12. Tie, J.-K.; Jin, D.-Y.; Stafford, D.W. Conserved loop cysteines of vitamin K epoxide reductase complex subunit 1-like 1 (VKORC1L1) are involved in its active site regeneration. *J. Biol. Chem.* **2014**, *289*, 9396–9407. [CrossRef] [PubMed]

13. Tie, J.-K.; Jin, D.-Y.; Stafford, D.W. Mycobacterium tuberculosis vitamin K epoxide reductase homologue supports vitamin K-dependent carboxylation in mammalian cells. *Antioxid. Redox Signal.* **2012**, *16*, 329–338. [CrossRef] [PubMed]

14. Li, W.; Schulman, S.; Dutton, R.J.; Boyd, D.; Beckwith, J.; Rapoport, T.A. Structure of a bacterial homologue of vitamin K epoxide reductase. *Nature* **2010**, *463*, 507–512. [CrossRef] [PubMed]

15. Furt, F.; van Oostende, C.; Widhalm, J.R.; Dale, M.A.; Wertz, J.; Basset, G.J.C. A bimodular oxidoreductase mediates the specific reduction of phylloquinone (vitamin K1) in chloroplasts. *Plant J. Cell Mol. Biol.* **2010**, *64*, 38–46. [CrossRef] [PubMed]

16. Wan, C.-M.; Yang, X.-J.; Du, J.-J.; Lu, Y.; Yu, Z.-B.; Feng, Y.-G.; Wang, X.-Y. Identification and characterization of SlVKOR, a disulfide bond formation protein from Solanum lycopersicum, and bioinformatic analysis of plant VKORs. *Biochem.* **2014**, *79*, 440–449. [CrossRef] [PubMed]

17. Sevier, C.S.; Kadokura, H.; Tam, V.C.; Beckwith, J.; Fass, D.; Kaiser, C.A. The prokaryotic enzyme DsbB may share key structural features with eukaryotic disulfide bond forming oxidoreductases. *Protein Sci. Publ. Protein Soc.* **2005**, *14*, 1630–1642. [CrossRef] [PubMed]

18. Sevier, C.S.; Kaiser, C.A. Conservation and diversity of the cellular disulfide bond formation pathways. *Antioxid. Redox Signal.* **2006**, *8*, 797–811. [CrossRef] [PubMed]

19. Wajih, N.; Hutson, S.M.; Wallin, R. Disulfide-dependent protein folding is linked to operation of the vitamin K cycle in the endoplasmic reticulum: A protein disulfide isomerase-VKORC1 redox enzyme complex appears to be responsible for vitamin K1 2,3-epoxide reduction. *J. Biol. Chem.* **2007**, *282*, 2626–2635. [CrossRef] [PubMed]

20. Rutkevich, L.A.; Williams, D.B. Vitamin K epoxide reductase contributes to protein disulfide formation and redox homeostasis within the endoplasmic reticulum. *Mol. Biol. Cell* **2012**, *23*, 2017–2027. [CrossRef] [PubMed]

21. Oldenburg, J.; Müller, C.R.; Rost, S.; Watzka, M.; Bevans, C.G. Comparative genetics of warfarin resistance. *Hamostaseologie* **2014**, *34*, 143–159. [CrossRef] [PubMed]

22. Goodstadt, L.; Ponting, C.P. Vitamin K epoxide reductase: homology, active site and catalytic mechanism. *Trends Biochem. Sci.* **2004**, *29*, 289–292. [CrossRef] [PubMed]

23. Robertson, H.M. Genes encoding vitamin-K epoxide reductase are present in Drosophila and trypanosomatid protists. *Genetics* **2004**, *168*, 1077–1080. [CrossRef] [PubMed]

24. Dutton, R.J.; Boyd, D.; Berkmen, M.; Beckwith, J. Bacterial species exhibit diversity in their mechanisms and capacity for protein disulfide bond formation. *Proc. Natl. Acad. Sci. USA* **2008**, *105*, 11933–11938. [CrossRef] [PubMed]

25. Heras, B.; Shouldice, S.R.; Totsika, M.; Scanlon, M.J.; Schembri, M.A.; Martin, J.L. DSB proteins and bacterial pathogenicity. *Nat. Rev. Microbiol.* **2009**, *7*, 215–225. [CrossRef] [PubMed]

26. Bader, M.; Muse, W.; Ballou, D.P.; Gassner, C.; Bardwell, J.C. Oxidative protein folding is driven by the electron transport system. *Cell* **1999**, *98*, 217–227. [CrossRef]

27. Reedstrom, C.K.; Suttie, J.W. Comparative distribution, metabolism, and utilization of phylloquinone and menaquinone-9 in rat liver. *Biol. Med.* **1995**, *209*, 403–409. [CrossRef]

28. Collins, M.D.; Jones, D. Distribution of isoprenoid quinone structural types in bacteria and their taxonomic implication. *Microbiol. Rev.* **1981**, *45*, 316–354. [PubMed]

29. Inaba, K.; Murakami, S.; Suzuki, M.; Nakagawa, A.; Yamashita, E.; Okada, K.; Ito, K. Crystal structure of the DsbB-DsbA complex reveals a mechanism of disulfide bond generation. *Cell* **2006**, *127*, 789–801. [CrossRef] [PubMed]

30. Shixuan, L.; Wei, C.; Fowle Grider, R.; Guomin, S.; Weikai, L. Structures of an intramembrane vitamin K epoxide reductase homolog reveal control mechanisms for electron transfer. *Nat. Commun.* **2014**, *5*, 3110.

31. Schwarz, R.; Seibel, P.N.; Rahmann, S.; Schoen, C.; Huenerberg, M.; Müller-Reible, C.; Dandekar, T.; Karchin, R.; Schultz, J.; Müller, T. Detecting species-site dependencies in large multiple sequence alignments. *Nucleic Acids Res.* **2009**, *37*, 5959–5968. [CrossRef] [PubMed]
32. Geer, L.Y.; Domrachev, M.; Lipman, D.J.; Bryant, S.H. CDART: Protein homology by domain architecture. *Genome Res.* **2002**, *12*, 1619–1623. [CrossRef] [PubMed]
33. Finn, R.D.; Bateman, A.; Clements, J.; Coggill, P.; Eberhardt, R.Y.; Eddy, S.R.; Heger, A.; Hetherington, K.; Holm, L.; Mistry, J.; *et al.* Pfam: The protein families database. *Nucleic Acids Res.* **2014**, *42*, D222–D230. [CrossRef] [PubMed]
34. Katoh, K.; Standley, D.M. MAFFT multiple sequence alignment software version 7: Improvements in performance and usability. *Mol. Biol. Evol.* **2013**, *30*, 772–780. [CrossRef] [PubMed]
35. Waterhouse, A.M.; Procter, J.B.; Martin, D.M.; Clamp, M.; Barton, G.J. Jalview Version 2—A multiple sequence alignment editor and analysis workbench. *Bioinformatics* **2009**, *25*, 1189–1191. [CrossRef] [PubMed]
36. Milne, I.; Lindner, D.; Bayer, M.; Husmeier, D.; McGuire, G.; Marshall, D.F.; Wright, F. TOPALi v2: A rich graphical interface for evolutionary analyses of multiple alignments on HPC clusters and multi-core desktops. *Bioinforma. Oxf. Engl.* **2009**, *25*, 126–127. [CrossRef] [PubMed]
37. Nguyen, L.-T.; Schmidt, H.A.; von Haeseler, A.; Minh, B.Q. IQ-TREE: A fast and effective stochastic algorithm for estimating maximum-likelihood phylogenies. *Mol. Biol. Evol.* **2015**, *32*, 268–274. [CrossRef] [PubMed]
38. Guindon, S.; Dufayard, J.-F.; Lefort, V.; Anisimova, M.; Hordijk, W.; Gascuel, O. New algorithms and methods to estimate maximum-likelihood phylogenies: Assessing the performance of PhyML 3.0. *Syst. Biol.* **2010**, *59*, 307–321. [CrossRef] [PubMed]
39. Stamatakis, A. RAxML version 8: A tool for phylogenetic analysis and post-analysis of large phylogenies. *Bioinforma. Oxf. Engl.* **2014**, *30*, 1312–1313. [CrossRef] [PubMed]
40. Minh, B.Q.; Nguyen, M.A.T.; von Haeseler, A. Ultrafast approximation for phylogenetic bootstrap. *Mol. Biol. Evol.* **2013**, *30*, 1188–1195. [CrossRef] [PubMed]
41. Letunic, I.; Bork, P. Interactive Tree Of Life (iTOL): An online tool for phylogenetic tree display and annotation. *Bioinforma. Oxf. Engl.* **2007**, *23*, 127–128. [CrossRef] [PubMed]
42. Berezin, C.; Glaser, F.; Rosenberg, J.; Paz, I.; Pupko, T.; Fariselli, P.; Casadio, R.; Ben-Tal, N. ConSeq: The identification of functionally and structurally important residues in protein sequences. *Bioinform. Oxf. Engl.* **2004**, *20*, 1322–1324. [CrossRef] [PubMed]
43. Ashkenazy, H.; Erez, E.; Martz, E.; Pupko, T.; Ben-Tal, N. ConSurf 2010: Calculating evolutionary conservation in sequence and structure of proteins and nucleic acids. *Nucleic Acids Res.* **2010**, *38*, W529–W533. [CrossRef] [PubMed]
44. Lo, A.; Cheng, C.-W.; Chiu, Y.-Y.; Sung, T.-Y.; Hsu, W.-L. TMPad: An integrated structural database for helix-packing folds in transmembrane proteins. *Nucleic Acids Res.* **2011**, *39*, D347–D355. [CrossRef] [PubMed]
45. Zhou, Y.; Cierpicki, T.; Jimenez, R.H.F.; Lukasik, S.M.; Ellena, J.F.; Cafiso, D.S.; Kadokura, H.; Beckwith, J.; Bushweller, J.H. NMR solution structure of the integral membrane enzyme DsbB: Functional insights into DsbB-catalyzed disulfide bond formation. *Mol. Cell* **2008**, *31*, 896–908. [CrossRef] [PubMed]
46. Sali, A.; Blundell, T.L. Comparative protein modelling by satisfaction of spatial restraints. *J. Mol. Biol.* **1993**, *234*, 779–815. [CrossRef] [PubMed]
47. Emsley, P.; Cowtan, K. Coot: Model-building tools for molecular graphics. *Acta Crystallogr. D Biol. Crystallogr.* **2004**, *60*, 2126–2132. [CrossRef] [PubMed]
48. Zhang, Y. I-TASSER server for protein 3D structure prediction. *BMC Bioinform.* **2008**, *9*, 40. [CrossRef] [PubMed]
49. Davis, I.W.; Leaver-Fay, A.; Chen, V.B.; Block, J.N.; Kapral, G.J.; Wang, X.; Murray, L.W.; Arendall, W.B.; Snoeyink, J.; Richardson, J.S.; *et al.* MolProbity: All-atom contacts and structure validation for proteins and nucleic acids. *Nucleic Acids Res.* **2007**, *35*, W375–W383. [CrossRef] [PubMed]
50. Senes, A.; Gerstein, M.; Engelman, D.M. Statistical analysis of amino acid patterns in transmembrane helices: The GxxxG motif occurs frequently and in association with beta-branched residues at neighboring positions. *J. Mol. Biol.* **2000**, *296*, 921–936. [CrossRef] [PubMed]
51. Stevens, T.J.; Arkin, I.T. Substitution rates in alpha-helical transmembrane proteins. *Protein Sci. Publ. Protein Soc.* **2001**, *10*, 2507–2517. [CrossRef]

52. Raczko, A.M.; Bujnicki, J.M.; Pawlowski, M.; Godlewska, R.; Lewandowska, M.; Jagusztyn-Krynicka, E.K. Characterization of new DsbB-like thiol-oxidoreductases of Campylobacter jejuni and Helicobacter pylori and classification of the DsbB family based on phylogenomic, structural and functional criteria. *Microbiol. Read. Engl.* **2005**, *151*, 219–231. [CrossRef] [PubMed]

53. Rishavy, M.A.; Usubalieva, A.; Hallgren, K.W.; Berkner, K.L. Novel insight into the mechanism of the vitamin K oxidoreductase (VKOR): Electron relay through Cys43 and Cys51 reduces VKOR to allow vitamin K reduction and facilitation of vitamin K-dependent protein carboxylation. *J. Biol. Chem.* **2011**, *286*, 7267–7278. [CrossRef] [PubMed]

54. Doolittle, W.F. Phylogenetic classification and the universal tree. *Science* **1999**, *284*, 2124–2128. [CrossRef] [PubMed]

55. Schaap, P. Guanylyl cyclases across the tree of life. *Fron. Biosci.* **2005**, *10*, 1485–1498. [CrossRef]

56. Lake, J.A.; Skophammer, R.G.; Herbold, C.W.; Servin, J.A. Genome beginnings: Rooting the tree of life. *Philos. Trans. R. Soc. Lond B. Biol. Sci.* **2009**, *364*, 2177–2185. [CrossRef] [PubMed]

57. Gribaldo, S.; Brochier, C. Phylogeny of prokaryotes: Does it exist and why should we care? *Res. Microbiol.* **2009**, *23*, 23. [CrossRef] [PubMed]

58. Nakayama, T.; Archibald, J.M. Evolving a photosynthetic organelle. *BMC Biol.* **2012**, *10*, 35. [CrossRef] [PubMed]

59. Nowack, E.C.M.; Melkonian, M.; Glöckner, G. Chromatophore genome sequence of Paulinella sheds light on acquisition of photosynthesis by eukaryotes. *Curr. Biol. CB* **2008**, *18*, 410–418. [CrossRef] [PubMed]

60. Marin, B.; Nowack, E.C.M.; Melkonian, M. A plastid in the making: Evidence for a second primary endosymbiosis. *Protist* **2005**, *156*, 425–432. [CrossRef] [PubMed]

61. Singh, A.K.; Bhattacharyya-Pakrasi, M.; Pakrasi, H.B. Identification of an atypical membrane protein involved in the formation of protein disulfide bonds in oxygenic photosynthetic organisms. *J. Biol. Chem.* **2008**, *283*, 15762–15770. [CrossRef] [PubMed]

62. Matagrin, B.; Hodroge, A.; Montagut-Romans, A.; Andru, J.; Fourel, I.; Besse, S.; Benoit, E.; Lattard, V. New insights into the catalytic mechanism of vitamin K epoxide reductase (VKORC1)—The catalytic properties of the major mutations of rVKORC1 explain the biological cost associated to mutations. *FEBS Open Bio.* **2013**, *3*, 144–150. [CrossRef] [PubMed]

63. Fasco, M.J.; Preusch, P.C.; Hildebrandt, E.; Suttie, J.W. Formation of hydroxyvitamin K by vitamin K epoxide reductase of warfarin-resistant rats. *J. Biol. Chem.* **1983**, *258*, 4372–4380. [PubMed]

64. Rost, S.; Pelz, H.-J.; Menzel, S.; MacNicoll, A.D.; León, V.; Song, K.-J.; Jäkel, T.; Oldenburg, J.; Müller, C.R. Novel mutations in the VKORC1 gene of wild rats and mice—A response to 50 years of selection pressure by warfarin? *BMC Genet.* **2009**, *10*, 4. [CrossRef] [PubMed]

65. Kapadia, M.; Rolston, K.V.I.; Han, X.Y. Invasive streptomyces infections: Six cases and literature review. *Am. J. Clin. Pathol.* **2007**, *127*, 619–624. [CrossRef] [PubMed]

66. Berkner, K.L. Vitamin K-dependent carboxylation. *Vitam. Horm.* **2008**, *78*, 131–156. [PubMed]

67. Note 1: Readers interested in viewing features summarized in Figure 5 for the all-atoms molecular models of hVKORC1 and hVKORC1L1 can download these from the Protein Model DataBase (https://bioinformatics.cineca.it/PMDB/main.php, PMDB identifiers PM0075969, PM007). The NMR structure for DsbB (PDB entry 2K74, model 1) can be downloaded from the RCSB Protein Data Bank (http://www.rcsb.org/pdb/home/home.do).

68. White, S.H. Biophysical dissection of membrane proteins. *Nature* **2009**, *459*, 344–346. [CrossRef] [PubMed]

69. Wallin, E.; von Heijne, G. Genome-wide analysis of integral membrane proteins from eubacterial, archaean, and eukaryotic organisms. *Protein Sci.* **1998**, *7*, 1029–1038. [CrossRef] [PubMed]

70. Lundstrom, K. Structural genomics and drug discovery. *J. Cell Mol. Med.* **2007**, *11*, 224–238. [CrossRef] [PubMed]

71. Oberai, A.; Ihm, Y.; Kim, S.; Bowie, J.U. A limited universe of membrane protein families and folds. *Protein Sci.* **2006**, *15*, 1723–1734. [CrossRef] [PubMed]

72. Vitkup, D.; Melamud, E.; Moult, J.; Sander, C. Completeness in structural genomics. *Nat. Struct. Biol.* **2001**, *8*, 559–566. [CrossRef] [PubMed]

73. Zhang, Y. Protein structure prediction: When is it useful? *Curr. Opin. Struct. Biol.* **2009**, *19*, 1–11. [CrossRef] [PubMed]

74. Schwede, T.; Sali, A.; Honig, B.; Levitt, M.; Berman, H.M.; Jones, D.; Brenner, S.E.; Burley, S.K.; Das, R.; Dokholyan, N.V.; *et al.* Outcome of a workshop on applications of protein models in biomedical research. *Structure* **2009**, *17*, 151–159. [CrossRef] [PubMed]

75. Adams, P.D.; Afonine, P.V.; Grosse-Kunstleve, R.W.; Read, R.J.; Richardson, J.S.; Richardson, D.C.; Terwilliger, T.C. Recent developments in phasing and structure refinement for macromolecular crystallography. *Curr. Opin. Struct. Biol.* **2009**, *21*, 21. [CrossRef] [PubMed]

76. Barbar, E.; Lehoux, J.G.; Lavigne, P. Toward the NMR structure of StAR. *Mol. Cell Endocrinol.* **2009**, *300*, 89–93. [CrossRef] [PubMed]

77. Bax, A. Weak alignment offers new NMR opportunities to study protein structure and dynamics. *Protein Sci.* **2003**, *12*, 1–16. [CrossRef] [PubMed]

78. Rost, B. Twilight zone of protein sequence alignments. *Protein Eng.* **1999**, *12*, 85–94. [CrossRef] [PubMed]

79. Forrest, L.R.; Tang, C.L.; Honig, B. On the accuracy of homology modeling and sequence alignment methods applied to membrane proteins. *Biophys. J.* **2006**, *91*, 508–517. [CrossRef] [PubMed]

80. Malojcić, G.; Owen, R.L.; Grimshaw, J.P.A.; Glockshuber, R. Preparation and structure of the charge-transfer intermediate of the transmembrane redox catalyst DsbB. *FEBS Lett.* **2008**, *582*, 3301–3307. [CrossRef] [PubMed]

81. Inaba, K.; Murakami, S.; Nakagawa, A.; Iida, H.; Kinjo, M.; Ito, K.; Suzuki, M. Dynamic nature of disulphide bond formation catalysts revealed by crystal structures of DsbB. *Embo J.* **2009**, *28*, 779–791. [CrossRef] [PubMed]

82. Vogel, C.; Morea, V. Duplication, divergence and formation of novel protein topologies. *Bioessays* **2006**, *28*, 973–978. [CrossRef] [PubMed]

83. Grishin, N.V. Fold change in evolution of protein structures. *J. Struct. Biol.* **2001**, *134*, 167–185. [CrossRef] [PubMed]

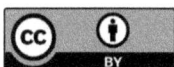

Review

VKORC1 and VKORC1L1: Why do Vertebrates Have Two Vitamin K 2,3-Epoxide Reductases?

Johannes Oldenburg [1,*], Matthias Watzka [1] and Carville G. Bevans [2]

[1] Institute of Experimental Haematology and Transfusion Medicine, University Clinic Bonn, Bonn 53105, Germany; E-Mail: matthias.watzka@ukb.uni-bonn.de

[2] Im Hermeshain 6, Frankfurt am Main 60388, Germany; E-Mail: bevans@jhu.edu

* Author to whom correspondence should be addressed; E-Mail: johannes.oldenburg@ukb.uni-bonn.de; Tel.: +49-228-287-15175; Fax: +49-228-287-14783.

Received: 18 May 2015 / Accepted: 15 July 2015 / Published: 30 July 2015

Abstract: Among all cellular life on earth, with the exception of yeasts, fungi, and some prokaryotes, VKOR family homologs are ubiquitously encoded in nuclear genomes, suggesting ancient and important biological roles for these enzymes. Despite single gene and whole genome duplications on the largest evolutionary timescales, and the fact that most gene duplications eventually result in loss of one copy, it is surprising that all jawed vertebrates (gnathostomes) have retained two paralogous VKOR genes. Both VKOR paralogs function as entry points for nutritionally acquired and recycled K vitamers in the vitamin K cycle. Here we present phylogenetic evidence that the human paralogs likely arose earlier than gnathostomes, possibly in the ancestor of crown chordates. We ask why gnathostomes have maintained these paralogs throughout evolution and present a current summary of what we know. In particular, we look to published studies about tissue- and developmental stage-specific expression, enzymatic function, phylogeny, biological roles and associated pathways that together suggest subfunctionalization as a major influence in evolutionary fixation of both paralogs. Additionally, we investigate on what evolutionary timescale the paralogs arose and under what circumstances in order to gain insight into the biological *raison d'être* for both VKOR paralogs in gnathostomes.

Keywords: evolution; subfunctionalization; paralog; vitamin K; VKOR; VKORC1; VKORC1L1

1. Introduction

Genomes of higher vertebrates possess two paralog genes, *VKORC1* and *VKORC1L1* (see Note 1 [1]), that encode enzymes unique in catalyzing de-epoxidation of vitamin K 2,3-epoxide (K>O), a product of post-translational modification of vitamin K-dependent (VKD) proteins [2,3]. VKD proteins are known to be essential for diverse physiological functions including hemostasis and coagulation [4, 5]; bone development and homeostasis [6–8]; vascular homeostasis, remodeling and calcification [9–13]; cellular growth, survival, and signaling [14,15]; metabolic homeostasis [16,17]; and fertility [18]. While the respective VKORC1 and VKORC1L1 protein primary sequences share ~50% identity and highly homologous function (Figure 1), it is surprising that both genes have been maintained with high fidelity throughout over 400 million years of vertebrate evolution [3,19] (See also Bevans *et al.* [20] in this Special Issue). In the following review, we point out structural and functional similarities and differences between both paralog enzymes and explore phylogenetic relationships in order to construct a hypothesis that addresses the question "Why do vertebrates have two vitamin K 2,3-epoxide reductase (VKOR) enzymes?".

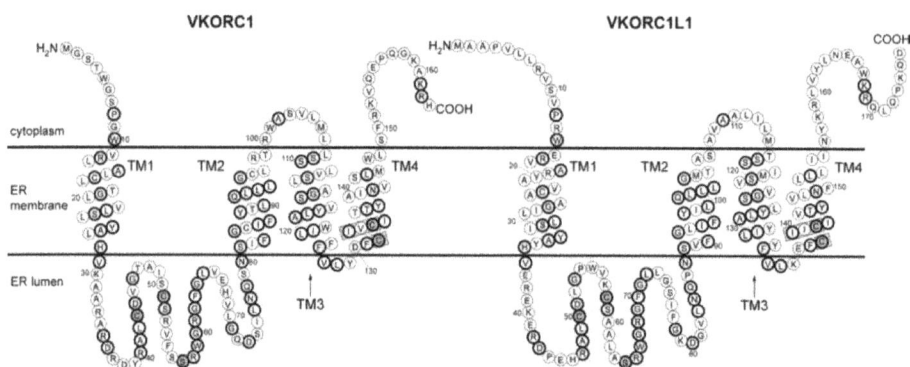

Figure 1. Primary protein sequence and predicted topology of human VKORC1 (left) and VKORC1L1 (right). Circles represent amino acid residues; bold circles indicate positions of sequence identity shared by both paralogs; green-filled circles, residues conserved among all VKOR family proteins; TM1–TM4, first through fourth transmembrane α-helices; gray-boxed regions, the catalytic CXXC active site motif.

1.1. Catalytic Function and Biological Roles of VKOR Family Enzymes

VKOR family homologs are expressed in the vast majority of the currently available sequenced genomes except those for all fungi and yeasts, and about half of the prokaryotic genomes available to-date, which almost always alternatively express DsbB oxidoreductases that function homologously to prokaryotic VKOR proteins [3,21–23] (See also Bevans *et al.* [20] in this Special Issue). Thus, VKOR homologs appear to have evolved very early in vertebrate evolutionary history and apparently carry out critical functions for most species, given their ubiquity and high degree of evolutionary conservation.

1.1.1. VKOR Enzymes Can Catalyze Multiple Reactions

Although the VKOR family is named for the first confirmed function of the human, rat and mouse orthologs [2,24], biochemical characterizations of non-vertebrate homologs reported to-date have indicated that they cannot catalyze VKOR activity, but alternatively catalyze vitamin K quinone reductase (VKR) or ubiquinone reductase activities [25–28]. To date, only one prokaryotic VKOR homolog from *Mycobacterium tuberculosis* has been demonstrated to possess VKOR activity *in vitro* when expressed in HEK 293 cells [27]. However, the native *M. tuberculosis* lipidome has been shown to possess only quinone and hydroquinone forms of menaquinones, but not menaquinone 2,3-epoxides [29], so it is not likely that the VKOR homolog of this bacterium catalyzes physiological VKOR activity *in vivo*. Subsequent to the initial reports identifying human VKORC1 by virtue of its VKOR de-epoxidase activity, the same enzyme was shown to additionally catalyze *in vitro* VKR activity that reduces vitamin K quinone (K) to vitamin K hydroquinone (KH$_2$) [30]. More recently, human VKORC1L1 was also confirmed to catalyze VKOR and VKR activities *in vitro* [31]. Thus, both vertebrate VKOR paralogs catalyze both VKOR and VKR enzymatic activities.

Four cysteine residues (human VKORC1 sequence numbering: Cys43, Cys51, Cys132, Cys135) are completely conserved among VKORC1 orthologs and are required for *in vivo* VKOR catalysis [27,32,33]. Only one *in vitro* study has investigated VKR enzymatic activity for VKORC1 and confirmed that Cys132 and Cys135 are required [30]. Additionally, a conserved serine or threonine (human VKORC1 sequence numbering: Ser57) has been shown to be essential for VKOR catalytic activity *in vitro* [32,34]. Based on sequence homology to the bacterial VKOR enzyme structure, the four redox-active cysteines are widely believed to be arranged in a double disulfide relay that shuttles reducing equivalents from ER-resident oxidoreductases, responsible for *de novo* oxidative protein folding (OPF), to membrane-soluble K>O [30,33–36]. Thus, VKORC1 accepts reducing equivalents from cysteine thiol groups of soluble oxidoreductase proteins in the ER lumen. Protein disulfide isomerase (PDI), TMX, TMX4 and ERp18, all with thioredoxin-like protein folds, have been implicated as physiological oxidoreductase partners by their ability to form intermolecular disulfide bonds with VKORC1 in cell culture experiments [36,37]. These ER-resident accessory oxidoreductases serve as the primary enzymes that interact with proteins and peptides undergoing oxidative folding by *de novo* disulfide formation [38]. Additionally, VKOR enzymes are the only OPF oxidoreductases that do not ultimately require molecular oxygen as the terminal electron acceptor by downstream enzymatic pathways, suggesting that the origin of these eukaryotic proteins may be very ancient, possibly having evolved before earth's atmosphere was substantially aerobic, and might predate the evolution of other enzymes involved in OPF in the ER including members of the Ero1, peroxiredoxin, and QSOX families [31,39].

1.1.2. Known Biological Roles for VKOR Family Enzymes

The first biological function attributed to VKORC1 was VKOR catalysis—the rate-limiting step in the classical vitamin K cycle [2,24,40,41]. In humans and other vertebrates, the vitamin K cycle drives post-translational modification of glutamic acid residues to form γ-carboxyglutamyl residues required for proper function of VKD proteins [42,43]. VKORC1 is the sole enzyme in vertebrates capable of sustaining sufficient VKOR activity to maintain hemostasis [42,44]. VKORC1L1 is apparently responsible for other functions as it cannot rescue VKORC1-specific production of VKD clotting factors in *vkorc1*$^{-/-}$ knock-out mice [44]. Newborn *vkorc1*$^{-/-}$ mice typically died within several days due to internal hemorrhage due to severe deficiency of γ-glutamyl carboxylated clotting factors. The lethal phenotype could be rescued by administration of large doses of vitamin K, similar to the rescue of the human VKCFD2 phenotype in patients homozygous for a VKORC1:Arg98Trp mutation [45]. Interestingly, with respect to hemostatic phenotype, heterozygous *vkorc1*$^{+/-}$ mice were indistinguishable from homozygous wild-type mice, suggesting that one wild-type *vkorc1* allele is sufficient for producing adequate levels of γ-glutamyl carboxylated VKD clotting factors to sustain normal development and growth. In contrast, with respect to bone morphology, eight-day old *vkorc1*$^{-/-}$ mice were found to have a pathological phenotype, whereby long bones were all found to be significantly shorter compared to those of homozygous wild-type *vkorc1* mice. In its fully γ-glutamyl carboxylated form, the VKD protein osteocalcin, secreted by osteoblast cells, has long been implicated in bone calcification and homeostasis [46]. Intriguingly, a recent study by Ferron *et al.* (2015) found that VKORC1L1 could not functionally substitute for VKORC1 in cultured osteoblast cells where VKORC1 expression level correlates with γ-glutamyl carboxylation of osteocalcin and modulation of its endocrine functions [47]. Thus, it appears that osteocalcin mediation of bone formation is a second example where VKORC1L1 cannot substitute for VKORC1-mediated biological function of a secreted VKD protein.

In addition to hemostatic functions of VKD clotting factors, other VKD proteins play crucial roles in bone growth and homeostasis [7,13], and recently were demonstrated to be necessary for inhibition of calcification in vasculature [9,10,12,48,49]. Vitamin K and VKD proteins have also been shown to protect oligodendrocytes and neurons from oxidative injury [50], function in cell signaling and growth [15,51], and support sphingomyelin synthesis and metabolism in nervous tissues [14].

A second important biological function was recently confirmed for VKORC1 as an acceptor of reducing equivalents from cysteines during oxidative protein folding in the ER [39]. This was independently confirmed by both siRNA silencing and warfarin knock-down of VKOR enzymatic activity in human hepatoma HepG2 cells after Ero1 α/β isoforms and peroxiredoxin IV (PRDX4) were first functionally silenced, demonstrating that VKORC1 alone can facilitate OPF.

That both vertebrate VKOR paralogs catalyze both VKOR and VKR reactions suggests that neofunctionalization of one of the evolved paralog enzymes, relative to the other retaining an ancestral function, has not occurred—at least with respect to catalytic reactions and substrates. Thus, further elucidation of biological functions for both enzymes may give clues to heretofore-unknown functional differences that might be the basis for selective pressure to conserve their otherwise redundant enzymatic activities in vertebrates. For example, there might be paralog-specific differences in which partner oxidoreductases pass reducing equivalents to each paralog or differences in tissue-specific or developmental stage-specific expression.

As a corollary to the above examples where VKORC1L1 cannot substitute for some of the biological functions of VKORC1 *in vivo*, we ask the question: Are there biological functions mediated by VKORC1L1 that VKORC1 cannot fulfill? Unfortunately, this question has not yet been experimentally addressed as it necessarily requires knock-down or knock-out of VKORC1L1 in cells or animal models that can be used to investigate its biological function. Recently, however, two lines of investigation have begun to focus on details of VKORC1L1 function.

First, a study by Westhofen *et al.* (2011) provided evidence from a number of different experimental perspectives. Expression of VKORC1L1 in HEK 293 T cells in the presence of vitamin K was found to promote vitamin K-dependent cell viability, elimination of intracellular reactive oxygen species and prevented oxidative damage to membrane proteins [31].

Second, a recent comprehensive study by Hammed *et al.* (2013) further measured and compared differential expression of vkorc1 and vkorc1l1 paralogs and tissue-specific VKOR activity of both paralogs in wild-type mice and the *vkorc1$^{-/-}$* mouse line originally reported by Spohn *et al.* (2009) [44,52]. Expression levels of vkorc1l1 in all tissues investigated were not different in *vkorc1$^{-/-}$* mice compared to mice with homozygous wild-type *vkorc1*. Thus, it appears that regulation of vkorc1l1 expression in mice is not sensitive to the level of vkorc1 expression, suggesting that the regulation of expression for both paralogs involves independent regulatory pathways. Furthermore, *in vitro* investigation of VKOR enzymatics for mouse and human VKOR paralog enzymes heterologously expressed in *Pichia pastoris* yielded surprising and unexpected results. While the Michaelis–Menton constants for $K_1 > O$ were determined to be similar for human VKORC1L1 and VKORC1 and for rat vkorc1l1 and vkorc1 (Table 1), the warfarin inhibition constants (K_i) for human VKORC1L1 and rat vkorc1l1 were found to be, respectively, 29-fold and 54-fold greater than for the respective VKORC1 and vkorc1 paralogs. Thus, it appears that both human and rat VKORC1L1 paralogs are ~1.5 orders of magnitude less warfarin sensitive than the respective VKORC1 paralogs. Based on these results, the study went on to show that tissue-specific expression of both paralogs contributes to overall level of VKOR activity (*i.e.*, tissue-specific VKOR activities of both paralogs are additive) and that the degree of warfarin sensitivity in various tissues is a function of the relative paralog expression ratio. Interestingly, by use of c-myc tagged expression constructs in *Pichia pastoris* cells, the authors were able to determine that the relative VKOR catalytic efficiency of rat vkorc1 is 30-fold greater than for rat vkorc1l1, while the VKOR catalytic efficiency of human VKORC1 is two-fold lower than that of human VKORC1L1. In summary, the study by Hammed *et al.* has demonstrated that VKORC1L1 is able to support VKOR activity and may constitute an alternative pathway that is able to substitute or partially complement for loss of VKORC1 function in various non-hepatic tissues of *vkorc1$^{-/-}$* mice.

1.1.3. Evolutionary Origins of the VKORC1 and VKORC1L1 Paralogs

Robertson (2004) previously suggested that an ancestral VKOR gene duplication likely occurred in early vertebrates and resulted in the extant human and other gnathostome VKOR paralogs [3]. This would be in agreement with the divergence of the common ancestor of the jawed vertebrates (gnathostomes) from urochordates and cephalochordates, as has been suggested for many other vertebrate protein paralog pairs [53]. In the article by Bevans *et al.* [20] in this special issue, a broad phylogenetic study of VKOR family homologs yielded strong support for distinct monophyletic clades comprising vertebrate VKORC1 and VKORC1L1 homologs. Thus, it is likely that the paralogs arose one time and quickly became fixed in the genomes of subsequently diverged early (crown) vertebrate lineages. That all extant gnathostome genomes sequenced to date include both paralog genes suggests that the functions of both paralogs are indispensable to vertebrate life. In order to more accurately confirm the divergence point of the last common ancestor of modern vertebrates with two VKOR family paralogs, we chose a series of index genomes sampling various evolutionary groupings that diverged before, during and after the last universal common ancestor of gnathostomes, many only very recently sequenced in draft form, to reconstruct a likely metazoan VKOR phylogeny (Figure 2).

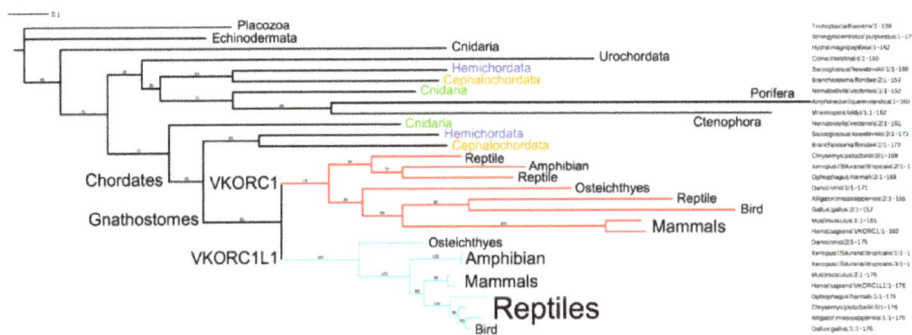

Figure 2. Reconstructed phylogeny (unrooted) for full-length sequences of index metazoans using PhyML with a WAG+I+G4 substitution model in the IQ-TREE ver1.2.3 server-based phylogenetics package with graphics generated using the iToL server (see Bevans *et al.* [20] in this Special Issue for details). Linnaean taxonomic names and primary sequence lengths are shown to the right; groupings shown on the left: Placozoa, basal invertebrate outgroup; Echinodermata and Hemichordata, basal deuterostomes belonging to the Ambulacaria; Cnidaria, basal metazoan invertebrates including jellyfish and sea anemonae; Urochordata, an invertebrate sister group to vertebrates; Porifera, basal non-metazoan animals including sponges; Ctenophora, basal non-bileterian metazoans including comb jellies; Cephalochordata, a basal chordate sister group to Olfactores which includes Urochordata and vertebrates; Chordates includes Cephalochordates, Tunicates (here represented by the Urochordate *Ciona intestinalis*) and Vertebrates; Gnathostomes are a subgroup of vertebrates with jaw bones that includes Chondrichthyes (sharks and rays—not included among the analyzed sequences; see Note 2 [54]) and Osteichthyes (bony fishes and tetrapods); VKORC1 and VKORC1L1 are paralog clades for Gnathostomes. Scale bar (upper left, labeled 0.1) represents single nucleotide substitution rate per million years; VKORC1 clade is represented by red lines; VKORC1L1 clade by cyan lines; numbers on branches are % support for 1000 bootstrap trees. VKOR paralogs encoded by non-gnathostome genomes are shown in blue (Hemichordata), orange (Cephalochordata) and green (Cnidaria) (see also Note 3 [55]).

As expected, we found high phylogenetic support for monophyletic VKORC1 and VKORC1L1 clades, which split uniformly for extant ganthostomes. Branch lengths for the VKORC1L1 clade (cyan) are relatively shorter than those for the VKORC1 clade (red), in agreement with earlier reports that primary sequences among VKORC1L1 orthologs are more highly conserved than for those among VKORC1 orthologs [2,3]. Reptilian VKORC1L1 orthologs appear on mixed branches with VKORC1L1 orthologs of amphibian, fish and bird as branch support for the VKORC1L1 clade is significantly weaker than for the VKORC1 clade. Surprisingly, for single genomes representing three non-gnathostome groups (Figure 2, indicated in blue, orange and green), we found pairs of VKOR paralogs where one paralog in each genome is inferred to be more similar to the gnathostome VKORs and the second paralogs for each genome are clustered together on a deeper-lying branch. However, inference support for the lower-lying branches (Figure 2, black lines) is considerably lower than the relatively high support for the gnathostome paralog clades. This is evident in the scrambled placement of representative non-gnathostome species in the tree that does not correlate well with the current consensus groupings on the Tree of Life (e.g., Echinodermata is placed on a low branch parallel to Placozoa, and chordate paralogs (Figure 2, blue and orange) are mixed with invertebrate

VKOR sequences on a single, deep branch (includes fourth through ninth sequences from the top). Notable results of our phylogenetic analysis include the VKOR paralog pairs of two invertebrate genomes (acorn worm, *Saccoglossus kowalevskii*; lancelet, *Branchiostoma floridae*) that are placed as basal deuterostomes, far deeper in the Tree of Life than vertebrates. This begs consideration that VKOR gene duplications may have occurred in these ancient invertebrate branches independent of the first whole genome duplication in gnathostomes, which, consistent with our inferred VKOR phylogeny, is the likeliest single event that resulted in the gnathostome paralogs. Similarly, the VKOR paralogs found in the Cnidarian sea anemone (*Nematostella vectensis*) may have arisen by a gene duplication unrelated to the gnathostome event. Whether these invertebrate genomes with VKOR paralog pairs represent isolated exceptions, or are evidence for deeper-rooted single gene duplication/loss events, will require more whole genome data from current and future sequencing efforts. In summary, our phylogenetic results suggest that the extant human VKOR paralogs VKORC1 and VKORC1L1 likely arose in an older common metazoan ancestor than the last universal common ancestor of gnathostomes, likely as early as the common ancestor of crown chordate groups.

2. Common Aspects of VKORC1 and VKORC1L1 Structure and Function

2.1. Gene and Protein Structural Organization

Parsing vertebrate *VKORC1* and *VKORC1L1* sequences in the NCBI Gene database confirmed both paralogs are organized into three exons of very similar lengths. Intron lengths vary considerably between the two paralogs with entire VKORC1L1 genes being typically 17–25 times longer than the respective VKORC1 paralogs (e.g., VKORC1: 2.3 kb mouse—human 3.5 kb; VKORC1L1: 40 kb mouse—86 kb human). In contrast, Robertson (2004) noted that three kinetoplast VKOR homologs, *Trypanosoma cruzi*, *T. brucei*, and *Leishmania major*, are encoded by single exon genes [3]. Pseudogenes found in the human, mouse and rat genomes have been previously reviewed in detail [3].

Inspection of vertebrate VKORC1 and VKORC1L1 full-length (isoform 1) protein sequences in the NCBI Proteins database revealed that most vertebrate VKORC1 orthologs are about 161–163 residues (Figure 3, yellow bars; range 160–163 residues), whereas VKORC1L1 sequences are predominantly 174–176 residues (Figure 3, cyan bars; range 161–190 residues). Most vertebrate VKORC1 ortholog primary sequences encompass a core domain of 153 residues (Figure 1, human VKORC1 residues Met1-Val153) with a *C*-terminus of variable length (7–14 residues). All VKORC1L1 sequences include an additional 3-residue insertion between corresponding human VKORC1 residues 10 and 11 (Figure 1, human VKORC1L1 residues Arg19-Tyr20-Ala21), effectively extending the length of the predicted 1st TMH by one α-helical turn and resulting in a core domain length of 152 residues (Figure 1, human VKORC1L1 residues Pro12-Leu163). The variable length *N*-termini of VKORC1L1 orthologs are 1–63 residues with the majority of orthologs having an *N*-terminal length of 11 residues. *C*-termini of VKORC1L1 orthologs are 8–13 residues with the majority having a length of 13 residues. Both VKORC1 and VKORC1L1 are localized to and retained in the ER [2,31], likely by a COP I-mediated mechanism of the *cis*-Golgi that recognizes known ER retention recognition sequences with adjacent pairs of positively charged amino acids in the *C*-termini of membrane-intrinsic proteins [56]. Recently, an additional ER retention motif in the short cytoplasmic loop connecting TMH2 and TMH3 of human VKORC1 has been identified [57].

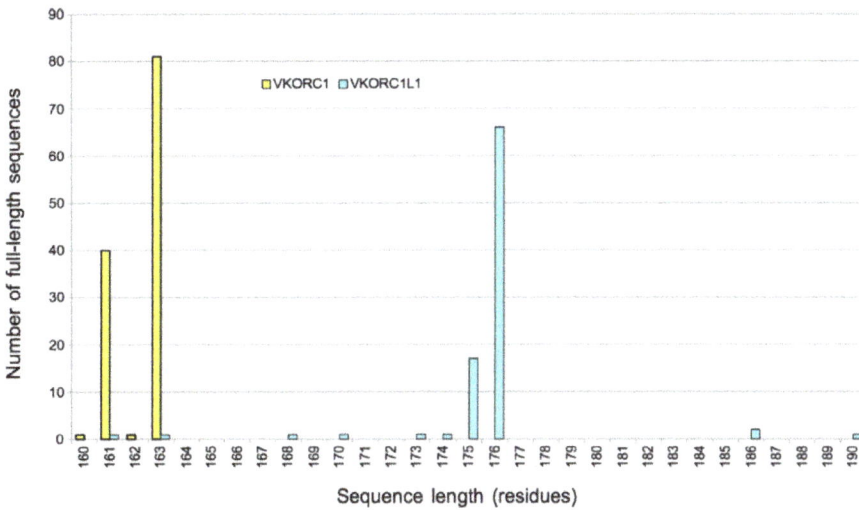

Figure 3. Histogram of vertebrate VKOR paralog sequence lengths in the NCBI Protein database. All sequences included were verified as full-length isoform 1 for VKORC1 (yellow bars) and VKORC1L1 (cyan bars).

Extramembraneous loops are of identical length among all sequenced vertebrate VKOR homologs. Thus, respective VKORC1 and VKORC1L1 proteins in vertebrates are expected to have highly homologous, evolutionarily conserved respective protein folds.

2.2. In Vitro VKOR Enzymatics—Substrates and Inhibitors

Although the first detailed enzymatic studies of VKOR activity in liver microsomes prepared from mice and rats commenced in 1984 [58–60], more recent studies, since 2011, characterizing the enzymatics of recombinantly produced human and rat VKORC1 and VKORC1L1 are just now gaining momentum among several active, independent research groups [31,52,61–68]. In order to form a comprehensive picture of our current understanding of VKOR enzymatics, we have summarized the basic results of these studies (Table 1). Of the dozen studies specifically addressing VKOR enzymatics, the initial three relied on rodent liver microsomal preparations as enzyme sources which, during preparation, substantially lose the ER lumenal oxidoreductases that are required for physiological VKOR activity *in vivo* [58]. In order to supply reducing equivalents to drive VKOR activity *in vitro*, DTT has been widely used since it was found to support VKOR activity (for a historical review of the DTT-driven *in vitro* VKOR assay, see [68]). Thus, in the DTT-driven VKOR assay, VKORC1 or VKORC1L1 catalyze reduction of K>O with concomitant oxidation of DTT. To achieve this, the enzymes function by a kinetic mechanism that alternates between two states where the active site CXXC motif cysteines are either oxidized (in the form of a disulfide bridge between them) or reduced [58,63,65,69]. Two different enzyme kinetic models have thus far been applied to VKOR studies—the "ping-pong" model takes enzymatic conversion of both substrates into account [58,63,65,68], while a simpler Michaelis–Menton single substrate kinetic model is based on enzymatic conversion of only the K>O substrate [31,52,59–62,64,66,67]. For the K>O single substrate model to be valid, the DTT substrate must be at saturating concentration in the VKOR assay a requisite condition for pseudo first-order kinetics [70]. Both kinetic models can yield valid enzymatic parameters (e.g., K_m, V_{max}, k_{cat}) from DTT-driven VKOR assay data. However, due to the fact that DTT competes with warfarin for binding to the enzymes, interpretation of warfarin dose-response data obtained using the DTT-driven VKOR assay has been extremely problematic [63,65,71,72]. For example, VKORC1 variants with single amino acid mutations that cause warfarin resistance in humans and rodents show dose-response data indicating warfarin susceptibility identical to wild-type VKORC1 [2,73]. This problem in *in vitro* assessment of resistance phenotypes for known VKORC1 warfarin-resistant variants has been recently overcome by use of alternative cell culture-based VKOR activity assays (see below) which yield warfarin resistance dose-response data in agreement with human and rodent resistance phenotypes. However, an advantage in continuing use of non-physiological reductant-driven VKOR assays lies in their ability to provide data suitable for detailed enzymatics and catalysis mechanism studies since, unlike in cell culture-based assays, the assay conditions can be strictly defined.

What we can generally conclude from VKOR enzymatics studies to-date includes (referring to Table 1): (1) wild-type VKORC1 and VKORC1L1 Michaelis-Menton constant (K_m) values determined for K>O substrates are in the low micromolar ($\sim$1–35 μM) range, while K_m for DTT and THPP reducing substrates are approximately millimolar (V_{max} values are not comparable between studies as they reflect a convolution of intrinsic enzyme turnover rate with the quantitative amount of enzyme used in the assay); (2) the enzymes to not appear to significantly discriminate between phylloquinone- and menaquinone-2,3-epoxide substrates; (3) for all warfarin resistance mutations studied, except for Tyr139 position mutations in rats, measured K_m values for K>O are considerably greater than for the respective wild-type enzymes, implying K>O substrate binding affinity is diminished by nearly all mutations; (4) the DTT-driven VKOR assay reveals warfarin-resistant *in vitro* phenotypes only for a very few mutations investigated (Table 1; last column, K_i values indicated in bold-face type are significantly increased with respect to the wild-type K_i in each study); and (5) both human and rat VKORC1L1 enzymes appear to be considerably less warfarin-sensitive than the respective VKORC1 enzymes. To-date, enzymatic studies of VKR catalytic function for VKORC1 and VKORC1L1 have not been reported. From enzymatic study of VKOR catalysis available so far for both VKORC1 and VKORC1L1, we are nudged towards the conclusion that there is no major difference in enzymatic function or substrate specificity between the vertebrate VKORC1 and VKORC1L1 paralogs.

Table 1. Summary of results from published VKORC1 and VKORC1L1 enzymatics studies.

Study	Enzyme	Species	K_m ($K_1 > O$) (μM)	K_m ($K_2 > O$) (μM)	K_m (DTT) (mM)	pH	K_m (THPP$_{Total}$) (μM)	K_i (warfarin) (μM)
Krettler *et al.* 2015 [65]	r VKORC1	human	**1.20**			7.4		0.32 ± 0.07
Goulois *et al.* 2015 [64]	r vkorc1	R. rattus	**15.9 ± 4.5**					
	r vkorc1	R. norvegicus				7.4	431	0.50 ± 0.01
	r vkorc1:Y25F	R. rattus	**15.9 ± 4.5**			7.4		**1.99**
Matagrin *et al.* 2014 [63]	r VKORC1	human				7.4		1.65
Hammed *et al.* 2013 [51]	r VKORC1	human	**21.5 ± 4.2**			7.4		1.8 ± 0.2
	r vkorc1	rat	**19.6 ± 1.6**			7.4		0.6 ± 0.04
	r VKORC1L1	human	**24.1 ± 3.0**			7.4		52.0 ± 3.0
	r vkorc1l1	rat	**35.0 ± 3.0**			7.4		32.6 ± 1.9
Matagrin *et al.* 2013 [61]	r vkorc1	rat	**7.2 ± 2.5**			7.4		
	r vkorc1:L120Q	rat	25.0 ± 4.0			7.4		
	r vkorc1:L128Q	rat	12.1 ± 1.0			7.4		
	r vkorc1:Y139C	rat	60.0 ± 6.0			7.4		
	r vkorc1:Y139F	rat	17.8 ± 4.5			7.4		
	r vkorc1:Y139S	rat	13.1 ± 1.3			7.4		
Bevans *et al.* 2013 [60]	r VKORC1	human	1.24		8.38	7.5		2.481
						7.5		2.633
						7.5		5.786
Hodroge *et al.* 2012 [59]	r VKORC1	human	**19.8 ± 4.5**			7.4		1.65 ± 0.79
	r VKORC1:A26P	human	57.4 ± 10.1			7.4		**18.43 ± 5.82**
	r VKORC1:A26T	human	18.7 ± 1.4			7.4		2.13 ± 0.56
	r VKORC1:L27V	human	22.8 ± 2.9			7.4		1.83 ± 0.62
	r VKORC1:H28Q	human	29.8 ± 4.6			7.4		0.65 ± 0.42
	r VKORC1:D36G	human	43.8 ± 0.2			7.4		0.74 ± 0.25
	r VKORC1:D36Y	human	23.6 ± 0.2			7.4		1.82 ± 0.70
	r VKORC1:A41S	human	65.9 ± 5.4			7.4		1.78 ± 0.02

31

Table 1. Cont.

Reference	Enzyme	Species			pH	
Hodroge et al. 2012 [59]	r VKORC1:V45A	human	26.9 ± 2.3		7.4	1.10 ± 0.04
	r VKORC1:V54L	human	102.5 ± 28.6		7.4	**7.95 ± 1.32**
	r VKORC1:S56F	human	23.2 ± 6.2		7.4	1.05 ± 0.82
	r VKORC1:R58G	human	71.0 ± 10.9		7.4	1.50 ± 0.36
	r VKORC1:W59C	human	179.7 ± 12.5		7.4	1.16 ± 0.20
	r VKORC1:H68Y	human	16.9 ± 2.8		7.4	**6.21 ± 0.85**
	r VKORC1:I123N	human	27.0 ± 2.1		7.4	**4.01 ± 1.01**
	r VKORC1:Y139H	human	9.2 ± 3.0		7.4	**5.91 ± 1.77**
	r vkorc1	rat	**7.20 ± 2.50**		7.4	0.50 ± 0.05
	vkorc1$^{wt/wt}$	rat	**8.40 ± 0.90**		7.4	0.72 ± 0.01
	r vkorc1:L120Q	rat			7.4	>100
Hodroge et al. 2011 [58]	r vkorc1:L128Q	rat			7.4	**4.0 ± 0.7**
	r vkorc1:Y139C	rat			7.4	>100
	r vkorc1:Y139F	rat	17.8 ± 4.5		7.4	>100
	vkorc1:Y139F+/+	rat	19.5 ± 4.0		7.4	**29.0 ± 4.1**
	r vkorc1:Y139S	rat			7.4	>100
Westhofen et al. 2011 [30]	r VKORC1	human	1.88 ± 0.13	1.55 ± 0.55	7.6	
	r VKORC1L1	human	4.15 ± 0.10	11.24 ± 0.23	7.6	
Lasseur et al. 2006 [57]	vkorc1$^{wt/wt}$	mouse	12.73 ± 0.93		7.4	5.97 ± 0.38
	vkorc1$^{W59G/W59G}$	mouse	15.31 ± 4.92		7.4	3.5 ± 0.27
Lasseur et al. 2005 [56]	vkorc1$^{wt/wt}$	rat	57.7 ± 12.5		7.4	0.72 ± 0.06
	vkorc1$^{Y139F/Y139F}$	rat	19.5 ± 4		7.4	**29 ± 4.1**
Hildebrandt et al. 1984 [55]	vkorc1$^{wt/wt}$	rat	10.0 ± 0.7 *	0.60 ± 0.03	8.8	
	vkorc1$^{wt/wt}$	rat	9.1 ± 0.13 *	0.54 ± 0.04	8.8	
	vkorc1:Y139S/Y139S	rat	4 *	0.16	8.8	
	vkorc1$^{wt/wt}$	rat	9	0.43	7.2	
	vkorc1:Y139S/Y139S	rat	6	0.29	7.2	

Symbols: r, (Enzyme column) recombinantly produced enzyme; * (K_m (K_1 > O) column), sodium cholate-solubilized and partially purified enzyme. All enzymes are wild-type unless indicated by a colon followed by a specific mutation; samples prepared from liver microsomes are indicated with a superscript where individual *VKORC1* alleles (separated by a slash) are indicated as (wild-type) or a specific mutation. Bold-face type in columns for Michaelis–Menten constants (K_m values) indicates values for wild-type enzymes. Bold-face type in the column for warfarin inhibition constants (K_i) indicates warfarin resistance phenotypes confirmed by *in vitro* measurement.

2.3. In Vitro Cell Culture-Based Assays of VKOR Activity

Recent studies have confirmed *in vitro* warfarin resistance phenotypes for known human VKORC1 mutations that are in agreement with reported *in vivo* resistance phenotypes [74]. Compared to warfarin IC_{50} values for wild-type warfarin-sensitive and warfarin-resistant human VKORC1 variants determined by Fregin *et al.* (2013) [75] and Czogalla *et al.* (2013) [76], warfarin IC_{50} values determined in the study of Tie *et al.* (2013) are all about an order of magnitude lower, but all of these studies ranked *in vitro* phenotype severity, with respect to specific mutations, identically [77]. Although the purpose of the study by Haque *et al.* (2014) was to investigate dose-response for warfarin and its hydroxylated metabolites, and did not investigate warfarin-resistant VKORC1 variants, the warfarin IC_{50} value obtained for wild-type human VKORC1 is greater than the values obtained in all of the other studies [78]. Directly compared, warfarin IC_{50} values reported by Fregin *et al.* (2013) and Haque *et al.* (2014) are 6.9-fold and 18.3- to 35.4-fold greater than the value reported by Tie *et al.* (2013) [75,77,78]. Variations in assay conditions between the studies that could account for the differences in warfarin dose-response have not yet been identified. One important difference between the non-physiological reductant-driven VKOR assays and the more physiological cell culture-based assays is that the former directly assess enzyme function, while the latter are actually indirect assays of enzyme function in that they each rely on the rate-limiting function of VKOR enzymes in the vitamin K cycle to ultimately enable intracellular γ-gutamyl carboxylation of VKD proteins heterologously coexpressed by the cells and secreted into the culture medium. Thus, while the effects of warfarin inhibition on the read-out VKD protein status can be directly attributed to warfarin's localized interaction with VKORC1 or VKORC1L1, there are likely many other influences on the secreted VKD status (e.g., due to choices of cell line, specific VKD reporter protein, expression vector, and variability in culture medium constituents especially in amounts of warfarin-binding serum albumin, *etc.*) that could have profound influence on the correspondence between applied warfarin dosage and secreted VKD protein response. Balancing these possible uncertainties are the opportunities to use these cell culture-based assays to explore the nature of the enzymes' biological functions. Thus, identification of native partner oxidoreductases that provide the physiological reducing equivalents to drive VKOR activity and characterizing their interactions with VKORC1 and VKORC1L1 in the ER lumen could be experimentally addressed. Similarly, studies could be designed to elucidate regulation of the respective gene transcription and protein expression for VKOR paralogs in cell lines representative of various native tissues and developmental stages. Cultured cell assays would also be useful in identification and assessment of new pharmacological lead compounds based on vitamin K or intended for use as oral anticoagulants with desired qualities superior to currently available warfarin and other 4-hydroxycoumarin derivatives.

3. Differences between VKORC1 and VKORC1L1 Paralogs

3.1. Tissue- and Developmental Stage-Specific Expression

It has been known for a long time that liver is the primary location of VKOR enzymatic activity essential to the vitamin K cycle and production and secretion of VKD coagulation factors [35,71]. In 2000, before the identification of the *VKORC1* and *VKORC1L1* genes, a study by Itoh and Onishi investigated developmental changes in VKOR enzymatic activity of human liver sampled from autopsied samples representing individuals from 12 weeks post-fertilization to 18 years of age [79]. They found hepatic VKOR activity was low (mean 100 nmol/15 min/g_{liver}) and possibly declined through prenatal week 30, then increased abruptly by prenatal week 35 (mean 200 nmol/15 min/g_{liver}) and thereafter remained constant through age 18. With the identification of both VKOR paralogs in 2004, recent discoveries of biological roles for non-coagulation factor VKD proteins, and elucidation of what cells and tissues are their primary sites of expression, an increasing number of studies have been focused on assessing tissue-specific expression distributions for both VKORC1 and VKORC1L1

(Table 2). With respect to developmental expression of vkorc1 in mouse, two studies provided some early insight. Ko *et al.* (1998) constructed a cDNA library from total mRNA prepared from 7.5-day post-conception mouse embryonic and extraembryonic cells and found no evidence of vkorc1 expression by RT-PCR analysis [80]. A subsequent mouse tissue expression study by Diez-Roux *et al.* (2011) used *in situ* RNA hybridization on whole embryo sections and found diffuse, weak expression of vkorc1 by 14.5 day post-fertilization embryos [81].

Two recent studies determined mouse VKOR paralog expression profiles for mouse tissues by relative mRNA expression quantitation using qRT-PCR of cDNA prepared from tissue-specific mRNAs. Hammed *et al.* (2013) measured vkorc1l1 expression in liver, lung, and testis of both C57BL/6 wild-type and *vkorc1$^{-/-}$* mice and in wild-type nine week-old OFA-Sprague Dawley rat brain, kidney, liver, lung and testis and rat osteosarcoma cell line ROS17/2.8 (Table 2) [52]. In mouse tissues, vkorc1l1 expression levels were highly similar between wild-type and *vkorc1$^{-/-}$* strains, suggesting distinctly independent regulation of expression for both VKOR paralogs. For all tissues investigated, vkorc1 expression was also found, but most predominantly in liver (10-fold greater than for vkorc1l1), whereas brain had greater vkorc1l1 expression relative to that for vkorc1. Other tissues had intermediate expression levels for both paralogs. For expression levels in rat liver, lung, brain, kidney and testis assessed at three, six and nine weeks post-partum, both paralogs showed minor variations that were not statistically significant except for vkorc1 expression in liver which peaked significantly at six weeks before declining at nine weeks. Taken together, these results explain why some extrahepatic tissues may have near physiological VKOR activities and down-stream VKD protein function in the presence of warfarin concentrations that effectively inhibit VKD clotting factor production in the liver. Another study by Caspers *et al.* (2015) similarly investigated VKOR paralog expression levels in 29 different tissues of CD1 wild-type mouse [82]. Expression levels for vkorc1 were found to be greatest in liver, lung and exocrine tissues including mammary, salivary and prostate glands, whereas vkorc1l1 expression was greatest in brain (Table 2). Taken together, results of both studies investigating rodent tissue expression patterns for both VKOR paralogs strongly suggests an emerging picture of independent regulation of the vitamin K cycle by differential expression of both VKOR paralog enzymes.

In zebrafish, Fernández *et al.* (2015) have assessed Vkorc1 and Vkorc1l1 expression by qPCR analysis during larval development and in adult tissues [83]. Vkorc1l1 was expressed at highest levels overall at the post-fertilization 4-cell stage and diminished by Prim-5 stage, remaining stable at later stages. Vkorc1 expression was detectable at the 4-cell stage, but peaked at 72–96 h post-fertilization followed by lower, stable levels at later stages. In adults, Vkorc1l1 was ubiquitously expressed in all tissues investigated (Table 2) with greatest levels in brain, muscle and ovary, while Vkorc1 was only detectable in about half of the surveyed tissues with elevated levels in brain, muscle and vertebra. Interestingly, no Vkorc1 expression could be detected in adult intestine, kidney, ovary, spleen and stomach. Using the ZFB1 cell line developed in a previous study [84], the authors found Vkorc1 and Vkorc1l1 to be significantly overexpressed during differentiation, but not during induction of extracellular matrix (ECM) mineralization, in cells cultured for 1 week. In cells cultured for three weeks, there was no significant difference between differentiating cells or cells induced to mineralize ECM. Taken together with results reported for ROS 17/2.8 osteoblast-like cells by Hammed *et al.* (2013), and moderate expression levels of both VKOR paralogs in vertebral tissue, the authors suggest that osteoblast differentiation may require increased vitamin K cycle turnover [51].

Since the initial draft of the human, mouse and rat genomes completed in 2000, 2002 and 2004, respectively, whole genome and proteome investigations have enabled large-scale, high through-put investigation of gene and protein expression levels in various tissues and cells [85]. Less than a year after the identification of both VKOR paralogs in 2004, high-density nucleotide arrays including *VKORC1* and *VKORC1L1* sequences were already being used to explore gene expression on a genomics scale. CHiP-Seq mRNA quantification studies including data for *VKORC1* and *VKORC1L1* have been published for frog, fruitfly, human, rat, mouse, pig, and zebrafish [86–90].

We recently recovered human and mouse VKOR paralog mRNA expression profiles based on chromatin immunoprecipitation (ChIP-seq) technology from a large, high through-put transcriptomics study by Su *et al.* (2004) available through the BioGPS database portal [86,91]. Their data includes VKORC1 and VKORC1L1 expression levels for 79 human and 61 mouse tissues from pooled samples of typically 1–10 individuals. For simplification, in Table 2 we summarize only results including tissues with the 10 highest VKORC1 and VKORC1L1 expression levels above mean values for all tissues (for comprehensive tissue data, see Figure S1, online Supplemental Material). For human and mouse, VKORC1L1 is uniformly expressed at or near median value for most all tissues and cells surveyed. From among those surveyed, only adipocytes, CD34+ cell lines (including monocytic lines) and B lymphoblasts exhibit statistically significant higher levels of VKORC1L1 expression than the median. Westhofen *et al.* (2011) previously pointed out that all three tissues/cell types generate intensely and protractedly elevated levels of ROS under physiological conditions, suggesting a role for VKORC1L1 in redox homeostasis [31]. BioGPS tissue-specific expression levels for *VKORC1* mRNA exhibit more highly varied differences than for *VKORC1L1*. Among tissues with the highest expression levels are liver, where most of the vitamin K-dependent blood-clotting factors are produced, and adipocytes, smooth muscle, thyroid, lung and pineal body.

Data from the GTEx Portal [92], a large-scale, high through-put human genomics project published earlier this year, has recently been mined for a study by Melé *et al.* (2015) on RNA-seq deep-sequenced transcriptomes of 175 individuals that covers 29 solid organ tissues, 11 brain subregions, whole blood and two standard cell lines [93]. We summarize the top six expressing tissues for each VKOR paralog in this study (Figure S2, online Supplemental Material) for comparison with data from other studies. Tissues with highest levels of VKORC1 (ENSG#167397) expression from the GTEx project data included aorta and coronary artery, liver, pituitary and gland, while VKORC1L1 (ENSG#196715) expression was found to be greatest in adipose tissue, mammary gland, lung and tibial nerve (Table 2). Interestingly, the study results indicated that gene activity, in general, differed substantially more across tissues than across individuals and expression patterns for both *VKORC1* and *VKORC1L1* follow this trend. Genes that changed expression (FDR < 0.05) with age across all GTEx study tissues included *VKORC1L1*, but not *VKORC1* [94].

Table 2. Summary of results from expression studies of human, mouse and rat VKORC1 and VKORC1L1.

Study	Itoh & Onishi 2000 [76] *	Su et al. 2004 [83] *	Hammed et al. 2013 [51]	Kim et al. 2014 [93]	Wilhelm et al. 2014 [94]	Caspers et al. 2015 [79]	Melé et al. 2015 [90] *	Fernández et al. 2015 [80] *
Species	Human	Human, Mouse	Mouse, Rat	Human	Human	Mouse	Human	Zebrafish
Method	VKOR activity assay	CHiP-Seq	mRNA	Mass Spectroscopy	Mass Spectroscopy	mRNA	mRNA	mRNA
Tissue/cell types	Liver (12 weeks post-fertilization to 18 years)	Adipocyte; Brain (whole); Colon	Brain	Adrenal gland; Colon; Esophagus	Adipocyte; Adrenal gland; Blood platelet; Bone; Brain; Breast; Cerebral cortex; Colon; Colonic epithelial cell	Adrenal gland; Bone; Brain; Mammary gland; Caecum; Colon; Diaphragm; Duodenum; Eye	Adipose-visceral (omentum); Adipose-subcutaneous; Aorta; Breast-mammary; Coronary artery	Operculum; Brain; Eye

Table 2. *Cont.*

Tissue/cell types	Liver (12 weeks post-fertilization to 18 years)	CD34+				
Fetal Brain Fetal Gut Fetal Heart Fetal Liver Fetal Ovary **Fetal Placenta Fetal Testis** Frontal cortex Gallbladder				Gall bladder		
Heart					Heart	
Hematopoietic B cells Hematopoietic CD4+ T cells Hematopoietic CD8+ T cells				Gut Heart Helper T-lymphocyte		
Hematopoietic Monocytes				**Monocyte**		
						Gills

Table 2. *Cont.*

Tissue/cell types							
Liver (12 weeks post-fertilization to 18 years)	Liver Lung 721 B-lymphoblasts Mast-cells-IgE Mast-cells-IgE+antigen-1 h Mast-cells-IgE+antigen-6 h Mega-erythrocyte-progenitor	Kidney Liver Lung	Hematopoietic NK cells Hematopoietic Platelets Kidney Liver Lung	Ileum epithelial cell Kidney Liver Lung Milk Myometrium Natural killer cell	Kidney Liver Lung Lymph node Masseter muscle Muscle Oesophagus	Liver Lung EBV transformed lymphocytes Nerve-tibial	Intestine Kidney Liver Muscle

---

Table 2. *Cont.*

Tissue/cell types	Liver (12 weeks post-fertilization to 18 years)							
Osteoblast-day 14 **Osteoblast-day 21** **Osteoblast-day 5**	**Rat osteosarcoma cell line ROS 17/2.8**		**Ovary** Pancreas	Osteosarcoma cell Ovary **Pancreas** **Pancreatic islet**		Ovary Pancreas	**Pituitary**	**Ovary**
Pineal body **Pituitary**			Prostate Rectum Retina	Placenta Prefrontal cortex Prostate gland Rectum **Retina**	**Prostate**			
Smooth-muscle			Spinal cord	Skin Spinal cord Stomach	**Salivary gland** Skin Soft tissue Stomach Spleen Testis			Skin
Thyroid	**Testis**		**Testis**	**Testis**				Stomach Spleen

Nutrients 2015, 7, 6250–6280

Table 2. *Cont.*

Tissue/cell types	Liver (12 weeks post-fertilization to 18 years)	Umbilical-cord		Urinary bladder	Urinary bladder	Tongue	Transformed fibroblasts
						Uterus	
						Vessels	
							Vertebra

Symbols: * only cells and tissues shown with significantly greater expression than mean levels for all cells/tissues included in large-scale study; bold type indicates cells/tissues with expression levels significantly above means for each study; yellow, high VKORC1L1 expression level; blue, high VKORC1 expression level; green high VKORC1 and VKORC1L1 coexpression.

40

Whole proteome studies using mass spectroscopic (MS) technologies have recently provided an opportunity to identify and quantitate intracellular pools of translated proteins across tissue types and populations of individuals [95]. Two recent MS proteomics studies include informative protein expression for human VKOR paralogs. Kim *et al.* (2014) systematically examined 30 different human tissues, including seven fetal tissues and six hematopoietic cell types from rapidly acquired postmortem samples from each of three donors [96]. Results for protein levels (~84% coverage of total predicted human proteome) of VKORC1 and VKORC1L1 from this study are available on the Human Proteome Map server [96]. VKORC1 proteolytic peptides (six 6–18 residue peptides representing 31% primary sequence coverage) were detected in six tissues including adrenal gland, monocytes, platelets, lung ovary and testes, while VKORC1L1 peptides (eleven 7–19 residue peptides representing 41% primary sequence coverage) were detected in fetal brain, placenta, testes and in adult lung (Table 2 lists all tissues in which VKOR paralog peptides were detected by MS). A similar MS proteomics study by Wilhelm *et al.* (2014) combined their own data from a similar number of tissues with >10,000 publicly available MS raw data files to generate a database encompassing 60 human tissues, 147 cell lines and 13 body fluids [97]. This study achieved a record 92% coverage of human proteome ORFs. VKORC1 (four 11–30 residue peptides representing 41.1% primary sequence coverage) was detected at higher than median expression levels only in monocytes, pancrease and retina, while VKORC1L1 (four 11–46 residue peptides representing 51.7% primary sequence coverage) was detected in higher than median expression levels only in brain. Compared to the results of Kim *et al.* (2014), this study had a very low detection efficiency for VKOR paralogs likely due to the much longer proteolytic fragments that were initially generated from tissue samples [96,97]. Comparing both MS studies to ChIP-seq method results (see above), it is clear that the MS-based techniques are still in their infancy as the number of tissues with detectable VKOR paralogs is low compared to the results from transcriptome studies. However, looking across all expression study results (Table 2), we find a general concurrence that VKORC1 is most highly expressed in liver, while VKORC1L1 is most highly expressed in brain.

3.2. Promoter Regions of VKORC1 and VKORC1L1 Genes

Since the coding regions of the *VKORC1* and *VKORC1L1* paralog genes are similarly organized and the respective expressed proteins are so highly conserved that their core domain sequence lengths, predicted folds, catalyzed reactions and substrate usage are essentially identical, we decided to survey existing published data for differences in non-coding regions of the genes for clues to why both paralogs have been preserved with complete fidelity in all extant (*i.e.*, sequenced to-date) vertebrate genomes. In a previously published study of human VKORC1L1 expression and function, we cited tissue-specific ChIP-seq gene expression data for both VKOR paralogs from the Functional ANnoTation Of the Mammalian genome phase 4 (FANTOM4) whole genome expression study [31,98]. For the purpose of exploring similarities and differences of the promoter regions for both human VKOR paralogs, we accessed deep-CAGE data using the FANTOM4 human genome viewer (Figure 4). FANTOM4 focused on the dynamics of transcription start site (TSS) usage in the myeloid cell line THP-1 [99]. We retrieved transcription start site (TSS) and predicted transcription factor binding site (TFBS) data for functionally expressed human *VKORC1* and *VKORC1L1* genes. In summary, *VKORC1* promoter organization is distinctly different from and relatively simpler than that for *VKORC1L1*. *VKORC1* uses four alternative TSSs spanning ~200 bp and 24 predicted TFBSs were identified around this region (Figure 4A, red arrows), while *VKORC1L1* uses seven alternative TSSs spanning ~150 bp with 53 predicted nearby TFBSs (Figure 4B, red arrows).

To predict putative binding sites for known TFBS motifs, a window of −300 to +100 bp flanking each promoter region was extracted, multiply aligned and the MotEvo algorithm applied [100]. Of the 52 predicted transcription regulators, 16 TFs were experimentally confirmed by systematic siRNA knock-down for the *VKORC1L1* promoter region, while only three TFs were found to bind the *VKORC1* promoter region (see Note 4 [101]) [98]. Taken together, these data support the notion that expression of each human VKOR paralog is apparently controlled by distinctly different transcriptional mechanisms, in agreement with previous study results for combined tissue expression levels and respective VKOR enzymatic activities in mice [52,82]. Furthermore, for *VKORC1*, there appear to be many predicted TFBSs in common with other hepatically expressed proteins, while predicted TFBSs for *VKORC1L1* are more similar to those from genes that express proteins with known house-keeping and homeostatic functions [31].

3.3. Human Coding Region Mutations

Naturally occurring coding region mutations for human, rat and mouse *VKORC1* genes mostly cause *in vivo* warfarin resistance phenotypes [73,74,102], and one human mutation causes VKCFD2, a severe deficiency in VKD clotting factors [2]. *VKORC1* mutations have been comprehensively reviewed elsewhere [103]. To gain insight into naturally occurring human *VKORC1L1* coding region mutations, we surveyed the NCBI dbVAR database, which includes combined whole genome sequence data for thousands of individuals, and found evidence for 21 total coding region SNPs in living adult humans of which seven are non-synonymous, one premature termination that shortens the C-terminus, and six synonymous variants that do not alter translated VKORC1L1 protein sequence. To date, no human *in vivo* phenotypes have been reported for VKORC1L1 non-wild type variants.

3.4. Commentary/Hypothesis: Why do Two VKOR Paralogs Persist in Vertebrates?

Here we summarize various conclusions drawn from the studies reviewed in this article and propose a novel hypothesis to explain why two VKOR paralogs with apparently identical enzymatic functions have persisted in vertebrates over ~400 million years of evolution. Rost *et al.* (2004) first noted that VKORC1L1 primary sequences are considerably more conserved among mammalian orthologs than the respective VKORC1 sequences [2]. Robertson (2004) suggested that the extant paralog genes likely arose in a common ancestor before the divergence of urochordates and vertebrates [3]. Phylogenetic analysis we present in this review suggests the last universal common ancestor (LUCA) of all extant metazoans with both VKOR paralogs was likely a crown chordate older than the LUCA of extant gnathostomes (Section 1.1.3. and Figure 2). Given aggregate evidence reviewed in this article that VKORC1 and VKORC1L1 enzymatic functions are virtually identical, but that regulation of developmental stage- and tissue-specific expression is the major notable difference between both paralogs, we further contemplate what other functional differences, at either the protein or biological pathway levels, could provide the required selection pressure to preserve both paralogs.

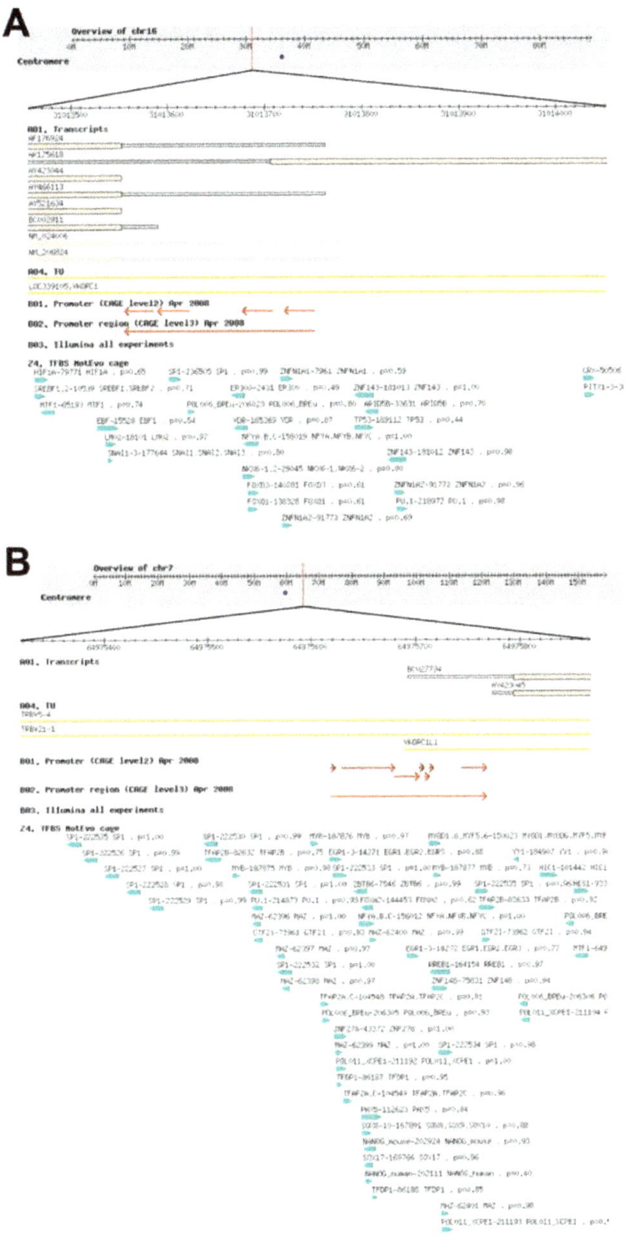

Figure 4. Overview of (top to bottom) chromosome maps (grey fields) showing genetic loci (vertical red lines), alternative mRNA transcripts (A01. Transcripts, tan bars), transcription start sequences (B01. Promoter (CAGE level 2, red arrows) and predicted transcription factor binding sites (24. TFBS MotEvo cage, blue arrows) for (**A**) human *VKORC1*; and (**B**) human *VKORC1L1*. Graphics are from the FANTOM4 Human (hg18) genome viewer (see Note 5 [104]).

Addressing this theme, Robertson (2004) commented, "...If this duplication follows the neofunctionalization model of gene duplication (Ohno, 1970) [105], then the rapid divergence of VKORC1 in vertebrates might suggest that its function related to vitamin K recycling might be the derived function, in which case the unknown VKORC1L1 function might better reflect the role of this protein in the other animals and trypanosomatids. Alternatively, if this duplication follows the subfunctionalization model of Lynch & Force (2000) [106], then both proteins might still be involved in vitamin K recycling; however, for some reason VKORC1 has been free to diverge more rapidly in vertebrates than has VKORC1L1..." It is clear from the evidence we review here that neofunctionalization cannot be the driving force for VKOR paralog maintenance, but that subfunctionalization, not of enzymatic function, but of developmental- and tissue-specific expression regulation, might be the basis for this unique preservation of paralogs. Furthermore, we can rationalize a biological need for this beginning with the evolution of aerobic heterotrophic organisms as the earth's atmosphere became increasingly oxygen-rich through photosynthesis. This led to evolution of multicellular animals and, eventually, vertebrates whose sizes increased over time [19,107]. Accordingly, closed circulatory systems of ever increasing volume and requiring increased cardiac capacity evolved leading to ever increasing circulatory pressure [108]. Parallel to these evolutionary developments in early metazoans, there arose the need for a robust hemostatic system and clotting capability to stem off bleeding through injury [109]. With all of this in mind, we propose that the regulatory mechanisms for VKOR paralog gene expression needed to keep pace with evolutionarily increasing circulatory volume and pressure, and so both VKOR paralogs were maintained in vertebrates due to selection pressure for distinct regulation of expression in non-coding regions of the genes. Thus, VKORC1L1 orthologs may have been maintained for more evolutionarily primitive housekeeping functions that might have included intracellular redox homeostasis and oxidative protein folding under anaerobic growth conditions [31,39]. In contrast, VKORC1 expression regulation has possibly evolved separately to sustain high systemic levels of secreted VKD proteins needed for maintaining large circulatory volume and pressure and also for development and homeostasis of a robust, calcified skeleton.

4. Conclusions and Future Perspectives

In this review, we have attempted to comprehensively summarize published results concerning structural and functional similarities and differences for VKORC1 and VKORC1L1 paralogs in extant metazoan genomes and to relate these to a rationale that explains why these proteins are evolutionarily maintained when their enzymatic functions are virtually identical. While it is presently clear that both enzymes are responsible for *de novo* reduction of K vitamins acquired from dietary sources, in addition to recycling oxidized forms of K vitamins to the respective reduced hydroquinone forms in the vitamin K cycle, evolutionary selection pressure has apparently maintained unique physiological functions for both paralogs by a tissue-specific "division of labor" under independent expression and regulatory controls.

In order to address important questions that remain about these paralogs, it will be necessary to more deeply investigate regulation of their expression with respect to cell and tissue type and developmental stage, to identify their functional intracellular protein partners, and to comprehensively identify and characterize new VKD proteins and the extent of the VKD proteome in individual species. We hope this review will stimulate discussion and cooperative investigation among researchers already

Nutrients **2015**, *7*, 6250–6280

engaged in vitamin K-related research areas as well as encourage researchers new to the field with expertise in complementary research methods.

Acknowledgments: This work was supported, in part, by funding from Baxter Germany GmbH (Johannes Oldenburg, Matthias Watzka), from Bayer AG for travel support and conference participation, and from the Deutsche Forschungsgemeinschaft (D.F.G.) grant Ol100 5-1 (Johannes Oldenburg, Matthias Watzka).

Author Contributions: Johannes Oldenburg, Matthias Watzka and Carville G. Bevans conceived and wrote the article. Carville G. Bevans provided literature and database analysis and figures.

Conflicts of Interest: The authors declare no conflict of interest.

References

1. Note 1: Official HUGO human gene designations are *VKORC1* and *VKORC1L1*; non-human orthologs are typically indicated using lower-case letters.
2. Rost, S.; Fregin, A.; Ivaskevicius, V.; Conzelmann, E.; Hörtnagel, K.; Pelz, H.J.; Lappegard, K.; Seifried, E.; Scharrer, I.; Tuddenham, E.G.D.; *et al.* Mutations in VKORC1 cause warfarin resistance and multiple coagulation factor deficiency type 2. *Nature* **2004**, *427*, 537–541. [CrossRef] [PubMed]
3. Robertson, H.M. Genes encoding vitamin-K epoxide reductase are present in Drosophila and trypanosomatid protists. *Genetics* **2004**, *168*, 1077–1080. [CrossRef] [PubMed]
4. Ferland, G. The vitamin K-dependent proteins: An update. *Nutr. Rev.* **1998**, *56*, 223–230. [CrossRef] [PubMed]
5. Willems, B.A.G.; Vermeer, C.; Reutelingsperger, C.P.M.; Schurgers, L.J. The realm of vitamin K dependent proteins: Shifting from coagulation toward calcification. *Mol. Nutr. Food Res.* **2014**, *58*, 1620–1635. [CrossRef] [PubMed]
6. Van Summeren, M.J.H.; van Coeverden, S.C.C.M.; Schurgers, L.J.; Braam, L.A.J.L.M.; Noirt, F.; Uiterwaal, C.S.P.M.; Kuis, W.; Vermeer, C. Vitamin K status is associated with childhood bone mineral content. *Br. J. Nutr.* **2008**, *100*, 852–858.
7. Gundberg, C.M.; Lian, J.B.; Booth, S.L. Vitamin K-dependent carboxylation of osteocalcin: Friend or foe? *Adv. Nutr. Bethesda Md.* **2012**, *3*, 149–157. [CrossRef] [PubMed]
8. Cancela, M.L.; Laizé, V.; Conceição, N. Matrix Gla protein and osteocalcin: From gene duplication to neofunctionalization. *Arch. Biochem. Biophys.* **2014**, *561*, 56–63. [CrossRef] [PubMed]
9. Laurance, S.; Lemarié, C.A.; Blostein, M.D. Growth arrest-specific gene 6 (gas6) and vascular hemostasis. *Adv. Nutr. Bethesda Md.* **2012**, *3*, 196–203. [CrossRef] [PubMed]
10. Shea, M.K.; Holden, R.M. Vitamin K status and vascular calcification: Evidence from observational and clinical studies. *Adv. Nutr. Bethesda Md.* **2012**, *3*, 158–165. [CrossRef] [PubMed]
11. Hegarty, J.M.; Yang, H.; Chi, N.C. UBIAD1-mediated vitamin K2 synthesis is required for vascular endothelial cell survival and development. *Dev. Camb. Engl.* **2013**, *140*, 1713–1719. [CrossRef] [PubMed]
12. Theuwissen, E.; Smit, E.; Vermeer, C. The role of vitamin K in soft-tissue calcification. *Adv. Nutr. Bethesda Md.* **2012**, *3*, 166–173. [CrossRef] [PubMed]
13. Cancela, M.L.; Conceicao, N.; Laize, V. Gla-rich protein, a new player in tissue calcification? *Adv. Nutr.* **2012**, *3*, 174–81. [CrossRef] [PubMed]
14. Ferland, G. Vitamin K and the nervous system: An overview of its actions. *Adv. Nutr. Bethesda Md.* **2012**, *3*, 204–212. [CrossRef] [PubMed]
15. Gely-Pernot, A.; Coronas, V.; Harnois, T.; Prestoz, L.; Mandairon, N.; Didier, A.; Berjeaud, J.M.; Monvoisin, A.; Bourmeyster, N.; de Frutos, P.G.; *et al.* An endogenous vitamin K-dependent mechanism regulates cell proliferation in the brain subventricular stem cell niche. *Stem Cells Dayt. Ohio* **2012**, *30*, 719–731. [CrossRef] [PubMed]
16. Lee, N.K.; Sowa, H.; Hinoi, E.; Ferron, M.; Ahn, J.D.; Confavreux, C.; Dacquin, R.; Mee, P.J.; McKee, M.D.; Jung, D.Y.; *et al.* Endocrine regulation of energy metabolism by the skeleton. *Cell* **2007**, *130*, 456–469. [CrossRef] [PubMed]
17. Ferron, M.; Hinoi, E.; Karsenty, G.; Ducy, P. Osteocalcin differentially regulates beta cell and adipocyte gene expression and affects the development of metabolic diseases in wild-type mice. *Proc. Natl. Acad. Sci. USA* **2008**, *105*, 5266–5270. [CrossRef] [PubMed]

18. Oury, F.; Sumara, G.; Sumara, O.; Ferron, M.; Chang, H.; Smith, C.E.; Hermo, L.; Suarez, S.; Roth, B.L.; Ducy, P.; *et al.* Endocrine regulation of male fertility by the skeleton. *Cell* **2011**, *144*, 796–809. [CrossRef] [PubMed]

19. Brazeau, M.D.; Friedman, M. The origin and early phylogenetic history of jawed vertebrates. *Nature* **2015**, *520*, 490–497. [CrossRef] [PubMed]

20. Bevans, C.G.; Krettler, C.; Reinhart, C.; Watzka, M.; Oldenburg, J. Phylogeny of the vitamin K 2,3-epoxide reductase (VKOR) family and evolutionary relationship to the disulfide bond formation protein B (DsbB) family. *Nutrients* **2015**, *7*, 6224–6249.

21. NCBI. Genome Information by Organism. Available online: http://www.ncbi.nlm.nih.gov/genome/browse/ (accessed on 30 April 2015).

22. NCBI. Bioproject Grid. Available online: http://www.ncbi.nlm.nih.gov/bioproject/browse/ (accessed on 30 April 2015).

23. Dutton, R.J.; Boyd, D.; Berkmen, M.; Beckwith, J. Bacterial species exhibit diversity in their mechanisms and capacity for protein disulfide bond formation. *Proc. Natl. Acad. Sci. USA* **2008**, *105*, 11933–11938. [CrossRef] [PubMed]

24. Li, T.; Chang, C.Y.; Jin, D.Y.; Lin, P.J.; Khvorova, A.; Stafford, D.W. Identification of the gene for vitamin K epoxide reductase. *Nature* **2004**, *427*, 541–544. [CrossRef] [PubMed]

25. Li, W.; Schulman, S.; Dutton, R.J.; Boyd, D.; Beckwith, J.; Rapoport, T.A. Structure of a bacterial homologue of vitamin K epoxide reductase. *Nature* **2010**, *463*, 507–512. [CrossRef] [PubMed]

26. Furt, F.; Oostende, C.; van Widhalm, J.R.; Dale, M.A.; Wertz, J.; Basset, G.J.C. A bimodular oxidoreductase mediates the specific reduction of phylloquinone (vitamin K_1) in chloroplasts. *Plant J. Cell Mol. Biol.* **2010**, *64*, 38–46. [CrossRef] [PubMed]

27. Tie, J.K.; Jin, D.Y.; Stafford, D.W. Mycobacterium tuberculosis vitamin K epoxide reductase homologue supports vitamin K-dependent carboxylation in mammalian cells. *Antioxid. Redox Signal.* **2012**, *16*, 329–338. [CrossRef] [PubMed]

28. Wan, C.M.; Yang, X.J.; Du, J.J.; Lu, Y.; Yu, Z.B.; Feng, Y.G.; Wang, X.Y. Identification and characterization of SlVKOR, a disulfide bond formation protein from Solanum lycopersicum, and bioinformatic analysis of plant VKORs. *Biochem. Biokhimiia* **2014**, *79*, 440–449. [CrossRef] [PubMed]

29. Collins, M.D.; Jones, D. Distribution of isoprenoid quinone structural types in bacteria and their taxonomic implication. *Microbiol. Rev.* **1981**, *45*, 316–354. [PubMed]

30. Jin, D.Y.; Tie, J.K.; Stafford, D.W. The conversion of vitamin K epoxide to vitamin K quinone and vitamin K quinone to vitamin K hydroquinone uses the same active site cysteines. *Biochemistry* **2007**, *46*, 7279–7283. [CrossRef] [PubMed]

31. Westhofen, P.; Watzka, M.; Marinova, M.; Hass, M.; Kirfel, G.; Müller, J.; Bevans, C.G.; Müller, C.R.; Oldenburg, J. Human vitamin K 2,3-epoxide reductase complex subunit 1-like 1 (VKORC1L1) mediates vitamin K-dependent intracellular antioxidant function. *J. Biol. Chem.* **2011**, *286*, 15085–15094. [CrossRef] [PubMed]

32. Goodstadt, L.; Ponting, C.P. Vitamin K epoxide reductase: Homology, active site and catalytic mechanism. *Trends Biochem. Sci.* **2004**, *29*, 289–292. [CrossRef] [PubMed]

33. Rishavy, M.A.; Usubalieva, A.; Hallgren, K.W.; Berkner, K.L. Novel insight into the mechanism of the vitamin K oxidoreductase (VKOR): Electron relay through Cys43 and Cys51 reduces VKOR to allow vitamin K reduction and facilitation of vitamin K-dependent protein carboxylation. *J. Biol. Chem.* **2011**, *286*, 7267–7278. [CrossRef] [PubMed]

34. Rost, S.; Fregin, A.; Hünerberg, M.; Bevans, C.G.; Müller, C.R.; Oldenburg, J. Site-directed mutagenesis of coumarin-type anticoagulant-sensitive VKORC1: Evidence that highly conserved amino acids define structural requirements for enzymatic activity and inhibition by warfarin. *Thromb. Haemost.* **2005**, *94*, 780–786. [PubMed]

35. Siegfried, C.M. Solubilization of vitamin K epoxide reductase and vitamin K-dependent carboxylase from rat liver microsomes. *Biochem. Biophys. Res. Commun.* **1978**, *83*, 1488–1495. [CrossRef]

36. Wajih, N.; Hutson, S.M.; Wallin, R. Disulfide-dependent protein folding is linked to operation of the vitamin K cycle in the endoplasmic reticulum. A protein disulfide isomerase-VKORC1 redox enzyme complex appears to be responsible for vitamin K1 2,3-epoxide reduction. *J. Biol. Chem.* **2007**, *282*, 2626–2635. [CrossRef] [PubMed]

37. Schulman, S.; Wang, B.; Li, W.; Rapoport, T.A. Vitamin K epoxide reductase prefers ER membrane-anchored thioredoxin-like redox partners. *Proc. Natl. Acad. Sci. USA* **2010**, *107*, 15027–15032. [CrossRef] [PubMed]

38. Depuydt, M.; Messens, J.; Collet, J.F. How proteins form disulfide bonds. *Antioxid. Redox Signal.* **2011**, *15*, 49–66. [CrossRef] [PubMed]

39. Rutkevich, L.A.; Williams, D.B. Vitamin K epoxide reductase contributes to protein disulfide formation and redox homeostasis within the endoplasmic reticulum. *Mol. Biol. Cell* **2012**, *23*, 2017–2027. [CrossRef] [PubMed]

40. Wajih, N.; Hutson, S.M.; Owen, J.; Wallin, R. Increased production of functional recombinant human clotting factor IX by baby hamster kidney cells engineered to overexpress VKORC1, the vitamin K 2,3-epoxide-reducing enzyme of the vitamin K cycle. *J. Biol. Chem.* **2005**, *280*, 31603–31607. [CrossRef] [PubMed]

41. Chu, P.H.; Huang, T.Y.; Williams, J.; Stafford, D.W. Purified vitamin K epoxide reductase alone is sufficient for conversion of vitamin K epoxide to vitamin K and vitamin K to vitamin KH$_2$. *Proc. Natl. Acad. Sci. USA* **2006**, *103*, 19308–19313. [CrossRef] [PubMed]

42. Oldenburg, J.; Bevans, C.G.; Müller, C.R.; Watzka, M. Vitamin K epoxide reductase complex subunit 1 (VKORC1): The key protein of the vitamin K cycle. *Antioxid. Redox Signal.* **2006**, *8*, 347–353. [CrossRef] [PubMed]

43. Oldenburg, J.; Marinova, M.; Müller-Reible, C.; Watzka, M. The vitamin K cycle. *Vitam. Horm.* **2008**, *78*, 35–62. [PubMed]

44. Spohn, G.; Kleinridders, A.; Wunderlich, F.T.; Watzka, M.; Zaucke, F.; Blumbach, K.; Geisen, C.; Seifried, E.; Müller, C.; Paulsson, M.; *et al.* VKORC1 deficiency in mice causes early postnatal lethality due to severe bleeding. *Thromb. Haemost.* **2009**, *101*, 1044–1050. [CrossRef] [PubMed]

45. Oldenburg, J.; von Brederlow, B.; Fregin, A.; Rost, S.; Wolz, W.; Eberl, W.; Eber, S.; Lenz, E.; Schwaab, R.; Brackmann, H.H.; *et al.* Congenital deficiency of vitamin K dependent coagulation factors in two families presents as a genetic defect of the vitamin K-epoxide-reductase-complex. *Thromb. Haemost.* **2000**, *84*, 937–941. [PubMed]

46. Price, P.A. Vitamin K-dependent formation of bone Gla protein (osteocalcin) and its function. *Vitam. Horm.* **1985**, *42*, 65–108. [PubMed]

47. Ferron, M.; Lacombe, J.; Germain, A.; Oury, F.; Karsenty, G. GGCX and VKORC1 inhibit osteocalcin endocrine functions. *J. Cell Biol.* **2015**, *208*, 761–776. [CrossRef] [PubMed]

48. Chatrou, M.L.L.; Reutelingsperger, C.P.; Schurgers, L.J. Role of vitamin K-dependent proteins in the arterial vessel wall. *Hämostaseologie* **2011**, *31*, 251–257. [CrossRef] [PubMed]

49. Chatrou, M.L.L.; Winckers, K.; Hackeng, T.M.; Reutelingsperger, C.P.; Schurgers, L.J. Vascular calcification: The price to pay for anticoagulation therapy with vitamin K-antagonists. *Blood Rev.* **2012**, *26*, 155–166. [CrossRef] [PubMed]

50. Li, J.; Lin, J.C.; Wang, H.; Peterson, J.W.; Furie, B.C.; Furie, B.; Booth, S.L.; Volpe, J.J.; Rosenberg, P.A. Novel role of vitamin K in preventing oxidative injury to developing oligodendrocytes and neurons. *J. Neurosci. Off. J. Soc. Neurosci.* **2003**, *23*, 5816–5826.

51. Varnum, B.C.; Young, C.; Elliott, G.; Garcia, A.; Bartley, T.D.; Fridell, Y.W.; Hunt, R.W.; Trail, G.; Clogston, C.; Toso, R.J. Axl receptor tyrosine kinase stimulated by the vitamin K-dependent protein encoded by growth-arrest-specific gene 6. *Nature* **1995**, *373*, 623–626. [CrossRef] [PubMed]

52. Hammed, A.; Matagrin, B.; Spohn, G.; Prouillac, C.; Benoit, E.; Lattard, V. VKORC1L1, an enzyme rescuing the vitamin K 2,3-epoxide reductase activity in some extrahepatic tissues during anticoagulation therapy. *J. Biol. Chem.* **2013**, *288*, 28733–28742. [CrossRef] [PubMed]

53. Holland, P.W.; Garcia-Fernàndez, J.; Williams, N.A.; Sidow, A. Gene duplications and the origins of vertebrate development. *Dev. Camb. Engl. Suppl.* **1994**, 125–133.

54. Note 2: The *Callorhinchus milii* (Australian ghostshark) genome, published in 2014, represents cartilagenous fishes among gnathostomes and includes entries of two VKOR family proteins. One apparently complete sequence (176 residues, NCBI genomic sequence entry XP_007894765.1, confirmed as transcriptome entry AFP01110.1) is homologous to vertebrate VKORC1L1 orthologs, while the second sequence (142 residues, NCBI genomic sequence entry XP_007894766.1) appears to be incomplete and possibly a concatenation of the 30 residue *N*-terminal sequence of a VKORC1 ortholog together with a *C*-terminal 112 residue sequence that

is identical to that of the putative VKORC1L1 paralog. Thus, the currently available data are inconclusive, but suggest that *Callorhinchus milii* possesses two VKOR paralogs.

55. Note 3: The genome of *Petromyzon marinus* (Japanese sea lamprey), published in 2011, represents the jawless vertebrates (Cyclostomata) and currently has no NCBI sequence entries. However, a BLAST search performed on the currently available lamprey genome (http://jlampreygenome.imcb.a-star.edu.sg, accessed 26 April 2015) using the human VKORC1 sequence returned only one partially homologous sequence (gene designation JL2487, 206 residues with no initial methionine, E-value 2e-22) with 57% identity to the human VKORC1 sequence from residue 11 through 95 and including the conserved loop cysteines and serine. However, the conserved active site CXXC motif is entirely absent from this sequence, suggesting an incorrect sequence assembly. Thus, no VKOR family homologs could be identified from the currently available lamprey genome data.

56. Vincent, M.J.; Martin, A.S.; Compans, R.W. Function of the KKXX Motif in Endoplasmic Reticulum Retrieval of a Transmembrane Protein Depends on the Length and Structure of the Cytoplasmic Domain. *J. Biol. Chem.* **1998**, *273*, 950–956. [CrossRef] [PubMed]

57. Czogalla, K.J.; Biswas, A.; Rost, S.; Watzka, M.; Oldenburg, J. The Arg98Trp mutation in human VKORC1 causing VKCFD2 disrupts a di-arginine-based ER retention motif. *Blood* **2014**, *124*, 1354–1362. [CrossRef] [PubMed]

58. Hildebrandt, E.F.; Preusch, P.C.; Patterson, J.L.; Suttie, J.W. Solubilization and characterization of vitamin K epoxide reductase from normal and warfarin-resistant rat liver microsomes. *Arch. Biochem. Biophys.* **1984**, *228*, 480–492. [CrossRef]

59. Lasseur, R.; Longin-Sauvageon, C.; Videmann, B.; Billeret, M.; Berny, P.; Benoit, E. Warfarin resistance in a French strain of rats. *J. Biochem. Mol. Toxicol.* **2005**, *19*, 379–385. [CrossRef] [PubMed]

60. Lasseur, R.; Grandemange, A.; Longin-Sauvageon, C.; Berny, P.; Benoit, E. Heterogeneity of the coumarin anticoagulant targeted vitamin K epoxide reduction system. Study of kinetic parameters in susceptible and resistant mice (Mus musculus domesticus). *J. Biochem. Mol. Toxicol.* **2006**, *20*, 221–229. [CrossRef] [PubMed]

61. Hodroge, A.; Longin-Sauvageon, C.; Fourel, I.; Benoit, E.; Lattard, V. Biochemical characterization of spontaneous mutants of rat VKORC1 involved in the resistance to antivitamin K anticoagulants. *Arch. Biochem. Biophys.* **2011**, *515*, 14–20. [CrossRef] [PubMed]

62. Hodroge, A.; Matagrin, B.; Moreau, C.; Fourel, I.; Hammed, A.; Benoit, E.; Lattard, V. VKORC1 mutations detected in patients resistant to vitamin K antagonists are not all associated with a resistant VKOR activity. *J. Thromb. Haemost. JTH* **2012**, *10*, 2535–2543. [CrossRef] [PubMed]

63. Bevans, C.G.; Krettler, C.; Reinhart, C.; Tran, H.; Koßmann, K.; Watzka, M.; Oldenburg, J. Determination of the warfarin inhibition constant K_i for vitamin K 2,3-epoxide reductase complex subunit-1 (VKORC1) using an *in vitro* DTT-driven assay. *Biochim. Biophys. Acta* **2013**, *1830*, 4202–4210. [CrossRef] [PubMed]

64. Matagrin, B.; Hodroge, A.; Montagut-Romans, A.; Andru, J.; Fourel, I.; Besse, S.; Benoit, E.; Lattard, V. New insights into the catalytic mechanism of vitamin K epoxide reductase (VKORC1)—The catalytic properties of the major mutations of rVKORC1 explain the biological cost associated to mutations. *FEBS Open Bio* **2013**, *3*, 144–150. [CrossRef] [PubMed]

65. Bevans, C.G.; Krettler, C.; Reinhart, C.; Tran, H.; Koßmann, K.; Watzka, M.; Oldenburg, J. Corrigendum to "Determination of the warfarin inhibition constant K_i for vitamin K 2,3-epoxide reductase complex subunit-1 (VKORC1) using an *in vitro* DTT-driven assay" [BBAGEN (2013) 4202–4210]. *Biochim. Biophys. Acta BBA—Gen. Subj.* **2014**, *1840*, 2382–2384. [CrossRef]

66. Matagrin, B.; Montagut-Romans, A.; Damin, M.; Lemaire, M.; Popowycz, F.; Benoit, E.; Lattard, V. Identification of VKORC1 genotype leading to resistance to tecarfarin. *J. Clin. Pharmacol.* **2014**, *54*, 896–900. [CrossRef] [PubMed]

67. Goulois, J.; Chapuzet, A.; Lambert, V.; Chatron, N.; Tchertanov, L.; Legros, L.; Benoît, E.; Lattard, V. Evidence of a target resistance to antivitamin K rodenticides in the roof rat Rattus rattus: Identification and characterization of a novel Y25F mutation in the Vkorc1 gene. *Pest Manag. Sci.* **2015**. [CrossRef]

68. Krettler, C.; Bevans, C.G.; Reinhart, C.; Watzka, M.; Oldenburg, J. Tris(3-hydroxypropyl)phosphine is superior to DTT for *in vitro* assessment of vitamin K 2,3-epoxide reductase activity. *Anal. Biochem.* **2015**, *474*, 89–94. [CrossRef] [PubMed]

69. Preusch, P.C.; Brummet, S.R. Steady-state kinetics of microsomal vitamin K epoxide reduction. In Current Advances in Vitamin K Research, Proceedings of the Seventeenth Steenbock Symposium, University of Wisconsin, Madison, WI, USA, 21–25 June 1987; Suttie, J.W., Ed.; Elsevier: New York, NY, USA, 1988; pp. 75–82.

70. Cornish-Bowden, A. *Fundamental of Enzyme Kinetics*; Butterworth & Co (Publishers) Ltd.: London, UK, 1979.

71. Whitlon, D.S.; Sadowski, J.A.; Suttie, J.W. Mechanism of coumarin action: Significance of vitamin K   epoxide reductase inhibition. *Biochemistry* **1978**, *17*, 1371–1377. [CrossRef] [PubMed]

72. Silverman, R.B.; Oliver, J.S. 2-(Fluoromethyl)-3-phytyl-1,4-naphthoquinone and its 2,3-epoxide. Inhibition of vitamin K epoxide reductase. *J. Med. Chem.* **1989**, *32*, 2138–2141. [CrossRef] [PubMed]

73. Rost, S.; Pelz, H.J.; Menzel, S.; MacNicoll, A.D.; León, V.; Song, K.J.; Jäkel, T.; Oldenburg, J.; Müller, C.R. Novel mutations in the VKORC1 gene of wild rats and mice—A response to 50 years of selection pressure by warfarin? *BMC Genet.* **2009**, *10*, 4. [CrossRef] [PubMed]

74. Watzka, M.; Geisen, C.; Bevans, C.G.; Sittinger, K.; Spohn, G.; Rost, S.; Seifried, E.; Müller, C.R.; Oldenburg, J. Thirteen novel VKORC1 mutations associated with oral anticoagulant resistance: Insights into improved patient diagnosis and treatment. *J. Thromb. Haemost. JTH* **2011**, *9*, 109–118. [CrossRef] [PubMed]

75. Fregin, A.; Czogalla, K.J.; Gansler, J.; Rost, S.; Taverna, M.; Watzka, M.; Bevans, C.G.; Müller, C.R.; Oldenburg, J. A new cell culture-based assay quantifies vitamin K 2,3-epoxide reductase complex subunit 1 function and reveals warfarin resistance phenotypes not shown by the dithiothreitol-driven VKOR assay. *J. Thromb. Haemost. JTH* **2013**, *11*, 872–880. [CrossRef] [PubMed]

76. Czogalla, K.J.; Biswas, A.; Wendeln, A.C.; Westhofen, P.; Müller, C.R.; Watzka, M.; Oldenburg, J. Human VKORC1 mutations cause variable degrees of 4-hydroxycoumarin resistance and affect putative warfarin binding interfaces. *Blood* **2013**, *122*, 2743–2750. [CrossRef] [PubMed]

77. Tie, J.K.; Jin, D.Y.; Tie, K.; Stafford, D.W. Evaluation of warfarin resistance using transcription activator-like effector nucleases-mediated vitamin K epoxide reductase knockout HEK293 cells. *J. Thromb. Haemost. JTH* **2013**, *11*, 1556–1564. [CrossRef] [PubMed]

78. Haque, J.; McDonald, M.; Kulman, J.; Rettie, A.E. A cellular system for quantitation of vitamin K cycle activity: Structure-activity effects on vitamin K antagonism by warfarin metabolites. *Blood* **2013**, *123*, 582–589. [CrossRef] [PubMed]

79. Itoh, S.; Onishi, S. Developmental changes of vitamin K epoxidase and reductase activities involved in the vitamin K cycle in human liver. *Early Hum. Dev.* **2000**, *57*, 15–23. [CrossRef]

80. Ko, M.S.; Threat, T.A.; Wang, X.; Horton, J.H.; Cui, Y.; Wang, X.; Pryor, E.; Paris, J.; Wells-Smith, J.; Kitchen, J.R.; *et al.* Genome-wide mapping of unselected transcripts from extraembryonic tissue of 7.5-day mouse embryos reveals enrichment in the *t*-complex and under-representation on the X chromosome. *Hum. Mol. Genet.* **1998**, *7*, 1967–1978. [CrossRef] [PubMed]

81. Diez-Roux, G.; Banfi, S.; Sultan, M.; Geffers, L.; Anand, S.; Rozado, D.; Magen, A.; Canidio, E.; Pagani, M.; Peluso, I.; *et al.* A high-resolution anatomical atlas of the transcriptome in the mouse embryo. *PLoS Biol.* **2011**, *9*, e1000582. [CrossRef] [PubMed]

82. Caspers, M.; Czogalla, K.J.; Liphardt, K.; Müller, J.; Westhofen, P.; Watzka, M.; Oldenburg, J. Two enzymes catalyze vitamin K 2,3-epoxide reductase activity in mouse: VKORC1 is highly expressed in exocrine tissues while VKORC1L1 is highly expressed in brain. *Thromb. Res.* **2015**, *135*, 977–983. [CrossRef] [PubMed]

83. Fernández, I.; Vijayakumar, P.; Marques, C.; Cancela, M.L.; Gavaia, P.J.; Laizé, V. Zebrafish vitamin K epoxide reductases: Expression *in vivo*, along extracellular matrix mineralization and under phylloquinone and warfarin *in vitro* exposure. *Fish Physiol. Biochem.* **2015**, *41*, 745–759. [CrossRef] [PubMed]

84. Vijayakumar, P.; Laizé, V.; Cardeira, J.; Trindade, M.; Cancela, M.L. Development of an *in vitro* cell system from zebrafish suitable to study bone cell differentiation and extracellular matrix mineralization. *Zebrafish* **2013**, *10*, 500–509. [CrossRef] [PubMed]

85. Zou, D.; Ma, L.; Yu, J.; Zhang, Z. Biological Databases for Human Research. *Genomics Proteomics Bioinform.* **2015**, *13*, 55–63. [CrossRef] [PubMed]

86. Su, A.I.; Wiltshire, T.; Batalov, S.; Lapp, H.; Ching, K.A.; Block, D.; Zhang, J.; Soden, R.; Hayakawa, M.; Kreiman, G.; *et al.* A gene atlas of the mouse and human protein-encoding transcriptomes. *Proc. Natl. Acad. Sci. USA* **2004**, *101*, 6062–6067. [CrossRef] [PubMed]

87. Blaveri, E.; Kelly, F.; Mallei, A.; Harris, K.; Taylor, A.; Reid, J.; Razzoli, M.; Carboni, L.; Piubelli, C.; Musazzi, L.; *et al.* Expression profiling of a genetic animal model of depression reveals novel molecular pathways underlying depressive-like behaviours. *PLoS ONE* **2010**, *5*, e12596. [CrossRef] [PubMed]

88. Freeman, T.C.; Ivens, A.; Baillie, J.K.; Beraldi, D.; Barnett, M.W.; Dorward, D.; Downing, A.; Fairbairn, L.; Kapetanovic, R.; Raza, S.; *et al.* A gene expression atlas of the domestic pig. *BMC Biol.* **2012**, *10*, 90. [CrossRef] [PubMed]

89. Lui, J.C.K.; Andrade, A.C.; Forcinito, P.; Hegde, A.; Chen, W.; Baron, J.; Nilsson, O. Spatial and temporal regulation of gene expression in the mammalian growth plate. *Bone* **2010**, *46*, 1380–1390. [CrossRef] [PubMed]

90. Forcinito, P.; Andrade, A.C.; Finkielstain, G.P.; Baron, J.; Nilsson, O.; Lui, J.C. Growth-inhibiting conditions slow growth plate senescence. *J. Endocrinol.* **2011**, *208*, 59–67. [CrossRef] [PubMed]

91. Wu, C.; Orozco, C.; Boyer, J.; Leglise, M.; Goodale, J.; Batalov, S.; Hodge, C.L.; Haase, J.; Janes, J.; Huss, J.W.; *et al.* BioGPS: An extensible and customizable portal for querying and organizing gene annotation resources. *Genome Biol.* **2009**, *10*, R130. [CrossRef] [PubMed]

92. The GTEx Consortium; Ardlie, K.G.; Deluca, D.S.; Segre, A.V.; Sullivan, T.J.; Young, T.R.; Gelfand, E.T.; Trowbridge, C.A.; Maller, J.B.; Tukiainen, T.; *et al.* The Genotype-Tissue Expression (GTEx) pilot analysis: Multitissue gene regulation in humans. *Science* **2015**, *348*, 648–660. [CrossRef] [PubMed]

93. Melé, M.; Ferreira, P.G.; Reverter, F.; de Luca, D.S.; Monlong, J.; Sammeth, M.; Young, T.R.; Goldmann, J.M.; Pervouchine, D.D.; Sullivan, T.J.; *et al.* The human transcriptome across tissues and individuals. *Science* **2015**, *348*, 660–665. [CrossRef] [PubMed]

94. Benjamini, Y.; Hochberg, Y. Controlling the False Discovery Rate: A Practical and Powerful Approach to Multiple Testing. *J. R. Stat. Soc. Ser. B Methodol.* **1995**, *57*, 289–300.

95. Thelen, J.J.; Miernyk, J.A. The proteomic future: Where mass spectrometry should be taking us. *Biochem. J.* **2012**, *444*, 169–181. [CrossRef] [PubMed]

96. Kim, M.S.; Pinto, S.M.; Getnet, D.; Nirujogi, R.S.; Manda, S.S.; Chaerkady, R.; Madugundu, A.K.; Kelkar, D.S.; Isserlin, R.; Jain, S.; *et al.* A draft map of the human proteome. *Nature* **2014**, *509*, 575–581. [CrossRef] [PubMed]

97. Wilhelm, M.; Schlegl, J.; Hahne, H.; Moghaddas Gholami, A.; Lieberenz, M.; Savitski, M.M.; Ziegler, E.; Butzmann, L.; Gessulat, S.; Marx, H.; *et al.* Mass-spectrometry-based draft of the human proteome. *Nature* **2014**, *509*, 582–587. [CrossRef] [PubMed]

98. Ravasi, T.; Suzuki, H.; Cannistraci, C.V.; Katayama, S.; Bajic, V.B.; Tan, K.; Akalin, A.; Schmeier, S.; Kanamori-Katayama, M.; Bertin, N.; *et al.* An atlas of combinatorial transcriptional regulation in mouse and man. *Cell* **2010**, *140*, 744–752. [CrossRef] [PubMed]

99. FANTOM Consortium; Suzuki, H.; Forrest, A.R.R.; van Nimwegen, E.; Daub, C.O.; Balwierz, P.J.; Irvine, K.M.; Lassmann, T.; Ravasi, T.; Hasegawa, Y.; *et al.* The transcriptional network that controls growth arrest and differentiation in a human myeloid leukemia cell line. *Nat. Genet.* **2009**, *41*, 553–562.

100. Arnold, P.; Erb, I.; Pachkov, M.; Molina, N.; van Nimwegen, E. MotEvo: Integrated Bayesian probabilistic methods for inferring regulatory sites and motifs on multiple alignments of DNA sequences. *Bioinform. Oxf. Engl.* **2012**, *28*, 487–494. [CrossRef] [PubMed]

101. Note 4: Data for *VKORC1* and *VKORC1L1* from EdgeExpress DB; http://fantom.gsc.riken.jp/4/edgeexpress/view/#5540409 and #5561011, accessed on 1 May 2015.

102. Pelz, H.J.; Rost, S.; Hünerberg, M.; Fregin, A.; Heiberg, A.C.; Baert, K.; MacNicoll, A.D.; Prescott, C.V.; Walker, A.S.; Oldenburg, J.; *et al.* The genetic basis of resistance to anticoagulants in rodents. *Genetics* **2005**, *170*, 1839–1847. [CrossRef] [PubMed]

103. Oldenburg, J.; Müller, C.R.; Rost, S.; Watzka, M.; Bevans, C.G. Comparative genetics of warfarin resistance. *Hämostaseologie* **2014**, *34*, 143–159. [CrossRef] [PubMed]

104. Note 5: Data for *VKORC1* and *VKORC1L1* can be viewed at http://fantom.gsc.riken.jp/4/gev/gbrowse/hg18/; accessed on 1 May 2010.

105. Ohno, S. *Evolution by Gene Duplication*; Allen & Unwin: London, UK; Springer-Verlag: New York, NY, USA, 1970.

106. Lynch, M.; Force, A. The probability of duplicate gene preservation by subfunctionalization. *Genetics* **2000**, *154*, 459–473. [PubMed]

107. Holland, N.D.; Holland, L.Z.; Holland, P.W.H. Scenarios for the making of vertebrates. *Nature* **2015**, *520*, 450–455. [CrossRef] [PubMed]

Nutrients **2015**, *7*, 6250–6280

108. Diogo, R.; Kelly, R.G.; Christiaen, L.; Levine, M.; Ziermann, J.M.; Molnar, J.L.; Noden, D.M.; Tzahor, E. A new heart for a new head in vertebrate cardiopharyngeal evolution. *Nature* **2015**, *520*, 466–473. [CrossRef] [PubMed]

109. Doolittle, R.F. Coagulation in vertebrates with a focus on evolution and inflammation. *J. Innate Immun.* **2011**, *3*, 9–16. [CrossRef] [PubMed]

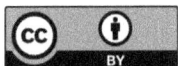

nutrients

MDPI

Article

Dietary Vitamin K Intake Is Associated with Cognition and Behaviour among Geriatric Patients: The CLIP Study

Justine Chouet [1], Guylaine Ferland [2], Catherine Féart [3,4], Yves Rolland [5], Nancy Presse [2], Kariane Boucher [2], Pascale Barberger-Gateau [3,4], Olivier Beauchet [1] and Cedric Annweiler [1,6,*]

[1] Department of Neuroscience, Division of Geriatric Medicine, Angers University Hospital; Angers University Memory Clinic; UPRES EA 4638, University of Angers, UNAM, Angers F-49933, France;
  E-Mails: justine.chouet@gmail.com (J.C.); OlBeauchet@chu-angers.fr (O.B.)
[2] Centre de recherche, Institut Universitaire de Gériatrie de Montréal, Montréal, QC H3W 1W5, Canada;
  E-Mails: guylaine.ferland@umontreal.ca (G.F.); nancy.presse@umontreal.ca (N.P.);
  kariane.boucher@gmail.com (K.B.)
[3] Université Bordeaux, ISPED, Centre INSERM U897-Epidemiologie-Biostatistique, Bordeaux F-33000, France;
  E-Mails: catherine.feart@isped.u-bordeaux2.fr (C.F.);
  Pascale.Barberger-Gateau@isped.u-bordeaux2.fr (P.B.-G.)
[4] INSERM, ISPED, INSERM U897-Epidemiologie-Biostatistique, Bordeaux F-33000, France
[5] Department of Geriatric Medicine, Institut du Vieillissement, University Hospital; INSERM U1027, Toulouse F-31400, France; E-Mail: rolland.y@chu-toulouse.fr
[6] Robarts Research Institute, Department of Medical Biophysics, Schulich School of Medicine and Dentistry, the University of Western Ontario, London, ON N6A 5B7, Canada
* Author to whom correspondence should be addressed; E-Mail: CeAnnweiler@chu-angers.fr;
  Tel.: +33-241355486; Fax: +33-241354894.

Received: 15 June 2015 / Accepted: 24 July 2015 / Published: 12 August 2015

Abstract: Our objective was to determine whether dietary vitamin K intake was associated with cognition and behavior among older adults. 192 consecutive participants $\geq$65 years, recruited in the cross-sectional CLIP (Cognition and LIPophilic vitamins) study, were separated into two groups according to the tertiles of dietary phylloquinone intake (*i.e.*, lowest third below 207 μg/day *versus* the other two thirds combined). Daily dietary phylloquinone intake was estimated from 50-item interviewer-administered food frequency questionnaire. Cognition was assessed with Mini-Mental State Examination (MMSE); behaviour with Frontotemporal Behavioral Rating Scale (FBRS). Age, gender, social problems, education, body mass index (BMI), comorbidities, history of stroke, use vitamin K antagonists, inadequate fatty fish intake, serum thyroid-stimulating hormone (TSH), vitamin B12, albumin, and estimated glomerular filtration rate were used as confounders. Compared to participants in the lowest third of dietary phylloquinone intake ($n = 64$), those with higher intake had higher (*i.e.*, better) mean MMSE score (22.0 ± 5.7 *versus* 19.9 ± 6.2, $p = 0.024$) and lower (*i.e.*, better) FBRS score (1.5 ± 1.2 *versus* 1.9 ± 1.3, $p = 0.042$). In multivariate linear regressions, log dietary phylloquinone intake was positively associated with MMSE score (adjusted $\beta = 1.66$, $p = 0.013$) and inversely associated with FBRS score (adjusted $\beta = -0.33$, $p = 0.037$). Specifically, log dietary phylloquinone intake correlated negatively with FBRS subscore of physical neglect ($r = -0.24$, $p = 0.001$). Higher dietary phylloquinone intake was associated with better cognition and behavior among older adults.

Keywords: cognition; behavior; diet; older adults; vitamin K

1. Introduction

Vitamin K is a fat-soluble substance found mainly in green vegetables and some vegetable oils. Vitamin K is classically known for its role as a coenzyme in the biological activation of seven proteins involved in blood coagulation [1]. Recently, a role for vitamin K has been demonstrated in target organs, such as the central nervous system (CNS) [2–10]. At the neuronal level, vitamin K is involved in the synthesis of sphingolipids—a major constituent of the myelin sheath and neuronal membranes—and the biological activation of vitamin K-dependent proteins (VKDPs) involved in neuronal physiology and survival [2,3]. Insufficient levels of vitamin K may, instead, cause neuropathological dysfunction [4]. Accordingly, an epidemiological study has reported a significant association between higher serum phylloquinone concentration (*i.e.*, vitamin K_1) and better verbal episodic memory performance in older adults [5]. Similarly, we found that the use of vitamin K antagonists (VKAs), which deplete the active form of vitamin K, was associated with cognitive impairment [6] and a lower volume of gray matter in the hippocampus [7] among geriatric patients. Taken together, these results suggest the importance of adequate (*i.e.*, high enough) vitamin K levels for optimal cognition in older adults [11]. To date, no randomized controlled trial has explored the benefits of vitamin K supplementation to maintain or improve cognition and related behavioral disorders in older adults. Before conducting such an expensive and time-consuming trial, it seems important and contributory to determine whether the intake of vitamin K relates to cognitive and behavioral performance in older adults.

We had the opportunity to examine the association between dietary vitamin K intake and cognitive behavioral performance in a sample of geriatric patients: the CLIP (Cognition and LIPophilic vitamins) cohort. Our objective was to determine whether dietary vitamin K intake was associated with cognitive and behavioral performance among geriatric patients.

2. Materials and Methods

2.1. Participants

We studied in- and outpatients aged 65 and over, consecutively recruited in the CLIP study. The CLIP study is an observational cross-sectional study designed to examine the relationships between neurocognition and lipophilic vitamins among all patients consecutively hospitalized or seen in consultation in the geriatric acute care unit of the University Hospital of Angers, France, from February to April 2014. After giving their informed consent for research, included participants received a full medical examination consisting of structured questionnaires, a standardized clinical examination, and a blood test. The study was conducted in accordance with the ethical standards set forth in the Helsinki Declaration (1983). The entire study protocol was approved by the local ethical committee (No. 2014-33).

2.2. Explanatory Variable: Dietary Intake of Vitamin K

Dietary vitamin K intake was estimated from a semi-quantitative food frequency questionnaire (FFQ) [12]. The 50-item FFQ used here was specifically designed to determine the daily dietary phylloquinone intake during the previous 12 months. It comprises 50 food items identified as important contributors to phylloquinone intake (e.g., spinach, iceberg lettuce, collards, and broccoli) and items with very high phylloquinone content ($\geqslant$500 μg/usual portion). The FFQ was interviewer-administered in 30 min by questioning the patients and/or their relatives, when applicable. Estimated phylloquinone intake was calculated for each food item by multiplying the amount of phylloquinone for that food item by the selected frequency and serving size (calculated as 0.5 for smaller than, and 1.5 for larger than the suggested portion), and all values were added to provide an estimate in μg/day of each participant's daily phylloquinone intake. The vitamin K FFQ shows good relative agreement with five-day food records (κ = 0.60, $p < 0.001$) [12]. In the present analysis, the participants were categorized into two groups based on the first tertile of the dietary phylloquinone intake: those in the lowest third of dietary phylloquinone intake below 207 μg/day, and those in the other two thirds combined of dietary phylloquinone intake above 207 μg/day.

2.3. Dependent Variables: Neuropsychiatric Measures

Cognition was assessed by one neuropsychologist blinded from participants' vitamin K intake using the Mini-Mental State Examination (MMSE) [13], in the absence of delirium identified with the Confusion Assessment Method [14]. The MMSE is a well-established measure of global cognitive performance in older adults composed of five sections (orientation, registration, attention-calculation, recall, and language). Scores range between 30 and 0 (worst). It shows good test-retest and inter-rater reliability and performs satisfactorily against more detailed measures of cognitive function [13].

Behavior was assessed at the same time as the MMSE using the Frontotemporal Behavioral Rating Scale (FBRS) [15]. The FBRS indicates the presence of symptoms of four domains of behavioral disturbances (*i.e.*, self-control disorder, physical neglect, mood disorders and loss of general interest). Each domain is scored 1 if at least 1 symptom is present, and 0 if no symptoms are present. The total FBRS score ranges from 0 (normal) to 4 (worst). The FBRS is easy to perform and has demonstrated good test-retest reliability [15].

2.4. Covariables

Age, gender, social problems, education level, body mass index, comorbidity burden, history of stroke, use of VKAs, regular fatty fish and eggs intakes, serum concentrations of thyroid-stimulating hormone (TSH), vitamin B12, albumin, and estimated glomerular filtration rate (*i.e.*, creatinine clearance, eGFR) are covariates related to diet and cognitive behavioral performance and were used as potential confounders. Evaluation of education level was based on self-report. Participants who passed at least the Elementary School Recognition Certificate were considered to have high education level. Social problems were defined by a geriatrician (yes/no) as the existence of social and/or familial isolation with consequent difficulties to stay in the usual place of life. Comorbidity burden was estimated with the Cumulative Illness Rating Scale-Geriatrics score (CIRS-G) (range 0–60, worst) [16]. History of stroke was sought by questioning the patients, the family physicians, and the patients' files. Stroke was defined according to the World Health Organization criteria as rapidly developed signs of focal or global disturbance of cerebral function lasting longer than 24 h, with no apparent nonvascular cause [17]. In case of clinical suspicion, computed tomography or magnetic resonance imaging scan was necessary to confirm the diagnosis and to distinguish among ischemic stroke and intracranial hemorrhage. The regular use of VKAs was systematically noted from the primary care physicians' prescriptions and sought by questioning the patients and their relatives, whatever the type of VKA used (*i.e.*, warfarin, acenocoumarol, or fluindione), the indication, length of treatment, and history of international normalized ratio (INR). The regular intake of fatty fish and eggs (*i.e.*, dietary sources of vitamin D and omega-3 polyunsaturated fatty acids (*n*-3 PUFAs), both linked to cognition) was sought using a standardized question: "Do you eat fatty fish at least once a week and/or eggs several times per week?" and was coded as low (*i.e.*, answer "No") or adequate (*i.e.*, answer "Yes"), as previously published [18]. Finally, the serum concentrations of TSH, vitamin B12, albumin and creatinine were measured using automated standard laboratory methods at the University Hospital of Angers, France, and eGFR was calculated using the Cockcroft-Gault formula $(((140 - \text{age}_{\text{years}}) \times \text{weight}_{\text{kg}} / \text{creatinine}_{\mu\text{mol/L}}) \times 1.04$ for females, and $\times 1.25$ for males).

2.5. Statistical Analysis

The participants' characteristics were summarized using means and standard deviations or frequencies and percentages, as appropriate. Statistics were performed on logarithmically-transformed values for the dietary phylloquinone intake to improve the symmetry of the non-Gaussian distribution.

Firstly, comparisons of participants' characteristics according to the dietary phylloquinone intake (*i.e.*, the lowest third *versus* the other two thirds combined) were performed using Student's *t*-test or the Chi-square test, as appropriate. Secondly, the mean difference of neuropsychiatric scores was calculated between participants in the lowest third *versus* the other two thirds combined of dietary phylloquinone intake. Thirdly, multiple linear regressions were used to examine the associations of log dietary phylloquinone intake (independent variable) with the MMSE score and the FBRS score (dependent variables), while adjusting for potential confounders. Separate analyses were conducted for each dependent variable. Finally, we examined the correlation between log dietary phylloquinone intake and each subscore of the FBRS. Lastly, we performed a sensitivity analysis after removing the participants who used VKA ($n = 31$). *p*-Values < 0.05 were considered significant. All statistics were performed using SPSS (v19.0, IBM corporation, Chicago, IL, USA) and RevMan (v5.1, Nordic Cochrane Centre, Copenhagen, Denmark).

3. Results

Among 192 included participants (mean $\pm$ standard deviation, 82.8 $\pm$ 7.1years; 62.5% female; 63.4% inpatient), the mean dietary phylloquinone intake estimated using a validated food frequency questionnaire (FFQ) [12] was 319.9 $\pm$ 196.3 µg/day. Sixty-four participants were in the lowest third of dietary phylloquinone intake, *i.e.*, below 207 µg/day (Table 1). The mean Mini-Mental State Examination score (MMSE) score was 21.4 $\pm$ 5.9 [13], and the mean Frontotemporal Behavioral Rating Scale (FBRS) score was 1.6 $\pm$ 1.2 [15]. Participants in the other two thirds combined of dietary phylloquinone intake had better MMSE and FBRS scores than those in the lowest third (respectively, 22.0 $\pm$ 5.7 *versus* 19.9 $\pm$ 6.2 with $p = 0.024$, and 1.5 $\pm$ 1.2 *versus* 1.9 $\pm$ 1.3 with $p = 0.042$) (Table 1). The between-group mean difference of MMSE score was -2.14 (95% confidence interval (CI): -3.95; -0.33), and that of FBRS score was 0.39 (95% CI: 0.01; 0.77) (Figure 1).

Neuropsychatric scores	Mean difference [95% CI]	
MMSE score	-2.14 [-3.95, -0.33]	
FBRS score	-0.39 [-0.77, -0.01]	

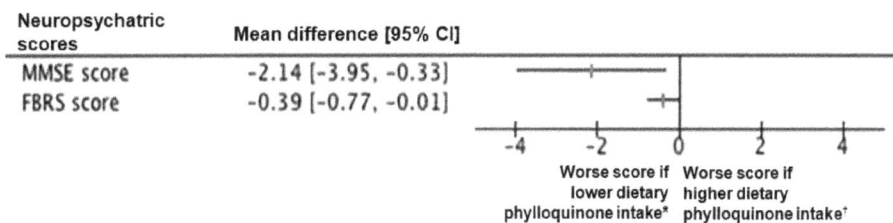

Figure 1. Forest plot for the mean difference of neuropsychiatric scores according to the dietary phylloquinone intake. Horizontal lines correspond to the 95% confidence interval (CI). The vertical line corresponds to a mean difference of 0.00, equivalent to no between-group difference. FBRS: Frontotemporal Behavioral Rating Scale; MMSE: Mini-Mental State Examination; *: lowest third of dietary phylloquinone intake below 206.97 µg/day; †: two other thirds combined of dietary phylloquinone intake.

Table 1. Baseline characteristics of 192 participants by dietary phylloquinone intake.

	Total Cohort (n = 192)	Dietary Phylloquinone Intake *		p-Value
		<207 µg/day (n = 64)	≥ 207 µg/day (n = 128)	
Demographical measures				
Age, years	82.8 ± 7.1	83.7 ± 5.9	82.4 ± 7.7	0.227
Female gender, n (%)	120 (62.5)	43 (67.2)	77 (60.2)	0.343
Social problems, n (%)	21 (10.9)	10 (15.6)	11 (8.6)	0.141
High education level [†], n (%)	152 (79.2)	51 (79.7)	101 (78.9)	0.900
Clinical measures				
Body mass index, kg/m^2	26.2 ± 5.4	25.8 ± 4.9	26.4 ± 5.6	0.492
CIRS-G score, /60	8.3 ± 4.0	9.0 ± 4.4	8.0 ± 3.8	0.118
History of stroke, n (%)	29 (15.2)	10 (15.6)	19 (15.0)	0.904
Use of vitamin K antagonists, n (%)	31 (16.1)	11 (17.2)	20 (15.6)	0.781
Dietary intake of phylloquinone, µg/day	319.9 ± 196.3	125.3 ± 52.1	417.1 ± 167.4	**<0.001**
Low dietary intake of fatty fish and eggs [‡], n (%)	23 (12.2)	9 (14.8)	14 (10.9)	0.453
Neuropsychiatric measures				
MMSE score, /30	21.4 ± 5.9	19.9 ± 6.2	22.0 ± 5.7	**0.024**
FBRS score, /4	1.6 ± 1.2	1.9 ± 1.3	1.5 ± 1.2	**0.042**
Serum measures				
TSH concentration, mIU/L	1.6 ± 1.8	1.5 ± 1.2	1.7 ± 2.0	0.440
Vitamin B12 concentration, ng/L	444.3 ± 266.2	478.5 ± 375.8	427.4 ± 190.6	0.228
Albumin concentration, g/L	34.9 ± 5.5	33.0 ± 5.7	35.9 ± 5.2	**0.001**
Estimated glomerular filtration rate, mL/min	53.7 ± 21.9	50.8 ± 18.2	55.1 ± 23.5	0.217

Data presented as mean ± standard deviation when applicable. CIRS-G: Cumulative Illness Rating Scale for Geriatrics; FBRS: Frontotemporal Behavioral Rating Scale; MMSE: Mini-Mental State Examination; TSH: thyroid stimulating hormone; *: lower dietary phylloquinone intake defined as the lowest third (*i.e.*, below 206.97 µg/day); higher dietary phylloquinone intake defined as the other two thirds combined (*i.e.*, above 206.97 µg/day); [†]: Elementary School Recognition Certificate passed; [‡]: Answer "No" to the question "Do you eat fatty fish at least once a week and/or eggs several times per week?"; *p*-values < 0.05 indicated in bold.

Results of multiple linear regression models were reported in Table 2. We observed a positive association between log dietary phylloquinone intake and the MMSE score (β = 1.66, *p* = 0.013), and an inverse association with the FBRS score (β = −0.33, *p* = 0.037). Higher education level and higher serum concentrations of thyroid-stimulating hormone (TSH) and albumin were also associated with higher (*i.e.*, better) MMSE score, but none was associated with the FBRS score (Table 2).

Finally, Table 3 reports the correlations between the log dietary phylloquinone intake and the subscores of the FBRS. Log dietary intake of phylloquinone correlated negatively with the subscore of physical neglect (*r* = −0.24, *p* = 0.001), but not with the subscores of self-control disorders (*p* = 0.060), mood disorders (*p* = 0.196) and loss of general interest (*p* = 0.699).

Table 2. Fully adjusted linear regressions examining the association between the dietary phylloquinone intake (independent variable) and the MMSE and FBRS scores * (dependent variables), adjusted for potential confounders (*n* = 192).

	Neuropsychiatric Measures					
	MMSE Score			FBRS Score		
	β	(95% CI)	*p*-value	β	(95% CI)	*p*-value
Log dietary phylloquinone intake	1.66	(0.36; 2.95)	0.013	−0.33	(−0.63; −0.02)	0.037
Age	−0.22	(−0.39; −0.06)	0.009	0.02	(−0.03; 0.06)	0.450
Female gender	−0.63	(−2.46; 1.19)	0.492	−0.01	(−0.47; 0.44)	0.953
Social problems	2.75	(−0.31; 5.82)	0.078	0.10	(−0.63; 0.83)	0.792
High education level [†]	2.52	(0.27; 4.77)	**0.029**	−0.11	(−0.67; 0.45)	0.691
Body mass index	0.02	(−0.18; 0.23)	0.842	0.02	(−0.04; 0.07)	0.561
CIRS-G score	−0.14	(−0.41; 0.13)	0.312	0.03	(−0.04; 0.09)	0.441
History of stroke	−1.56	(−4.26; 1.13)	0.253	0.38	(−0.27; 1.02)	0.248
Use of vitamin K antagonists	−0.07	(−2.69; 2.56)	0.628	−0.10	(−0.75; 0.56)	0.773
Low dietary intake of fatty fish and eggs [‡]	−0.09	(−2.83; 2.65)	0.948	0.63	(−0.06; 1.31)	0.072
TSH concentration	0.76	(0.02; 1.49)	**0.044**	0.06	(−0.13; 0.24)	0.556
Vitamin B12 concentration	−0.00	(−0.01; 0.00)	0.513	0.00	(0.00; 0.00)	0.281
Albumin concentration	0.24	(0.04; 0.43)	**0.018**	0.01	(−0.04; 0.06)	0.698
Estimated glomerular filtration rate	−0.02	(−0.07; 0.04)	0.567	−0.01	(−0.02; 0.01)	0.242

β: coefficient of regression corresponding to a change of cognitive score; CI: confidence interval; CIRS-G: Cumulative Illness Rating Scale for Geriatrics; FBRS: Frontotemporal Behavioral Rating Scale; MMSE: Mini-Mental State Examination; TSH: Thyroid Stimulating Hormone; *: Separate models were used for each dependent variable; [†]: Elementary School Recognition Certificate passed; [‡]: Answer "No" to the question "Do you eat fatty fish at least once a week and/or eggs several times per week?"; β significant (*i.e.*, *p* < 0.05) indicated in bold.

Table 3. Correlation matrix of the dietary phylloquinone intake with the subscores of the Frontotemporal Behavioural Rating Scale.

Characteristics	1.	2.	3.	4.	5.
1. Log dietary phylloquinone intake	-	−0.14	−0.24 **	−0.09	−0.03
2. Self-control disorders		-	0.16 *	0.29 ***	0.32 ***
3. Physical neglect			-	0.14	0.25 ***
4. Mood disorders				-	0.35 ***
5. Lower general interest					-

*: *p* < 0.05 (2-tailed); **: *p* < 0.01 (2-tailed); ***: *p* < 0.001 (2-tailed).

Lastly, the sensitivity analysis found unaltered results after removing all participants who used VKA (*n* = 31). Of the 161 remaining participants, those in the lowest third of dietary phylloquinone intake had worse MMSE score (19.9 ± 6.0 *versus* 22.4 ± 5.8, *p* = 0.016) and FBRS score (1.9 ± 1.3 *versus* 1.5 ± 1.2, *p* = 0.035) than those in the other two thirds combined. Log dietary phylloquinone intake was linearly associated with the MMSE score (β = 1.83 (95% CI: 0.46; 3.20), *p* = 0.009) and with the FBRS score (β = −0.34 (95% CI: −0.66; −0.01), *p* = 0.041). Log dietary phylloquinone intake correlated negatively with the subscores of physical neglect (*r* = −0.24, *p* = 0.003) and self-control disorders (*r* = −0.17, *p* = 0.037), but not with mood disorders (*p* = 0.127) and loss of general interest (*p* = 0.978).

4. Discussion

The main finding of this cross-sectional study is that, irrespective of all measured potential confounders, increased dietary phylloquinone intake was associated with better cognition and behavior among geriatric patients. Specifically, compared to those in the lowest third of dietary phylloquinone intake, participants with higher dietary phylloquinone intake had 2.1 points more on the MMSE (*i.e.*, better) and 0.4 points less on the FBRS (*i.e.*, better).

These findings are consistent with the emerging epidemiological literature on vitamin K and cognition. Specifically, previous studies have reported that the serum concentration of phylloquinone was lower among patients with Alzheimer's disease (AD) compared to cognitively healthy controls [8], and that higher serum phylloquinone concentration was associated with better verbal episodic memory performance [5]. In line with this, we recently found that the use of VKAs, a drug class that generates a relative state of vitamin K deficiency, was associated among geriatric patients with greater prevalence of cognitive disorders [6], and with lower volume of gray matter in the brain, including in the hippocampus [7]. Here, we found no association between the use of VKAs and the global cognitive performance used as a quantitative variable. Several explanations can be proposed to account for this divergence: first, the potential lack of power of the present study that was not originally designed to assess the covariate VKA; second, the use of the cognitive performance as a continuous variable, unlike the previous study [6], which was focused on the cognitive impairment as a categorical variable; third, the lack of specification on the length of treatment and stability of the INR, which could influence the potential cognitive effect of VKAs. Of note, removing from the analysis the participants who were taking VKAs regularly did not alter our results, which strengthened the possibility of a specific link between dietary vitamin K intake and cognition. To the best of our knowledge, only two case-control studies have specifically examined the intake of phylloquinone in relation to cognition [9,10]. Shatenstein *et al.* found that that the mean dietary phylloquinone intake was persistently two-fold less in 36 community-dwelling patients with early-stage AD followed during 18 months in the Nutrition-Memory Study compared to 58 cognitively healthy control subjects (55.5 $\pm$ 54.3 *versus* 104.5 $\pm$ 83.7 with $p < 0.001$ at baseline) [9]. Consistently, Presse *et al.* found, in an additional analysis of the Nutrition-Memory Study cohort, that 31 cases with mild-to-moderate AD had lower dietary phylloquinone intake compared to 31 age- and gender-matched cognitively-healthy control subjects (37 μg/day *versus* 70 μg/day, $p < 0.0001$), even after adjusting for energy intakes ($p = 0.0003$) [10]. Additional indirect evidence stems from two cohort studies in which the high consumption of green leafy and cruciferous vegetables, rich in vitamin K, was associated with slower rates of age-related cognitive decline [19,20]. Compared to these studies, we did not use diet records to estimate the dietary phylloquinone intake, but a FFQ. Nevertheless, despite this methodological divergence, we observed that the higher the dietary phylloquinone intake, the better the cognitive performance and the lower the behavioural disorders. Specifically, we found a correlation of dietary phylloquinone intake with self-control disorders and physical neglect, but not with mood disorders and loss of interest (Table 3). In other words, the intake of phylloquinone does not appear to be related to emotional and affect regulation, but rather to behavioral disorders in relation with the cognitive sphere, which was confirmed by the finding of a direct association between dietary phylloquinone intake and MMSE score.

The mechanism linking dietary phylloquinone intake with cognition and behavior is not fully elucidated. Causality cannot be inferred from our cross-sectional study. It is possible that worse cognitive performance and greater behavioral disorders precipitate loss of functional autonomy with consequent poorer access to vitamin K-rich food. For instance, lower consumption of green vegetables, a major source of phylloquinone, has been reported in participants with AD compared to cognitively healthy participants [10]. In addition, the association of dietary phylloquinone intake with neuropsychiatric performance could be explained in a more general way by an overall healthy diet, which could also reflect generally healthy lifestyles. However, the latter assumptions should be mitigated here by the fact that the mean BMI of 26.2 kg/m^2 in our study indicated overweight according to the National Heart, Lung, and Blood Institute [21], and because there was no BMI difference between participants in the lowest third of phylloquinone intake and those in the highest thirds ($p = 0.492$, Table 1). Moreover the associations of dietary phylloquinone intake with the MMSE score and the FBRS score were significant even after adjustment for BMI and albumin concentration (Table 2). A scenario of reverse causation is plausible and should be considered. Evidence precisely supports a role for vitamin K in the CNS. Vitamin K modulates the synthesis and metabolism of sphingolipids, which are key players in neuronal proliferation, differentiation, senescence, cell-cell interaction, and transformation [2,3]. Recent research has linked alterations in sphingolipid metabolism to the aging process and neurodegenerative disorders such as AD [3]. In parallel, two VKDPs, Gas6 (growth arrest-specific gene 6) and protein S, are also closely associated with the CNS functioning [2,3]. Gas6 is involved in chemotaxis, mitogenesis, cell growth, and myelination, and has further been shown to rescue cortical neurons from amyloid β-induced apoptosis, a hallmark of AD [22]. Protein S offers neuronal protection during ischemic/hypoxic injury, both *in vivo* and *in vitro* [23]. Vitamin K may also protect neurons from *N*-methyl-D-aspartate-induced toxicity and apoptosis [24]. Finally, other authors have proposed that insufficient vitamin K could contribute to the pathogenesis of AD through a link to the apolipoprotein Eε4 allele, an established risk factor for AD that is also associated with lower vitamin K levels [11]. ApoE genotype was not determined in our cohort, which precludes testing this assumption. All these data suggest that the less available the vitamin K is, the less protected and effective the CNS may be, with subsequently greater risks of brain changes, cognitive decline, and behavioral disorders.

The strengths of our study include the originality of the research question on a highly common condition in older adults, the standardized collection of data from a single research center, the assessment of the dietary phylloquinone intake over preceding 12 months based on a validated tool, the assessment of both cognitive and behavioral outcomes, and the detailed description of the participants' characteristics allowing the use of regression models to measure adjusted associations. Regardless, a number of limitations should be acknowledged. First, due to the limited number of 192 in- and outpatients, our study may lack power and the participants may be not representative of the population of all seniors. Second, our study is cross-sectional at present, which precludes inferring causality. Third, the FFQ was validated on a Canadian population [12], and it is likely that the eating habits of our elderly patients were not strictly the same as those of North Americans. Moreover, it is noticeable that FFQs tend to overestimate intakes [25,26]. Nonetheless, the FFQ used in the present study presents a very good relative agreement with results from 24 h dietary recalls in healthy older adults [12]. It is also possible that the dietary phylloquinone intake may have been poorly estimated by interviewing patients with cognitive disorders. However, to avoid this bias, we double-checked information whenever possible from formal or informal carers. Fourth, although we were able to control for important characteristics that could modify the associations, residual potential confounders such as the determination of energy and homocysteine intakes or the determination of ApoE genotype, might still be present. Fifth, limitations include the use of the MMSE and FBRS tools, which may exhibit ceiling effects and limited sensitivity to subtle abnormalities [27]. In future studies, the screening for cognitive disorders should use other outcomes, e.g., comparing episodic memory or executive functions according to dietary phylloquinone intakes.

5. Conclusions

In conclusion, we report a clinically and statistically significant association between increased dietary phylloquinone intake and better cognition and behavior among geriatric patients. There is a strong need for novel effective preventive and therapeutic strategies for cognitive decline and dementia. The potential role of vitamin K in the development of dementia is therefore of substantial interest. Further prospective nutrition studies and clinical trials are needed to clarify whether older adults with higher dietary vitamin K intake are less likely to experience cognitive and behavioral declines than those with lower intake, and whether enhancing vitamin K intake could improve, or prevent, this process.

Acknowledgments: The authors thank Elena De Neree Tot Babberich, Clemence Gourdeau, Simon Pointel, Bruno Lemarchant, from Medical School, University of Angers, UNAM, Angers F-49933, France, for their help in collecting the participants' data and food records.

Author Contributions: Cedric Annweiler has full access to the data in the study and takes responsibility for the integrity of the data and the accuracy of the data analyses. Study concept and design: Cedric Annweiler;

Acquisition of data: Justine Chouet, Kariane Boucher, Nancy Presse, Guylaine Ferland and Cedric Annweiler; Analysis and interpretation of data: Justine Chouet and Cedric Annweiler; Drafting of the manuscript: Justine Chouet and Cedric Annweiler; Critical revision of the manuscript for important intellectual content: Guylaine Ferland, Catherine Féart, Yves Rolland, Nancy Presse, Kariane Boucher, Pascale Barberger-Gateau, and Olivier Beauchet; Statistical expertise: Cedric Annweiler and Catherine Féart; Administrative, technical, or material support: Cedric Annweiler; Study supervision: Cedric Annweiler.

Conflicts of Interest: The authors declare no conflict of interest.

References

1. Suttie, J.W. *Vitamin K in Health and Disease*; CRC Press: Boca Raton, FL, USA, 2009.
2. Ferland, G. Vitamin K, an emerging nutrient in brain function. *Biofactors* **2012**, *38*, 151–157. [CrossRef] [PubMed]
3. Ferland, G. Vitamin K and the nervous system: An overview of its actions. *Adv. Nutr.* **2012**, *3*, 204–212. [CrossRef] [PubMed]
4. Hall, J.G.; Pauli, R.M.; Wilson, K.M. Maternal and fetal sequelae of anticoagulation during pregnancy. *Am. J. Med.* **1980**, *68*, 122–140. [CrossRef]
5. Presse, N.; Belleville, S.; Gaudreau, P.; Greenwood, C.E.; Kergoat, M.J.; Morais, J.A.; Payette, H.; Shatenstein, B.; Ferland, G. Vitamin K status and cognitive function in healthy older adults. *Neurobiol. Aging* **2013**, *34*, 2777–2783. [CrossRef] [PubMed]
6. Annweiler, C.; Ferland, G.; Barberger-Gateau, P.; Brangier, A.; Rolland, Y.; Beauchet, O. Vitamin K antagonists and cognitive impairment: Results from a cross-sectional pilot study among geriatric patients. *J. Gerontol. A Biol. Sci. Med. Sci.* **2015**, *70*, 97–101. [CrossRef] [PubMed]
7. Annweiler, C.; Denis, S.; Duval, G.; Ferland, G.; Bartha, R.; Beauchet, O. Use of vitamin K antagonists and brain volumetry in seniors: Preliminary results from the GAIT study. *J. Gerontol. A Biol. Sci. Med. Sci.* **2015**. (in press).
8. Sato, Y.; Honda, Y.; Hayashida, N.; Iwamoto, J.; Kanoko, T.; Satoh, K. Vitamin K deficiency and osteopenia in elderly women with Alzheimer's disease. *Arch. Phys. Med. Rehabil.* **2005**, *86*, 576–581. [CrossRef] [PubMed]
9. Shatenstein, B.; Kergoat, M.J.; Reid, I. Poor nutrient intakes during 1-year follow-up with community-dwelling older adults with early stage Alzheimer dementia compared to cognitively intact matched controls. *J. Am. Diet Assoc.* **2007**, *107*, 2091–2099. [CrossRef] [PubMed]
10. Sato, Y.; Honda, Y.; Hayashida, N.; Iwamoto, J.; Kanoko, T.; Satoh, K. Low vitamin K intakes in community-dwelling elders at an early stage of Alzheimer's disease. *J. Am. Diet Assoc.* **2008**, *108*, 2095–2099.
11. Allison, A.C. The possible role of vitamin K deficiency in the pathogenesis of Alzheimer's disease and in augmenting brain damage associated with cardiovascular disease. *Med. Hypotheses* **2001**, *57*, 151–155. [CrossRef] [PubMed]
12. Presse, N.; Shatenstein, B.; Kergoat, M.J.; Ferland, G. Validation of a semi-quantitative food frequency questionnaire measuring dietary vitamin K intake in elderly people. *J. Am. Diet Assoc.* **2009**, *109*, 1251–1255. [CrossRef] [PubMed]
13. Folstein, M.F.; Folstein, S.E.; McHugh, P.R. Mini-mental state: a practical method for grading the cognitive state of patients for the clinician. *J. Psychiatr. Res.* **1975**, *12*, 189–198. [CrossRef]
14. Inouye, S.K.; van Dyck, C.H.; Alessi, C.A.; Balkin, S.; Siegal, A.P.; Horwitz, R.I. Clarifying confusion: The confusion assessment method. A new method for detection of delirium. *Ann. Intern. Med.* **1990**, *113*, 941–948. [CrossRef] [PubMed]
15. Lebert, F.; Pasquier, F.; Souliez, L.; Petit, H. Frontotemporal behavioral scale. *Alzheimer Dis. Assoc. Disord.* **1998**, *12*, 335–339. [CrossRef] [PubMed]
16. Linn, B.S.; Linn, M.W.; Gurel, L. Cumulative illness rating scale. *J. Am. Geriatr. Soc.* **1968**, *16*, 622–626. [CrossRef] [PubMed]
17. Hatano, S. Experience from a multicentre stroke register: A preliminary report. *Bull World Health Organ.* **1976**, *54*, 541–553. [PubMed]
18. Chevallereau, G.; Gleyses, X.; Roussel, L.; Hamdan, S.; Beauchet, O.; Annweiler, C. Proposal and validation of a quick question to rate the influence of diet in geriatric epidemiological studies on vitamin D. *Int. J. Vitam. Nutr. Res.* **2013**, *83*, 254–258. [CrossRef] [PubMed]

19. Kang, J.H.; Ascherio, A.; Grodstein, F. Fruit and vegetable consumption and cognitive decline in aging women. *Ann. Neurol.* **2005**, *57*, 713–720. [CrossRef] [PubMed]

20. Morris, M.C.; Evans, D.A.; Tangney, C.C.; Bienias, J.L.; Wilson, R.S. Associations of vegetable and fruit consumption with age-related cognitive change. *Neurology* **2006**, *67*, 1370–1376. [CrossRef] [PubMed]

21. Clinical guideline on the identification, evaluation, and treatment of overweight and obesity in adults: The evidence report. National Heart, Lung, and Blood Institute (online), 1998. Available online: http://www.nhlbi.nih.gov/guidelines/obesity/ob_gdlns.png (accessed on 6 August 2014).

22. Yagami, T.; Ueda, K.; Asakura, K.; Okamura, N.; Sakaeda, T.; Sakaguchi, G.; Itoh, N.; Hashimoto, Y.; Nakano, T.; Fujimoto, M.; *et al.* Effect of Gas6 on secretory phospholipase A(2)-IIA-induced apoptosis in cortical neurons. *Brain Res.* **2003**, *985*, 142–149. [CrossRef]

23. Liu, D.; Guo, H.; Griffin, J.H.; Fernandez, J.A.; Zlokovic, B.V. Protein S confers neuronal protection during ischemic/hypoxic injury in mice. *Circulation* **2003**, *107*, 1791–1796. [CrossRef] [PubMed]

24. Zhong, Z.; Wang, Y.; Guo, H.; Sagare, A.; Fernández, J.A.; Bell, R.D.; Barrett, T.M.; Griffin, J.H.; Freeman, R.S.; Zlokovic, B.V.; *et al.* Protein S protects neurons from excitotoxic injury by activating the TAM receptor Tyro3-phosphatidylinositol 3-kinase-Akt pathway through its sex hormone-binding globulin-like region. *J. Neurosci.* **2010**, *30*, 15521–15534. [CrossRef] [PubMed]

25. Booth, S.L.; Suttie, J.W. Dietary intake and adequacy of vitamin K. *J. Nutr.* **1998**, *128*, 785–788. [PubMed]

26. Holmes, M.V.; Hunt, B.J.; Shearer, M.J. The role of dietary vitamin K in the management of oral vitamin K antagonists. *Blood Rev.* **2012**, *26*, 1–14. [CrossRef] [PubMed]

27. Spencer, R.J.; Wendell, C.R.; Giggey, P.P.; Katzel, L.I.; Lefkowitz, D.M.; Siegel, E.L.; Waldstein, S.R. Psychometric limitations of the mini-mental state examination among nondemented older adults: An evaluation of neurocognitive and magnetic resonance imaging correlates. *Exp. Aging Res.* **2013**, *39*, 382–397. [CrossRef] [PubMed]

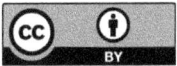

nutrients

MDPI

Review

Structural Modeling Insights into Human VKORC1 Phenotypes

Katrin J. Czogalla [1], Matthias Watzka [1,2] and Johannes Oldenburg [1,2,*]

[1] Institute of Experimental Hematology and Transfusion Medicine, University Clinic Bonn, Bonn 53105, Germany; E-Mails: katrin.czogalla@ukb.uni-bonn.de (K.J.C.); matthias.watzka@ukb.uni-bonn.de (M.W.)
[2] Center for Rare Diseases Bonn (ZSEB), University Clinic Bonn, Bonn 53127, Germany
* Author to whom correspondence should be addressed; E-Mail: johannes.oldenburg@ukb.uni-bonn.de; Tel.: +49-228-287-15175; Fax: +49-228-287-15176.

Received: 20 May 2015 / Accepted: 6 August 2015 / Published: 14 August 2015

Abstract: Vitamin K 2,3-epoxide reductase complex subunit 1 (VKORC1) catalyses the reduction of vitamin K and its 2,3-epoxide essential to sustain γ-carboxylation of vitamin K-dependent proteins. Two different phenotypes are associated with mutations in human VKORC1. The majority of mutations cause resistance to 4-hydroxycoumarin- and indandione-based vitamin K antagonists (VKA) used in the prevention and therapy of thromboembolism. Patients with these mutations require greater doses of VKA for stable anticoagulation than patients without mutations. The second phenotype, a very rare autosomal-recessive bleeding disorder caused by combined deficiency of vitamin K dependent clotting factors type 2 (VKCFD2) arises from a homozygous Arg98Trp mutation. The bleeding phenotype can be corrected by vitamin K administration. Here, we summarize published experimental data and *in silico* modeling results in order to rationalize the mechanisms of VKA resistance and VKCFD2.

Keywords: vitamin K epoxide reductase (VKOR); VKORC1; vitamin K; vitamin K 2,3-epoxide; warfarin; VKCFD2; molecular modeling; vitamin K antagonists

1. Introduction

Vitamin K 2,3-epoxide reductase complex subunit 1 (VKORC1) is the rate limiting enzyme of the vitamin K cycle [1,2]. VKORC1 is located in the endoplasmic reticulum (ER) membrane and catalyses reduction of vitamin K 2,3-epoxide (K > O) to vitamin K quinone (K) and further to vitamin K hydroquinone (KH_2) [3]. Vitamin K reduction to KH_2 is essential for the enzyme γ-glutamyl carboxylase (GGCX) to modify vitamin K-dependent (VKD) proteins at their Gla domains. During γ-carboxylation, KH_2 is oxidized to K > O. The K > O is reduced to vitamin K quinone and further to KH_2 by VKORC1, completing a recycling mechanism known as the vitamin K cycle [4]. A functional vitamin K cycle including VKORC1 and GGCX is required to enable physiological function of all VKD proteins. VKD proteins are involved in blood coagulation (coagulation factors FII, FVII, FIX, FX, Protein C, S, and Z) as well as in calcium homeostasis (matrix Gla protein, MGP; bone Gla protein, OST) [5,6]. There have been several additional VKD proteins reported to be involved in other pathways including cell-cycle regulation or with unknown functions [7].

Since the *VKORC1* gene was cloned in 2004, genetic analysis has revealed a number of mutations causing one of two different pathological phenotypes [8–10]. To date, 28 human *VKORC1* mutations have been identified that cause resistance to several vitamin K antagonists (VKA) that are used clinically as oral anticoagulants [11,12]. Patients with these mutations require higher VKA doses for stable anticoagulation. Other 4-hydroxycoumarin and indandione derivatives are used as rodenticides. Historically, warfarin has been the most common VKA used in the anticoagulant clinic or as a rodenticide, and it has been common terminology to describe patients and animals with resistance to any VKA as possessing "warfarin resistance" (WR). This convention will be used in this manuscript. Interestingly, there are also several rat and mouse VKORC1 mutations reported to cause WR that affect residues homologous to known warfarin resistance mutations in human VKORC1 (hVKORC1) [13,14].

In contrast, there is only one mutation known to result in the VKCFD2 phenotype. VKORC1:p.Arg98Trp causes diminished vitamin K epoxide reductase (VKOR) activity compared to that of the wild-type enzyme [15]. VKCFD2 patients exhibit severely diminished activities for the VKD coagulation factors and suffer spontaneous or surgery/injury induced bleeding episodes [16,17]. In addition to this haemorrhagic phenotype, abnormalities in epiphyseal growth have been reported in one case [18]. This phenotype is very rare. Worldwide, there are only four unrelated families known to be affected with VKCFD2 [16–18].

This review discusses features of the modeled structure of the human VKORC1 enzyme, putative amino acid sequences involved in warfarin binding, and motifs that influence ER-retention of the enzyme and proposed general mechanisms that can explain the respective phenotypes.

2. The Crystal Structure of *Synechococcus* VKOR—A Homolog to hVKORC1

The first X-ray crystallographic structure of *Synechococcus* sp. VKOR (synVKOR), a bacterial homolog of the hVKORC1 enzyme, was reported by Li *et al.* in 2010 [19]. This enzyme is composed of five transmembrane helices (TMs). The first four TMs form a bundle surrounding a quinone in its interior thereby comprising the catalytic core of synVKOR. The quinone substrate is close to the periplasmic side of the enzyme and in close proximity to the CXXC active site motif located in TM4. There is a long periplasmic loop between TM1 and TM2 that includes a 1/2 helix ("1/2 segment" in the original article) and a pair of cysteines (Cys50, Cys56) and a serine/threonine residue (Ser62) conserved among all VKOR homologs [20]. The fifth TM of synVKOR is located outside of the four-helix bundle and is connected via a C-terminal linker segment to a thioredoxin (Trx)-like domain. The Trx-like domain is the naturally fused redox partner of synVKOR. Li *et al.* [19] observed a disulfide bridge with strong electron density between Cys50 in the periplasmic loop of the VKOR domain and Cys209 of the Trx-like domain. Thus, the synVKOR structure suggests an electron transfer mechanism that shuttles reducing equivalents from the Trx-like domain, via the conserved cysteines in the loop, to the CXXC active site motif where the bound ubiquinone substrate becomes reduced to the hydroquinone form [21].

3. The Human VKORC1 Homology Model

In the absence of high-resolution X-ray crystallographic or NMR structures of hVKORC1, creation of a homology model based on the synVKOR structure provides an opportunity to gain structure-based insights into hVKORC1 function. Several *in silico* algorithms revealed conflicting topology predictions of either a 3TM, 4TM or 5TM structure for *hVKORC1* [8,9,11,22–24]. There are also conflicting experimental data supporting 3TM or 4TM topologies [25–27]. Nevertheless, all VKOR homologues share conserved functional residues at homologous positions which strongly suggest that all homologs share a common protein fold and topology with respect to the lipid membrane in which they are embedded.

4. Conserved Amino Acid Residues of Human VKORC1

VKORC1 homologues are found in plants, bacteria, archaea and mammals but not in yeast and fungi [20,28,29]. All VKOR homolog enzymes possess a CXXC motif in the active site, essential for reduction of quinone substrates [3,20,30–32]. The cysteines of the CXXC motif form a disulfide bridge that becomes reduced for catalytic activity. There are two additional cysteines (Cys43 and Cys51) that can form a disulfide bond and a conserved serine at amino acid position 57 (or either threonine in some VKORC1 homologues) in the large loop of hVKORC1 [3,19,30,32,33]. These four cysteines and the serine/threonine are absolutely conserved and define proteins of the VKOR family.

Nutrients **2015**, *7*, 6837–6851

The CXXC motif is located in the last TM and is oriented towards the ER lumen in both 3TM and 4TM models for hVKORC1 (Figure 1). All published reports show complete loss of VKOR activity if one of the cysteines in the CXXC motif is mutated (Cys132 and Cys135, Table 1) [3,19,30,31]. These data clearly demonstrate that the CXXC motif is the active center essential for substrate reduction. The functional role of the conserved cysteines in the large loop, Cys43 and Cys51, is not completely clear. Due to their localisation Cys43 and Cys51 are also called "loop cysteines". Of the two topology models, studies proposing the 4TM model claim that the loop cysteines are essential for *in vivo* VKOR activity [27,33], whereas studies supporting the 3TM model argue that they are not necessary [3,26,34]. The main difference between both models is the orientation of the N-terminus, the first TM, and the large loop. In the 3TM model, the loop is located in the cytoplasm, whereas in the 4TM model, the loop is in the ER lumen (Figure 1). In the 4TM model, the loop cysteines are required for electron transfer from redox partners located in the ER lumen to reduce the CXXC motif. This postulated electron transfer pathway is necessary for catalytic VKOR activity and is also present in bacterial VKOR homologues. In synVKOR, the disulfide bridge formed between the loop cysteines is reduced by a periplasmic Trx-like redox partner naturally fused to the VKOR core protein. In vertebrates, this natural fused redox partner is missing. Therefore, Trx-like domain containing proteins are thought to reduce the loop cysteines in vertebrates. Candidate partner oxidoreductases include protein disulfide isomerases (PDIs) that are either separate globular proteins in the ER lumen or type-I ER membrane-anchored proteins with redox-active cysteines facing the ER lumen [27,35]. Thus, electron transfer mediated by the loop cysteines is feasible for the 4TM model only, as most PDIs are resident in the ER lumen. However, for the 3TM model, PDIs would not be able to reduce the loop cysteines if the loop is located in the cytoplasm. Here, the two loop cysteines could not be essential for VKOR activity, and electron transfer would presumably take place through direct reduction of the CXXC motif. Thus, location of the loop cysteines in the ER lumen might not be a strict requirement for hVKORC1 function if the 3TM model were to be correct.

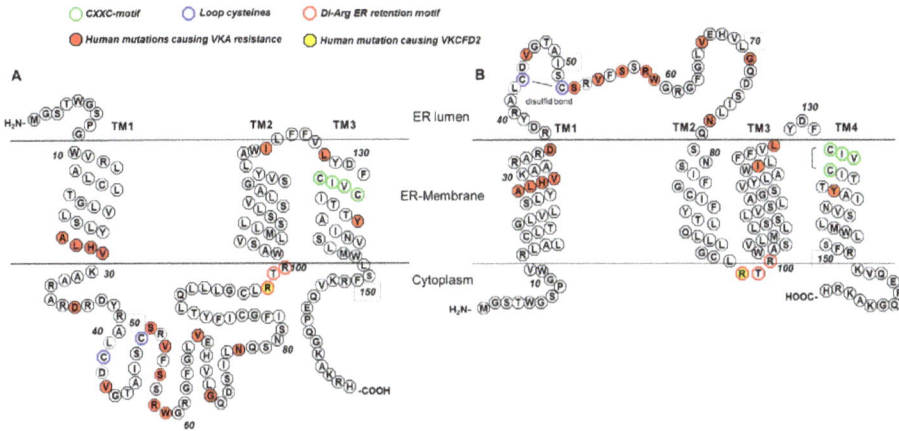

Figure 1. 3TM and 4TM topological models for hVKORC1 (modified from Tie *et al.*, 2012 [26]). In both models, conserved cysteines (Cys132 and Cys135 of the active center (CXXC motif), green; loop cysteines Cys43 and Cys51, blue) and Arg98_Arg100 of the di-arginine endoplasmic reticulum (ER) retention motif (red) are labeled with colored circles. Amino acid positions for which mutations were reported to be associated with either vitamin K antagonist (VKA) resistance or combined deficiency of vitamin K dependent clotting factors type 2 (VKCFD2) are marked by filled circles (mutations causing VKA resistance, red; VKCFD2 mutation, yellow). (**A**) Shows the putative topology for hVKORC1 as a 3 TM membrane-embedded protein with the loop located in the cytoplasm. The N-terminus is located in the ER lumen, whereas the C-terminus is in the cytoplasm. (**B**) Shows the putative 4TM topology for hVKORC1 with the loop containing the conserved cysteines Cys43 and Cys51 in the ER lumen with both termini located in the cytoplasm.

Table 1. Published activities for hVKORC1 conserved cysteines by various functional assays.

Publication	Rost *et al.* [30]	Jin *et al.* [3]	Rishavy *et al.* [33]	Tie *et al.* [26]	Tie *et al.* [34]	Tie *et al.* [36]
Type of VKOR assay	DTT-driven assay	DTT-driven assay	DTT-driven assay	Cell-based assay	DTT-driven assay/cell-based assay	Cell-based assay
Reductant	DTT	DTT	DTT/Trx/TrxR	-	-	-
Cell line	HEK293 cells	Sf9 cells	Sf21 cells	HEK293 cells	HEK293 cells	C1 + L1 DKO HEK cells
Cysteine residue variants:						
Cys43Ala	20%	25%	~85%/0%	<5%	25%/<5%	<5%
Cys43Ser	20%					
Cys51Ala		100%	~50%/0%	95%	100%/100%	105%
Cys51Ser	<5%					
Cys43Ala + Cys51Ala		112%		60%	85%/110%	90%
Cys43_Cys51del		85%			85%/60%	
Cys132Ala/Ser	<5%	0%			0%/0%	
Cys135Ala/Ser	<5%	0%			0%/0%	

This table shows the published vitamin K epoxide reductase (VKOR) activities of human vitamin K 2,3-epoxide reductase complex subunit 1 (hVKORC1) variants in which conserved cysteines were selectively mutated or deleted. In each published study the VKOR activities are presented as a percentage of the activity of the wild-type hVKORC1 reported in the same study. The table also lists the type of VKOR assay, reductant (dithiothreitol (DTT) or thioredoxin/thioredoxin reductase (Trx/TrxR)), and cell line (human embryonic kidney (HEK) cells, *Spodoptera frugiperda* (Sf21) cells, or double knock-out (DKO) HEK cells) used.

It follows from the arguments presented above that VKOR activity measurements of variants affecting the loop cysteines might provide important clues to elucidate the topology and structure of hVKORC1. Reduced activities for amino acid substitutions of loop cysteines would tend to support the 4TM model where loop cysteines would be essential for electron transfer. Alternatively, data revealing unaffected activity for these variants would favour the 3TM topology model where loop cysteines would not be required for CXXC motif reduction. Several research groups have published conflicting activity data regarding the loop cysteines supporting either the 3TM or 4TM topology (Table 1). Rost *et al.* [30] were the first to publish data regarding the loop cysteines of hVKORC1 investigated by the commonly used dithiothreitol (DTT)-driven VKOR assay. They demonstrated a reduction of VKOR activity to 5% for Cys51Ser and to 20% for Cys43Ser with respect to wild-type activity [30]. By contrast, Jin *et al.* published results revealing more than 100% activity for Cys51Ala compared to that of wild-type VKORC1. However, the Cys43Ala variant showed reduced activity to 25% which corresponds well to the data of Rost *et al.* for Cys43Ser. Interestingly, VKOR activity of a variant with both loop cysteines mutated was unaffected (Table 1) [3]. Rishavy *et al.* [33] modified this *in vitro* VKOR assay by replacing the non-physiological DTT with the reductant thioredoxin/thioredoxin reductase (Trx/TrxR). In their study, they demonstrated that VKOR activity assessed by the DTT-driven assay is prone to false positive results. They showed that membrane-permeable DTT directly reduces the active centre of hVKORC1, essentially bypassing the loop cysteines. Thus, the loop cysteine variants showed VKOR activity when DTT was used as reductant. When DTT was replaced by the membrane impermeable Trx/TrxR reductant, VKORC1 loop cysteine mutants did not show VKOR activity (Table 1) [33]. This strongly suggests that loop cysteines are essential for VKOR activity when driven by a biological oxidoreductase enzyme. However, the study was negatively critiqued regarding the relative concentration differences between DTT and Trx/TrxR concentrations used (millimolar for DTT *vs.* micromolar for Trx/TrxR) [22]. Alternatively, loop cysteine variants have been examined in one of the recently reported cell-based assays in which no detergent and extra reductants are used and VKOR activity is indirectly assessed in living cells. Two studies by Tie *et al.* [26,36] revealed very low VKOR activity for Cys43Ala (<5%), whereas Cys51Ala showed activity comparable to that of wild-type VKORC1. Again, they found that mutation of both loop cysteines did not affect VKOR activity (Table 1) [26,36].

Taken together, data from all research groups demonstrated reduction of VKOR activity for all variants affecting Cys43, independent of the type of assay used. However, results regarding activities of Cys51 variants are in disaccord as they range between 0% and 100% relative to wild-type VKOR activity. Moreover, these data do not unequivocally clarify whether or not the loop cysteines are essential for hVKORC1 activity and, thus, do not definitively support either the 3TM or 4TM model.

5. The 3TM VKORC1 Topology Model

The 3TM model is characterized by three transmembrane alpha-helices with a large cytoplasmic loop containing the conserved loop cysteines located between the first and second TMs. The C-terminus is located in the cytoplasm and the N-terminus in the ER lumen (Figure 1A). The 3TM model is supported by several *in silico* topology prediction algorithms and by experimental data from a fluorescence protease protection (FFP) assay of Tie *et al.* [26,37]. In this assay, VKORC1 enzyme was either C- or N-terminal tagged with the green fluorescent protein (GFP). After expression of both GFP tagged variants in HEK293 cells, a GFP digestion was performed using trypsin. The cells were treated before the digestion with digitonin to selectively permeabilize only the plasma membrane so that GFP tags located in the cytoplasm, but not in the ER lumen, become digested by the protease. The FFP assay results revealed a complete digestion of GFP for the C-terminal tagged VKORC1 protein after 90 s, whereas the N-terminal GFP-tagged VKORC1 continued to show a fluorescent signal even after 150 s. These data suggest that N- and C-termini are located on opposite sides of the ER membrane with the C-terminus in the cytoplasm. The N-terminus appears to be located in the ER lumen because it is protected from the proteolysis [26].

6. The 4TM VKORC1 Topology Model

The putative 4TM topology for hVKORC1 is composed of 4TM domains and includes the large ER lumenal loop between TM1 and TM2 with the two conserved loop cysteines. Both termini are located in the cytoplasm (Figure 1B). The CXXC motif is located in 4TM close to the ER lumen, equivalent to its placement in the third and final TM for the 3TM model. The crystal structure of the bacterial synVKOR enzyme strongly suggests a 4TM topology for hVKORC1. The membrane embedded four-helix bundle of synVKOR is homologous to hVKORC1 which shares ~24% primary sequence identity [19].

Wajih *et al.* [35] performed a knock-down of PDI expression by using siRNA silencing. This revealed reduced VKOR activity to 25% in HEK293 cells. In addition, they demonstrated by sodium dodecyl sulfate polyacrylamide gel electrophoresis (SDS-PAGE) that PDIs form a complex with VKORC1 [35]. This was the first convincing evidence that PDIs may be physiological redox partners for hVKORC1. Further immunoprecipitation data by Li *et al.* [27] confirmed which PDI family member interacts with hVKORC1 [27]. The interaction was only present if Cys51 of hVKORC1 and the second active site cysteine of the Trx-like domain of PDI were both mutated to alanine. These amino acid substitutions were necessary because the native cysteine pairs of VKORC1 and PDI are self-reducing during redox cycling and do not form stable disulfide bonds. As a result of the mutagenesis, the "donor" cysteine of PDI and the "acceptor" cysteine (Cys43) of hVKORC1 form a stable disulfide bond that remains oxidized during immunoprecipitation and detection. These results indicate that at least three PDIs identified can transfer electrons to the loop cysteines of hVKORC1. *In silico* modeling of hVKORC1 on the X-ray crystallographic structure of synVKOR also suggests a 4TM topology [19,23]. Additionally, *in silico* docking of warfarin on this model disclosed three putative binding interfaces. All human, as well as rodent, VKORC1 mutations associated with warfarin resistance are located in or close to these putative binding interfaces, supporting the plausibility of our *in silico* analysis (see detailed information in the next section) [23].

Taken together, data from the PDI knock-down, immunoprecipitation interaction studies, and *in silico* modeling of hVKORC1 with the identification of putative warfarin binding interfaces are largely consistent with a 4TM topology for hVKORC1 (Table 2).

Table 2. Overview of published experimental data supporting 3TM or 4TM topological models for hVKORC1.

Arguments for 3TM hVKORC1 Structure	Arguments for 4TM hVKORC1 Structure
Location of the C-Terminus of VKORC1 in the cytoplasm and of the N-Terminus in the ER-lumen; FFP assay [26]	siRNA knock-down of PDI located in the ER lumen results in reduced VKOR activity [35]
Cys51Ala exhibits VKOR activity = Cys51 is not required for VKOR activity, DTT and cell-based assays [3,26,36]	Cys43Ala/Ser and Cys51Ala/Ser exhibit no VKOR activity = Cys43 and Cys51 are required for VKOR activity, DTT and Trx/TrxR assays [30,33]
hVKOR model, prediction program TOPCONS [37]	Cys43 forms a disulfide bond with four PDIs, immunoprecipitation [27] 3.6 Å crystal structure of the bacterial homologue of VKOR from *Synechococcus* sp. in conjunction with multiple sequence alignments [19] hVKORC1 model based on crystal structure of synVKOR and putative warfarin binding interfaces that correspond to the reported WR mutations [23]

The left- and right-hand columns present brief summaries of the experimental data obtained from structural studies and assays of VKOR activity (together with literature citations) that support either the 3TM or 4TM topology for hVKORC1 respectively.

7. Warfarin Binding and Mutations Causing Warfarin Resistance

VKA such as warfarin, are direct inhibitors of VKORC1 and are used in the prevention and therapy of thromboembolic disorders [4,29]. It is widely believed that warfarin binds to VKORC1 irreversibly [38]. To date, genetic analysis of *VKORC1* has implicated a total of 28 mutations to be associated with WR in humans (Table 3) [8,11,12]. Affected patients require greater doses of VKA drugs for stable oral anticoagulation compared to wild-type VKORC1 probands. Some WR patients even exhibit an apparent complete resistance leading to ineffective control or to the abandonment of anticoagulation therapy with VKA [11,12].

Table 3. Comparison of warfarin inhibition for hVKORC1 variants determined by *in vitro* assays of vitamin K 2,3-epoxide reductase (VKOR) in cell fractions or in cultured cells.

hVKORC1 Variant	Mean Patient Dosage in HDT Multiples [Drug] for n = Number of Reported Patients [11]	Warfarin IC_{50} by DTT-Driven VKOR Assay [8,12]	Warfarin IC_{50} by Cell Based Assay [23]	Warfarin Phenotypes by Cell Based Assay [36]
Wild-type	1.0 [W, P] (n = 77)			
Ala26Pro	>3.0 [W] (n = 1)	11.2-fold increased K_i [12]	49.6-fold increased IC_{50}	n.d.
Ala26Thr	>2.0 [P] (n = 1)	sensitive as wt [12]	3.0-fold increased IC_{50}	n.d.
Leu27Val	>3.0 [F], 1.0 [W] (n = 1) *	sensitive as wt [12]	2.5-fold increased IC_{50}	n.d.
His28Gln	3.5 [P] (n = 1)	more sensitive than wt [12]	2.9-fold increased IC_{50}	n.d.
Val29Leu	2.0 [W] (n = 1)	absence of expression [12]/low VKOR activity and more sensitive than wt [8]	5.5-fold increased IC_{50}	n.d.
Ala34Pro	3.8 [W] (n = 1)	n.d.	n.d.	n.d.
Asp36Gly	3.0 [W] (n = 1)	more sensitive than wt [12]	3.2-fold increased IC_{50}	n.d.
Asp36Tyr	1.5–3.5 [W] (n = 10)	sensitive as wt [12]	3.8-fold increased IC_{50}	n.d.
Val45Ala	>2.0 [W] (n = 1)	low VKOR activity [8], more sensitive than wt [8,12]	6.2-fold increased IC_{50}	n.d.
Ser52Leu	>3.0 [P] (n = 1)	low VKOR activity, K_i determination not possible [12]	7.4-fold increased IC_{50}	moderate resistance
Ser52Trp	3.5 [P] (n = 1)	low VKOR activity, K_i determination not possible [12]	5.7-fold increased IC_{50}	sensitive as wt
Val54Leu	1.5–5.5 [W] (n = 2)	4.6-fold increased K_i [12]	4.5-fold increased IC_{50}	n.d.
Ser56Phe	>5.0 [P] (n = 1)	more sensitive than wt [12]	6.8-fold increased IC_{50}	n.d.
Arg58Gly	5.0 [W] (n = 1)	low VKOR activity [8], more sensitive than wt [8,12]	3.4-fold increased IC_{50}	n.d.
Trp59Arg	7.0 [P] (n = 1)	low VKOR activity, K_i determination not possible [12]	17.5-fold increased IC_{50}	high resistance
Trp59Cys	>3.5 [P] (n = 1)	more sensitive than wt [12]	7.6-fold increased IC_{50}	n.d.

Table 3. *Cont.*

hVKORC1 Variant	Mean Patient Dosage in HDT Multiples [Drug] for *n* = Number of Reported Patients [11]	Warfarin IC_{50} by DTT-Driven VKOR Assay [8,12]	Warfarin IC_{50} by Cell Based Assay [23]	Warfarin Phenotypes by Cell Based Assay [36]
Trp59Leu	>5.0 [P] (*n* = 1)	low VKOR activity, K_i determination not possible [12]	75.2-fold increased IC_{50}	high VKOR activity, high resistance
Val66Gly	2.5 [P] (*n* = 1)	low VKOR activity, K_i determination not possible [12]	2.8-fold increased IC_{50}	sensitive as wt
Val66Met	3.0–6.0 [W] (*n* = 7)	low VKOR activity, K_i determination not possible [12]	5.4-fold increased IC_{50}	sensitive as wt
Gly71Ala	>2.0 [P] (*n* = 1)	low VKOR activity, K_i determination not possible [12]	5.1-fold increased IC_{50}	sensitive as wt
Asn77Ser	>3.0 [P] (*n* = 1)	low VKOR activity, K_i determination not possible [12]	5.3-fold increased IC_{50}	moderate resistance
Asn77Tyr	3.5 [W] (*n* = 1)	low VKOR activity, K_i determination not possible [12]	3.9-fold increased IC_{50}	sensitive as wt
Ile123Asn	>7.0 [P] (*n* = 1)	2.4-fold increased K_i [12]	8.5-fold increased IC_{50}	n.d.
Leu128Arg	>4.0–7.0 [W] (*n* = 5)	low VKOR activity [8,12], K_i determination not possible [12]/more sensitive than wt [8]	49.7-fold increased IC_{50}	high VKOR activity, high resistance
Tyr139His	>3.0 [W] (*n* = 1)	3.6-fold increased K_i [12]	4.6-fold increased IC_{50}	n.d.

This table shows patient data as well as *in vitro* results from the DTT-driven and cell culture-based VKOR assays for VKORC1 variants reported to cause resistance to VKA. Patient data from Watzka *et al.* [11] and Hodroge *et al.* [12], with [P] = phenprocoumon, [W] = warfarin; HDT = High Dosage Threshold which is equivalent to the mean patient population dosage divided by that for the control group (homozygous wild-type *VKORC1* alleles with *VKORC1*:c.-1639GG haplotype). The patient marked with an asterisk (*) and Leu27Val mutation had additionally the CYP2C9*2*3 haplotype which results in a reduced warfarin dosage requirement to achieve a stable, therapeutic INR compared to patients with wild-type CYP2C9*1*1 haplotype. Variants investigated by the DTT-driven assay by Hodroge *et al.* [12] and Rost *et al.* [8] were summarized in one column, followed by data from Czogalla *et al.* [23] and Tie *et al.* [36]. n.d. = not determined.

Investigation by *in vitro* assays of these mutations is challenging and the results often do not correlate with patient phenotypes [39]. Rost *et al.* (2004) first investigated warfarin inhibition of six WR variants heterologously expressed in HEK293 cells using the DTT-driven VKOR assay but none of these mutations showed an *in vitro* resistance phenotype [8]. Similarly, Hodroge *et al.* (2012) expressed human WR variants in *Pichia pastoris* and found that only four of 25 mutations investigated revealed resistance phenotypes by the DTT-driven VKOR assay [12]. Nineteen variants were either non-functional or did not show a resistance phenotype [12]. Ten of the mutations that had essentially no *in vitro* VKOR activity in the study of Hodroge *et al.* (2012) [12] were re-examined by Tie *et al.* (2013) [36] using a cell-based assay. This assay indirectly reports activity of hVKORC1 using carboxylation of a coexpressed chimeric VKD protein in a HEK293 cell line constitutively knocked-out for both endogenous *VKORC1* and its paralog enzyme *VKORC1L1* [36]. For all the variants investigated, Tie *et al.* [36] detected VKOR activity as great as or greater than that of wild-type VKORC1. Five mutations exhibited a warfarin resistance phenotype by their cell culture-based assay, consistent with reported patient WR phenotypes [35]. However, five other WR mutations were not resistant to warfarin in their assay [36]. Hodroge *et al.* (2012) [12] and Tie *et al.* (2013) [36] both speculated that therapeutic doses of warfarin in these patients possibly have impact alternative enzyme targets other than the hVKORC1 mutated variants. In contrast, our group showed that all known hVKORC1 mutations associated with WR revealed *in vitro* WR phenotypes by a similar cell culture-based assay [23,39]. In all cases, we measured *in vitro* WR phenotypes ranging from mild to total resistance, in agreement with elevated patient dosages previously reported (Table 3) [11]. Discrepancies detected for WR phenotypes by the cell culture-based assays of Tie *et al.* [36] and of Czogalla *et al.* [23,39] might be explained by differences in the experimental setting. The genomic background of the HEK293T cell strains used was a wild-type in the study of Czogalla *et al.* [23] and a *VKORC1/VKORC1L1* double knock-out in the study of Tie *et al.* [36]. Additionally, our group [23,39] used wild-type FIX as a coexpressed VKD reporter protein to measure VKORC1 function, whereas Tie and co-workers [36] used a chimeric construct comprising protein C with its Gla domain replaced by that of FIX. Similar differences in the ability of DTT-based and cell culture-based assays to report *in vitro* WR phenotypes for mouse and rat VKORC1 have been reported [13,14,40].

To gain further insight into the binding and inhibitory action of warfarin, we performed *in silico* docking of warfarin on our model of hVKORC1. Molecular docking analysis revealed three putative warfarin binding interfaces on hVKORC1 comprising linear sequences of the ER-lumenal loop (Ser52-Phe55), and the first (Leu22-Lys30) and fourth (Phe131-Thr137) transmembrane helices of hVKORC1 [23]. Twenty-four human and nine rodent VKORC1 mutations confirmed to be WR are located at or near to the predicted binding interfaces. In addition, all amino acid substitutions causing WR, except for Tyr139His, were found to have their side chains on the ER lumenal side of the enzyme, thereby potentially influencing warfarin binding. Furthermore, our data suggest that warfarin might inhibit hVKORC1 in three possible ways. Firstly, binding of warfarin may interfere with the redox cycling of the disulfide bridge between the loop cysteines (Cys43 and Cys51). Secondly, warfarin binding might hinder the close approach of the reduced loop cysteines to the active centre of VKORC1 (CXXC motif). Thirdly, binding of warfarin might also hinder access of the K > O substrate to its binding pocket in the hVKORC1 active site. In summary, the insight gained through comparative modeling of hVKORC1 based on the synVKOR X-ray crystallographic structure has led to further investigation of the molecular mechanisms of warfarin inhibition of hVKORC1 and warfarin resistance.

8. VKCFD2

To date, there have been only three unrelated families reported with probands suffering from VKCFD2 who harbour homozygous VKORC1:p.Arg98Trp alleles [16,17]. Instead of WR, this mutation causes spontaneous bleedings due to reduced VKOR activity of 20%–60% compared to that for homozygous wild-type hVKORC1 individuals [8,16–18]. A previous study confirmed diminished, warfarin-sensitive VKOR activity of ~10%, relative to that of wild-type enzyme by the DTT-driven VKOR assay [30]. However, the haemorrhagic phenotype of these patients can be corrected by vitamin K administration which results in restoration of activities for the vitamin K-dependent clotting factors to normal ranges. Until recently, the pathophysiological mechanism underlying the single mutation causing VKCFD2 was unknown.

In a recent study, we modeled hVKORC1 and performed *in silico* analysis of the region of interest. We found that the Arg98Trp mutation might be part of a putative di-arginine ER retention motif [15]. To confirm these *in silico* results experimentally, different variants affecting Arg98 and/or Arg100 of the putative ER retention motif were expressed in HEK293T cells and analysed by fluorescence confocal microscopy. As expected, wild-type hVKORC1 was exclusively located in the ER, whereas all variants affecting the di-arginine ER retention motif revealed reduced ER localization to only 9% compared to that of wild-type hVKORC1. The naturally occurring variant Arg98Trp resulted in 20% ER-localization compared to that of the wild-type. We further observed that the protein variants affecting the di-arginine ER retention motif were directed to the cytoplasm. If the residual amount of hVKORC1:Arg98Trp in the ER is not functionally impaired with respect to VKOR activity, this would explain phenotype correction by vitamin K administration for VKCFD2 patients [41].

Interestingly, our identified di-arginine ER retention motif (Arg98_Arg100) is consistent with both the 3TM and 4TM topology models for hVKORC1. Di-arginine based ER retention motifs are generally present in cytosolic domains of proteins at approximately 16–46 A° from the lipid bilayer and allows for interaction with ER retention proteins [42,43]. This is observed for both hVKORC1 models, in which the guanidyl groups of Arg98 and Arg100 are exposed to the cytoplasm. In the 4TM model, these arginines are located in the small cytoplasm-exposed loop connecting TM2 with TM3 (Figure 1B) [42,43]. However, our results would also support the alternative 3TM model for hVKORC1 where the di-arginine ER retention motif would be located at the end of the large putative cytoplasmic loop just before the TM2 helix (Figure 1A).

9. Conclusions

The identification of the human *VKORC1* gene in 2004 was a major step towards understanding the molecular and genetic mechanisms of the vitamin K cycle. Since then, 28 mutations causing WR and a single mutation responsible for VKCFD2 have been identified and functionally confirmed by *in vitro* studies. *In silico* analysis has provided insight into structural requirements for warfarin binding and the pathophysiological mechanism of VKCFD2.

Acknowledgments: This work was supported, in part, by funding from BONFOR grant 2014-1-3 (KJC), Baxter Germany GmbH (JO, MW) and from the Deutsche Forschungsgemeinschaft (DFG) grant Ol100 5-1 (JO, MW).

Author Contributions: Katrin J. Czogalla, Matthias Watzka and Johannes Oldenburg conceived and wrote the article. Katrin J. Czogalla provided the figure and tables.

Conflicts of Interest: The authors declare no conflict of interest.

References

1. Wajih, N.; Sane, D.C.; Hutson, S.M.; Wallin, R. Engineering of a recombinant vitamin K-dependent gamma-carboxylation system with enhanced gamma-carboxyglutamic acid forming capacity: Evidence for a functional CXXC redox center in the system. *J. Biol. Chem.* **2005**, *280*, 10540–10547. [CrossRef] [PubMed]
2. Oldenburg, J.; Bevans, C.G.; Müller, C.R.; Watzka, M. Vitamin K epoxide reductase complex subunit 1 (VKORC1): The key protein of the vitamin K cycle. *Antioxid. Redox Signal.* **2006**, *8*, 347–353. [CrossRef] [PubMed]
3. Jin, D.-Y.; Tie, J.-K.; Stafford, D.W. The conversion of vitamin K epoxide to vitamin K quinone and vitamin K quinone to vitamin K hydroquinone uses the same active site cysteines. *Biochemistry* **2007**, *46*, 7279–7283. [CrossRef] [PubMed]
4. Oldenburg, J.; Marinova, M.; Müller-Reible, C.; Watzka, M. The vitamin K cycle. *Vitam. Horm.* **2008**, *78*, 35–62. [PubMed]
5. Gundberg, C.M.; Lian, J.B.; Booth, S.L. Vitamin K-dependent carboxylation of osteocalcin: Friend or foe? *Adv. Nutr.* **2012**, *3*, 149–157. [CrossRef] [PubMed]
6. Cancela, M.L.; Laizé, V.; Conceição, N. Matrix Gla protein and osteocalcin: From gene duplication to neofunctionalization. *Arch. Biochem. Biophys.* **2014**, *561*, 56–63. [CrossRef] [PubMed]
7. Ferland, G. Vitamin K and the nervous system: An overview of its actions. *Adv. Nutr.* **2012**, *3*, 204–212. [CrossRef] [PubMed]
8. Rost, S.; Fregin, A.; Ivaskevicius, V.; Conzelmann, E.; Hörtnagel, K.; Pelz, H.J.; Lappegard, K.; Seifried, E.; Scharrer, I.; Tuddenham, E.G.; *et al.* Mutations in VKORC1 cause warfarin resistance and multiple coagulation factor deficiency type 2. *Nature* **2004**, *427*, 537–541. [CrossRef] [PubMed]
9. Li, T.; Chang, C.Y.; Jin, D.Y.; Lin, P.J.; Khvorova, A.; Stafford, D.W. Identification of the gene for vitamin K epoxide reductase. *Nature* **2004**, *427*, 541–544. [CrossRef] [PubMed]
10. Fregin, A.; Rost, S.; Wolz, W.; Krebsova, A.; Muller, C.R.; Oldenburg, J. Homozygosity mapping of a second gene locus for hereditary combined deficiency of vitamin K-dependent clotting factors to the centromeric region of chromosome 16. *Blood* **2002**, *100*, 3229–3232. [CrossRef] [PubMed]
11. Watzka, M.; Geisen, C.; Bevans, C.G.; Sittinger, K.; Spohn, G.; Rost, S.; Seifried, E.; Müller, C.R.; Oldenburg, J. Thirteen novel VKORC1 mutations associated with oral anticoagulant resistance: Insights into improved patient diagnosis and treatment. *J. Thromb. Haemost.* **2011**, *9*, 109–118. [CrossRef] [PubMed]
12. Hodroge, A.; Matagrin, B.; Moreau, C.; Fourel, I.; Hammed, A.; Benoit, E.; Lattard, V. VKORC1 mutations detected in patients resistant to vitamin K antagonists are not all associated with a resistant VKOR activity. *J. Thromb. Haemost.* **2012**, *10*, 2535–2543. [CrossRef] [PubMed]
13. Pelz, H.-J.; Rost, S.; Hünerberg, M.; Fregin, A.; Heiberg, A.C.; Baert, K.; MacNicoll, A.D.; Prescott, C.V.; Walker, A.S.; Oldenburg, J.; *et al.* The genetic basis of resistance to anticoagulants in rodents. *Genetics* **2005**, *170*, 1839–1847. [CrossRef] [PubMed]

14. Rost, S.; Pelz, H.-J.; Menzel, S.; MacNicoll, A.D.; León, V.; Song, K.J.; Jäkel, T.; Oldenburg, J.; Müller, C.R. Novel mutations in the VKORC1 gene of wild rats and mice—A response to 50 years of selection pressure by warfarin? *BMC Genet.* **2009**, *10*, 4. [CrossRef] [PubMed]
15. Czogalla, K.J.; Biswas, A.; Rost, S.; Watzka, M.; Oldenburg, J. The Arg98Trp mutation in human VKORC1 causing VKCFD2 disrupts a di-Arginine-based ER retention motif. *Blood* **2014**, *124*, 1354–1362. [CrossRef] [PubMed]
16. Oldenburg, J.; von Brederlow, B.; Fregin, A.; Rost, S.; Wolz, W.; Eberl, W.; Eber, S.; Lenz, E.; Schwaab, R.; Brackmann, H.H.; *et al.* Congenital deficiency of vitamin K dependent coagulation factors in two families presents as a genetic defect of the vitamin K-epoxide-reductase-complex. *Thromb. Haemost.* **2000**, *84*, 937–941. [PubMed]
17. Marchetti, G.; Caruso, P.; Lunghi, B.; Pinotti, M.; Lapecorella, M.; Napolitano, M.; Canella, A.; Mariani, G.; Bernardi, F. Vitamin K-induced modification of coagulation phenotype in VKORC1 homozygous deficiency. *J. Thromb. Haemost.* **2008**, *6*, 797–803. [CrossRef] [PubMed]
18. Pauli, R.M.; Lian, J.B.; Mosher, D.F.; Suttie, J.W. Association of congenital deficiency of multiple vitamin K-dependent coagulation factors and the phenotype of the warfarin embryopathy: Clues to the mechanism of teratogenicity of coumarin derivatives. *Am. J. Hum. Genet.* **1987**, *41*, 566–583. [PubMed]
19. Li, W.; Schulman, S.; Dutton, R.J.; Boyd, D.; Beckwith, J.; Rapoport, T.A. Structure of a bacterial homologue of vitamin K epoxide reductase. *Nature* **2010**, *463*, 507–512. [CrossRef] [PubMed]
20. Goodstadt, L.; Ponting, C.P. Vitamin K epoxide reductase: Homology, active site and catalytic mechanism. *Trends Biochem. Sci.* **2004**, *29*, 289–292. [CrossRef] [PubMed]
21. Liu, S.; Cheng, W.; Fowle Grider, R.; Shen, G.; Li, W. Structures of an intramembrane vitamin K epoxide reductase homolog reveal control mechanisms for electron transfer. *Nat. Commun.* **2014**, *5*, 3110. [CrossRef] [PubMed]
22. Van Horn, W.D. Structural and functional insights into human vitamin K epoxide reductase and vitamin K epoxide reductase-like1. *Crit. Rev. Biochem. Mol. Biol.* **2013**, *48*, 357–372. [CrossRef] [PubMed]
23. Czogalla, K.J.; Biswas, A.; Wendeln, A.C.; Westhofen, P.; Müller, C.R.; Watzka, M.; Oldenburg, J. Human VKORC1 mutations cause variable degrees of 4-hydroxycoumarin resistance and affect putative warfarin binding interfaces. *Blood* **2013**, *122*, 2743–2750. [CrossRef] [PubMed]
24. Wu, S.; Liu, S.; Davis, C.H.; Stafford, D.W.; Kulman, J.D.; Pedersen, L.G. A hetero-dimer model for concerted action of vitamin K carboxylase and vitamin K reductase in vitamin K cycle. *J. Theor. Biol.* **2011**, *279*, 143–149. [CrossRef] [PubMed]
25. Tie, J.K.; Nicchitta, C.; von Heijne, G.; Stafford, D.W. Membrane topology mapping of vitamin K epoxide reductase by *in vitro* translation/cotranslocation. *J. Biol. Chem.* **2005**, *280*, 16410–16416. [CrossRef] [PubMed]
26. Tie, J.K.; Jin, D.Y.; Stafford, D.W. Human vitamin K epoxide reductase and its bacterial homologue have different membrane topologies and reaction mechanisms. *J. Biol. Chem.* **2012**, *287*, 33945–33955. [CrossRef] [PubMed]
27. Schulman, S.; Wang, B.; Li, W.; Rapoport, T.A. Vitamin K epoxide reductase prefers ER membrane-anchored thioredoxin-like redox partners. *Proc. Natl. Acad. Sci. USA* **2010**, *107*, 15027–15032. [CrossRef] [PubMed]
28. Robertson, H.M. Genes encoding vitamin-K epoxide reductase are present in Drosophila and trypanosomatid protists. *Genetics* **2004**, *168*, 1077–1080. [CrossRef] [PubMed]
29. Oldenburg, J.; Müller, C.R.; Rost, S.; Watzka, M.; Bevans, C.G. Comparative genetics of warfarin resistance. *Hamostaseologie* **2014**, *34*, 143–159. [CrossRef] [PubMed]
30. Rost, S.; Fregin, A.; Hünerberg, M.; Bevans, C.G.; Müller, C.R.; Oldenburg, J. Site-directed mutagenesis of coumarin-type anticoagulant-sensitive VKORC1: Evidence that highly conserved amino acids define structural requirements for enzymatic activity and inhibition by warfarin. *Thromb. Haemost.* **2005**, *94*, 780–786. [PubMed]
31. Du, J.J.; Zhan, C.Y.; Lu, Y.; Cui, H.R.; Wang, X.Y. The conservative cysteines in transmembrane domain of AtVKOR/LTO1 are critical for photosynthetic growth and photosystem II activity in Arabidopsis. *Front. Plant Sci.* **2015**, *6*, 238. [CrossRef] [PubMed]
32. Yang, X.J.; Cui, H.R.; Yu, Z.B.; Du, J.J.; Xu, J.N.; Wang, X.Y. Key amino acids of arabidopsis VKOR in the activity of phylloquinone reduction and disulfide bond formation. *Pro. Pept. Lett.* **2015**, *22*, 81–86. [CrossRef]

33. Rishavy, M.A.; Usubalieva, A.; Hallgren, K.W.; Berkner, K.L. Novel insight into the mechanism of the vitamin K oxidoreductase (VKOR): Electron relay through Cys43 and Cys51 reduces VKOR to allow vitamin K reduction and facilitation of vitamin K-dependent protein carboxylation. *J. Biol. Chem.* **2011**, *286*, 7267–7278. [CrossRef] [PubMed]

34. Tie, J.K.; Jin, D.Y.; Stafford, D.W. Mycobacterium tuberculosis vitamin K epoxide reductase homologue supports vitamin K-dependent carboxylation in mammalian cells. *Antioxid. Redox. Signal.* **2012**, *16*, 329–338. [CrossRef] [PubMed]

35. Wajih, N.; Hutson, S.M.; Wallin, R. Disulfide-dependent protein folding is linked to operation of the vitamin K cycle in the endoplasmic reticulum. A protein disulfide isomerase-VKORC1 redox enzyme complex appears to be responsible for vitamin K1 2,3-epoxide reduction. *J. Biol. Chem.* **2007**, *282*, 2626–2635. [CrossRef] [PubMed]

36. Tie, J.K.; Jin, D.Y.; Tie, K.; Stafford, D.W. Evaluation of warfarin resistance using transcription activator-like effector nucleases-mediated vitamin K epoxide reductase knockout HEK293 cells. *J. Thromb. Haemost.* **2013**, *11*, 1556–1564. [CrossRef] [PubMed]

37. Wu, S.; Tie, J.K.; Stafford, D.W.; Pedersen, L.G. Membrane topology for human vitamin K epoxide reductase. *J. Thromb. Haemost.* **2014**, *12*, 112–114. [CrossRef] [PubMed]

38. Fasco, M.J.; Principe, L.M.; Walsh, W.A.; Friedman, P.A. Warfarin inhibition of vitamin K 2,3-epoxide reductase in rat liver microsomes. *Biochemistry* **1983**, *22*, 5655–5660. [CrossRef] [PubMed]

39. Fregin, A.; Czogalla, K.J.; Gansler, J.; Rost, S.; Taverna, M.; Watzka, M.; Bevans, C.G.; Müller, C.R.; Oldenburg, J. A new cell culture-based assay quantifies vitamin K 2,3-epoxide reductase complex subunit 1 function and reveals warfarin resistance phenotypes not shown by the dithiothreitol-driven VKOR assay. *J. Thromb. Haemost.* **2013**, *11*, 872–880. [CrossRef] [PubMed]

40. Müller, E.; Keller, A.; Fregin, A.; Müller, C.R.; Rost, S. Confirmation of warfarin resistance of naturally occurring VKORC1 variants by coexpression with coagulation factor IX and in silico protein modelling. *BMC Genet.* **2014**, *15*, 17. [CrossRef] [PubMed]

41. Van Horn, W.D. VKORC1 ER mislocalization causes rare disease. *Blood* **2014**, *124*, 1215–1216. [CrossRef] [PubMed]

42. Michelsen, K.; Yuan, H.; Schwappach, B. Hide and run. Arginine-based endoplasmic-reticulum-sorting motifs in the assembly of heteromultimeric membrane proteins. *EMBO Rep.* **2005**, *6*, 717–722. [CrossRef] [PubMed]

43. Shikano, S.; Li, M. Membrane receptor trafficking: Evidence of proximal and distal zones conferred by two independent endoplasmic reticulum localization signals. *Proc. Natl. Acad. Sci. USA* **2003**, *100*, 5783–5788. [CrossRef] [PubMed]

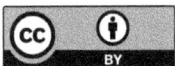

nutrients

MDPI

Article

High-Dose Menaquinone-7 Supplementation Reduces Cardiovascular Calcification in a Murine Model of Extraosseous Calcification

Daniel Scheiber [1,†], Verena Veulemans [1,†], Patrick Horn [1], Martijn L. Chatrou [2], Sebastian A. Potthoff [3], Malte Kelm [1,4], Leon J. Schurgers [2,†] and Ralf Westenfeld [1,†,*]

[1] Division of Cardiology, Pulmonology, and Vascular Medicine, Medical Faculty, University Duesseldorf, Duesseldorf 40225, Germany; E-Mails: daniel.scheiber@med.uni-duesseldorf.de (D.S.); verena.veulemanns@med.uni-duesseldorf.de (V.V.); patrick.horn@med.uni-duesseldorf.de (P.H.); malte.kelm@med.uni-duesseldorf.de (M.K.)

[2] Department of Biochemistry, Cardiovascular Research Institute Maastricht, Maastricht University, Maastricht 6229 ER, The Netherlands; E-Mails: m.chatrou@maastrichtuniversity.nl (M.L.C.); l.schurgers@maastrichtuniversity.nl (L.J.S.)

[3] Department of Nephrology, University Duesseldorf, Medical Faculty, Duesseldorf 40225, Germany; E-Mail: sebastian.potthoff@med.uni-duesseldorf.de

[4] Cardiovascular Research Institute Duesseldorf, University Duesseldorf, Medical Faculty, Duesseldorf 40225, Germany

* Author to whom correspondence should be addressed; E-Mail: ralf.westenfeld@med.uni-duesseldorf.de; Tel.: +49-211-8118800; Fax: +49-211-8118812.

† These authors contributed equally to this work.

Received: 15 May 2015 / Accepted: 6 August 2015 / Published: 18 August 2015

Abstract: Cardiovascular calcification is prevalent in the aging population and in patients with chronic kidney disease (CKD) and diabetes mellitus, giving rise to substantial morbidity and mortality. Vitamin K-dependent matrix Gla-protein (MGP) is an important inhibitor of calcification. The aim of this study was to evaluate the impact of high-dose menaquinone-7 (MK-7) supplementation (100 µg/g diet) on the development of extraosseous calcification in a murine model. Calcification was induced by 5/6 nephrectomy combined with high phosphate diet in rats. Sham operated animals served as controls. Animals received high or low MK-7 diets for 12 weeks. We assessed vital parameters, serum chemistry, creatinine clearance, and cardiac function. CKD provoked increased aortic (1.3 fold; $p < 0.05$) and myocardial (2.4 fold; $p < 0.05$) calcification in line with increased alkaline phosphatase levels (2.2 fold; $p < 0.01$). MK-7 supplementation inhibited cardiovascular calcification and decreased aortic alkaline phosphatase tissue concentrations. Furthermore, MK-7 supplementation increased aortic MGP messenger ribonucleic acid (mRNA) expression (10-fold; $p < 0.05$). CKD-induced arterial hypertension with secondary myocardial hypertrophy and increased elastic fiber breaking points in the arterial tunica media did not change with MK-7 supplementation. Our results show that high-dose MK-7 supplementation inhibits the development of cardiovascular calcification. The protective effect of MK-7 may be related to the inhibition of secondary mineralization of damaged vascular structures.

Keywords: menaquinone-7; vitamin K_2; cardiovascular calcification; matrix Gla-protein; chronic kidney disease

---

1. Introduction

Biological aging [1] and diseases like chronic kidney disease (CKD) [2] or diabetes mellitus [3] are associated with an increased incidence of cardiovascular calcification, an independent cardiovascular risk factor accompanied by enhanced morbidity and mortality [4].

Nutrients **2015**, *7*, 6991–7011

For decades vascular calcification (VC) was thought to be the consequence of passive precipitation of calcium (Ca) and phosphate (P) ions resulting from a supersaturated Ca × P product [5]. Today cardiovascular calcification is appreciated as an actively regulated, cell-mediated process characterized by the interaction of inductive and inhibitory proteins [6]. According to the anatomical localization, VC can be classified as intimal and medial calcification, although a clear-cut distinction is almost impossible in clinical practice [7]. Intimal calcification is linked to atherosclerosis and characterized by inflammatory accumulation of oxidized lipids [8]. Medial calcification develops independently of inflammation and lipid deposition along the elastic fibers. It is a typical consequence of aging and found in patients suffering from chronic kidney disease or diabetes mellitus [9–11]. Despite differences in etiology, the underlying pathophysiological mechanism of intimal and medial calcification is similar [6].

The vitamin K-dependent matrix Gla-protein (MGP) is a potent inhibitor of arterial calcification [12]. MGP was presented first in 1983 by Price and colleagues as a 14kD protein purified from bovine bone matrix [13]. That the function of MGP was mainly vascular became clear from MGP-deficient mice, all of which died within a few months of birth due to blood vessel rupture as a result of VC [14]. Likewise, humans with a hereditary dysfunctional MGP (Keutel syndrome) suffer from widely distributed extraosseous calcifications [15]. There are two posttranslational modifications in MGP: gamma-glutamate carboxylation and serine phosphorylation [16]. While the function of posttranslational MGP phosphorylation is not completely understood, Murshed and colleagues showed that MGP has to be carboxylated to prevent VC [17]. Diminished MGP carboxylation is associated with an increased tendency of calcification of the vasculature [18]. Analogous to vitamin K-dependent blood clotting factors (Factors II, VII, IX, X, and Protein C, S, and Z), the biological activity of MGP depends on the presence of vitamin K as cofactor [19]. Current medical treatment with vitamin K antagonists may, besides providing effective anticoagulation, also increase the risk for VC [20].

Patients with CKD are characterized by widespread extraosseous calcification. We as well as others have shown that CKD patients display vitamin K insufficiency, associated with elevated plasma concentrations of inactive MGP [21–23]. Increased plasma levels of inactive ucMGP are paralleled by enhanced morbidity and mortality in patients suffering from CKD, aortic stenosis, or congestive heart failure [22,24,25]. Supplementation with vitamin K results in a dose- and time-dependent decrease of ucMGP plasma levels [23,26,27]. So far, no trials reported "hard outcomes" such as VC in the context of CKD and vitamin K supplementation.

Fat-soluble vitamin K is an essential micronutrient [28]. There are two forms of vitamin K in nature: phylloquinone (vitamin K_1; VK_1) and the menaquinones (vitamin K_2; VK_2; MK-n). VK_1 is tightly bound to the chloroplast membrane of plants [29]. Menaquinones differ in side chains of varying length. They are described as MK-n, in which n denotes the number of unsaturated isoprenoid residues. MK-7 is produced by bacteria and is present in fermented foods such as cheese or sauerkraut [30]. In this study we used MK-7 because of its long half-life and good bioavailability. Two independent observational studies [31,32] described a protective cardiovascular effect of nutritional intake of menaquinones, whereas no effect was found for phylloquinone. This discrepancy in function was ascribed to the better availability and transport of long-chain menaquinones such as MK-7 as compared to VK_1. However, in animal models of warfarin-induced vascular calcification, the short chain menaquinone MK-4 was tested, which displayed greater potency in the inhibition of vascular calcification [33–35]. The MK-7 supplementation dose of 100 µg/g diet used in this present study was based on these MK-4 studies [33–35].

The aim of this study is to evaluate the impact of high-dose MK-7 supplementation on the development of cardiovascular calcification and the impact on cardiovascular function in a murine model of chronic kidney disease characterized by enhanced extraosseous calcification.

2. Materials and Methods

2.1. Animals and Diets

The animal study protocol was authorized by the responsible governmental office called *LANUV* ("Landesamt für Natur, Umwelt und Verbraucherschutz Nordrhein-Westfalen"; file reference 87-51.04.2010.A275). All experiments were executed according to the German animal welfare act in close cooperation with veterinaries of the Heinrich Heine University. We used 42 male Wistar rats aged 12 weeks with a body weight about 300 g at the beginning of the study protocol. Rats were kept in a climate-controlled room (22–24 °C, relative humidity 60%–80%) with a 12-hour light, 12-hour dark cycle. Food and water were given *ad libitum*.

Animals were divided into an interventional group undergoing 5/6 nephrectomy, receiving a high phosphate diet and into a control group undergoing sham operations. Half of each group received a high MK-7 diet, so that we distinguished between four different treatment groups receiving different diets (sniff-Spezialdiäten GmbH) (Table 1).

Pure synthetic MK-7 was provided by NattoPharma ASA (Hovik, Norway).

Table 1. Diets.

Control (Sham-OP)	
Co ($n = 10$)	Co-K$_2$ ($n = 10$)
Standard diet:	MK-7-supplemented standard diet:
0.36% Phosphate	0.36% Phosphate
0.6% Calcium	0.6% Calcium
0.5 µg/g VK$_1$	0.5 µg/g VK$_1$
0 MK-7	100 µg/g MK-7
Intervention (5/6-Nephrectomy + high phosphate diet)	
CKD ($n = 11$)	CKD-K$_2$ ($n = 11$)
High phosphate diet:	Phosphate- and MK-7-rich diet:
1.2% Phosphate	1.2% Phosphate
0.6% Calcium	0.6% Calcium
0.5 µg/g VK$_1$	0.5 µg/g VK$_1$
0 MK-7	100 µg/g MK-7

Animals were randomly distributed to four study groups, with two diets different in MK-7 and phosphate concentration. Animals in CKD and CKD-K$_2$ groups were 5/6 nephrectomized. Control animals were sham operated. Co = control group; Co-K$_2$ = MK-7-supplemented control group; CKD = intervention group; CKD-K$_2$ = MK-7-supplemented intervention group; MK-7 = menaquinone-7; VK$_1$ = vitamin K$_1$.

2.2. Study Design

All animals took part in a three-month study protocol. On the first day we measured blood pressure using a tail-cuff system. Blood samples were taken by retro orbital bleeding. Body weight was taken twice weekly. 5/6 nephrectomy was performed according to a surgical technique initially described by Perez-Ruiz [36]. Briefly, we performed right-sided nephrectomy and one week later following recovery from the initial surgery, rats underwent functional 2/3 nephrectomy of the remaining left kidney by careful ligation of the renal parenchyma. Controls underwent a similar two-step laparotomy exposing the kidneys but without nephrectomy. After three and eight weeks we repeated the measurements from the preoperative day. At the end of the study after three months we collected 24-hour urine samples from six animals in each group in metabolic cages. Animals were sacrificed under anesthesia by puncture of the vena cava inferior. Blood was collected for serum analyses. Heart, aorta, and kidney tissues were collected for further analyses.

2.3. Echocardiography

Echocardiography was performed as described previously [33]. Briefly, rats were anesthetized using Isoflurane and two-dimensional and M-mode measurements were accomplished using Vivid i, GE Healthcare (GE Healthcare, Buckinghamshire, England) with a 12 MHz probe. Animals were placed in the supine-lateral position with ECGs were obtained throughout the procedure. Parasternal long-axis and short-axis views of the left ventricle (LV) were obtained, ensuring that the mitral and aortic valves and apex were well visualized. Area fraction and wall area were determined by planimetry of end-diastolic and systolic volumes in parasternal short axis. Measurements of LV end-diastolic and end-systolic dimensions were obtained in M-mode at mid-papillary level from more than three beats and fractional shortening (FS) was calculated as FS (%) = ((LVIDd – LVIDs)/LVIDd) × 100, where LVID is LV internal diameter, s is systole, and d is diastole. Diastole is defined as the maximum measurable area; systole is defined as the minimum measurable area. Doppler flow spectrum of the ascending aorta was recorded from the suprasternal view. Peak velocity was measured, and the waveform was also traced to obtain a velocity time-integral calculation and peak gradient.

2.4. Blood/Urine Analyses

Blood and urine analyses were performed by Animal Blood Counter (Scil Animal Care Company GmbH, Viernheim, Germany) and in the Institute of Clinical Chemistry of University Hospital Düsseldorf.

2.5. Histology

Tissues were perfused with cold phosphate-buffered saline (PBS) solution by cannulation of left ventricle. Afterwards tissues were embedded in TissueTek (Sakura Finetek Europe B.V., Alphen aan den Rijn, the Netherlands) on dry ice for cryofixation, paraffin embedded, or placed in frozen nitrogen. Different histological and immunohistological stainings were performed and analyzed with a Leica DM4000 M RL microscope mounted with a Leica DFC 425C camera (Leica Mikrosysteme GmbH, Wetzlar, Germany). Quantitative measurements were performed with ImageJ software (National Institutes of Health, Bethesda, MD, USA).

2.6. qRT-PCR

Real-Time PCR mRNA was extracted using the commercial kits RNAlater and RNeasy (Qiagen, Hilden, Germany) with proteinase K digestion before RNA extraction to maximize mRNA yield. Integrity and amount of mRNA were analyzed by capillary electrophoresis (Agilent Bioanalyzer 2100; Agilent Technologies, Böblingen, Germany). Reverse transcription and real-time PCR were performed with Applied Biosystems 7500 Fast Real Time PCR System (Applied Biosystems, Foster City, CA, USA) according to the manufacturer's instructions. The expression level in untreated mice was arbitrarily assigned the value 1.0, and all other expression values were expressed as fold changes thereof. Values were analyzed using REST software tool (Quiagen, Hilden, Germany).

2.7. Statistics

We performed ANOVA with Bonferroni's *post hoc* analysis using GraphPad Prism 5 software (GraphPad, San Diego, CA, USA) to estimate the overall differences between experimental groups. Confidence intervals over 95% were regarded as significant.

3. Results

3.1. Experimental CKD

Combination of surgical 5/6 nephrectomy with supplementation of a high phosphate diet succeeded in mimicking key metabolic features of CKD. Serum creatinine levels were elevated by more than 50% in CKD and CKD-K_2 animals compared to controls (Table 2) (CKD *vs.* Co after 12 weeks, $p <$ 0.001). Likewise, blood urea nitrogen (BUN) concentrations were significantly elevated in the CKD groups (CKD *vs.* Co after 12 weeks, $p < 0.001$). 5/6 nephrectomy and phosphate supplementation affected phosphate concentrations in serum and urine: urine phosphate excretion was more than tripled in CKD animals compared to controls (CKD *vs.* Co after 12 weeks, $p < 0.001$) (Table 2) with an apparent hyperphosphatemia only in CKD but not in CKD-K_2 rats. There was no difference in hemoglobin or hematocrit concentration between the experimental groups (Table 2). Since severe renal impairment is associated with cachexia, we repetitively assessed body weight. All animals that were not fully grown at the start of the study gained weight during the 12 weeks of the experimental period. Control animals increased significantly more weight compared to CKD and CKD-K_2 animals (Figure 1) (CKD *vs.* Co after 12 weeks, $p < 0.01$).

Table 2. Serum and urine parameters after 12 weeks of study protocol.

Parameters	Co	Co-K_2	CKD	CKD-K_2
Serum creatinine (mg/dl)				
Week 12	0.3 ± 0	0.3 ± 0	0.5 ± 0	0.5 ± 0
BUN (mg/dl)				
Week 12	40 ± 2.2	42 ± 1.3	51 ± 2.9	50 ± 1.9
Serum phosphate (mmol/l)				
Week 12	1.8 ± 0.1	1.6 ± 0.1	2.2 ± 0.2	1.8 ± 0.1
Hb (g/dl)				
Week 12	15.0 ± 0.5	15.5 ± 0.2	15.5 ± 0.2	15.5 ± 0.1
Hkt (%)				
Week 12	45.8 ± 1.3	47.9 ± 0.9	44.0 ± 1.5	45.0 ± 0.3
Creatinine clearance (ml/min)				
Week 12	3.2 ± 0.6	2.5 ± 0.2	1.7 ± 0.2	1.8 ± 0.1
Urine phosphate excretion				
(mg/24 h)	33.1 ± 1	23.6 ± 3.6	82.8 ± 29.9	59.8 ± 7.5

BUN = blood urea nitrogen; K_2 = MK-7.

3.2. Cardiovascular Calcification

We directly assessed cardiovascular calcification by histology (von Kossa) and chemical analysis (AAS = atomic absorption spectroscopy) in the aorta, myocardium, and kidneys in the various treatment groups. AAS is a sensitive method for detecting total tissue calcium amount [37]. In the aortas we performed additional immunohistochemistry for alkaline phosphatase to evaluate the downstream effects of mineralization in terms of VSMC dedifferentiation.

Nutrients **2015**, *7*, 6991–7011

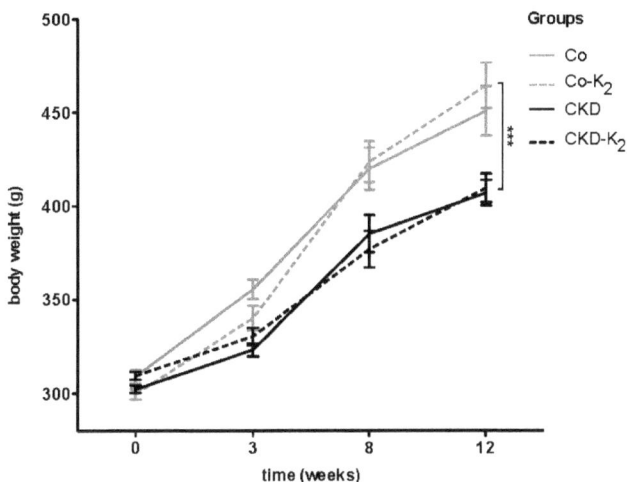

Figure 1. Body weight in grams (g). Body weight of animals was measured repetitively during 12 weeks of study protocol. Experimental animals were not fully grown at start of the experiment; however, all animals gained weight significantly. During the experiment, control animals (Co; Co-K_2) gained significantly more weight compared to CKD and CKD-K_2 animals. Co = control group; Co-K_2 = MK-7 supplemented control group; CKD = 5/6 nephrectomized group; CKD-K_2 = MK-7 supplemented 5/6 nephrectomized group; g = grams. Significant differences: *** $p < 0.001$.

Aorta: While von Kossa staining did not encounter calcification in any treatment group, we detected significant differences in the chemical calcium analysis applying AAS. Animals from the CKD group displayed an induction of aortic calcium content compared to controls by about 30% ($p < 0.05$). MK-7 supplementation abolished aortic calcification, thus CKD-K_2 rats displayed aortic calcium content indistinguishable from controls (Figure 2). In line with the calcium accumulation in the CKD group, we detected an intensified ALP staining in aortic tissue samples of CKD animals compared to control groups (CKD *vs.* Co, $p < 0.01$) and CKD-K_2 animals (Figure 3).

Myocardium: Similar to our observations in aortic tissue, we did not detect overt myocardial calcification by von Kossa staining in any treatment group. Applying chemical analysis by AAS, myocardial tissues of the CKD group displayed a 2.4-fold increased calcium concentration compared to controls (CKD *vs.* Co, $p < 0.05$). Again, MK-7 supplementation inhibited calcium accumulation in the CKD-K_2 rats with calcium tissue concentrations in the range of control rats (Figure 4).

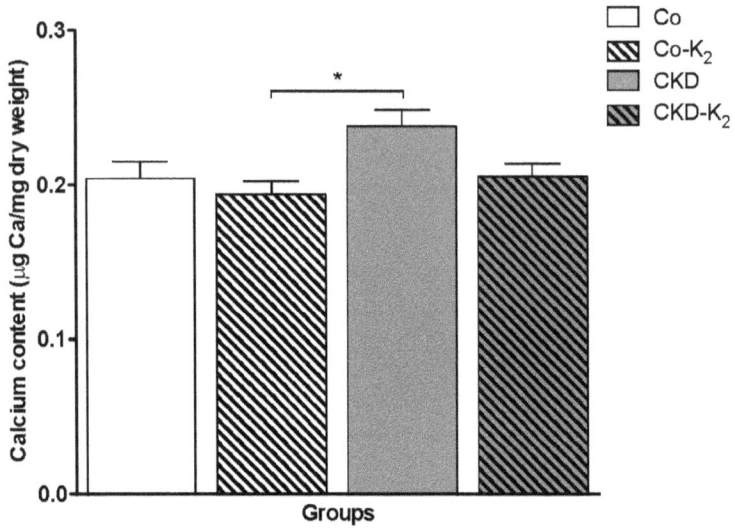

Figure 2. Aortic calcium content. Measurement of aortic calcium content was performed by atomic absorption spectrometry and expressed as µg Ca/mg dry weight tissue. CKD animals display a significant increase in aortic calcium content compared to Co-K$_2$ animals. Co = control group; Co-K$_2$ = MK-7 supplemented control group; CKD = 5/6 nephrectomized group; CKD-K$_2$ = MK-7 supplemented 5/6 nephrectomized group; mg = milligrams; µg = micrograms. Significant differences: * $p < 0.05$.

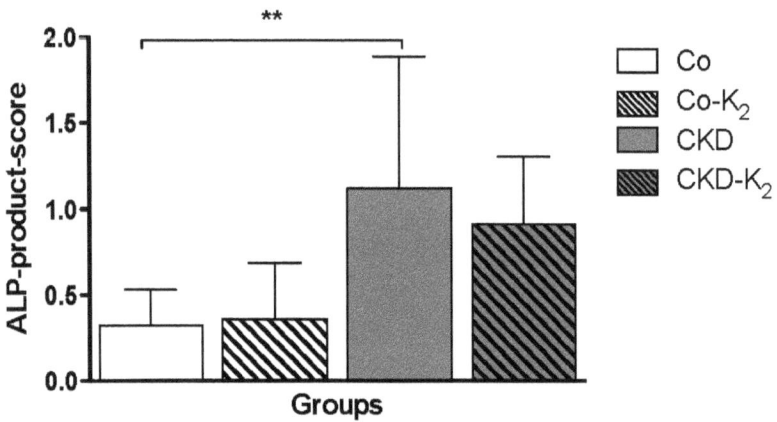

Figure 3. Alkaline phosphatase (ALP) in aortic tissues. ALP was measured to detect local vascular osteochondrogenic activity. Positive staining for ALP is expressed as product score: ALP-positive staining areal × intensity. ALP-product-score is significantly increased in CKD animals as compared to Co animals. Co = control group; Co-K$_2$ = MK-7 supplemented control group; CKD = 5/6 nephrectomized group; CKD-K$_2$ = MK-7 supplemented 5/6 nephrectomized group. Significant differences: ** $p < 0.01$.

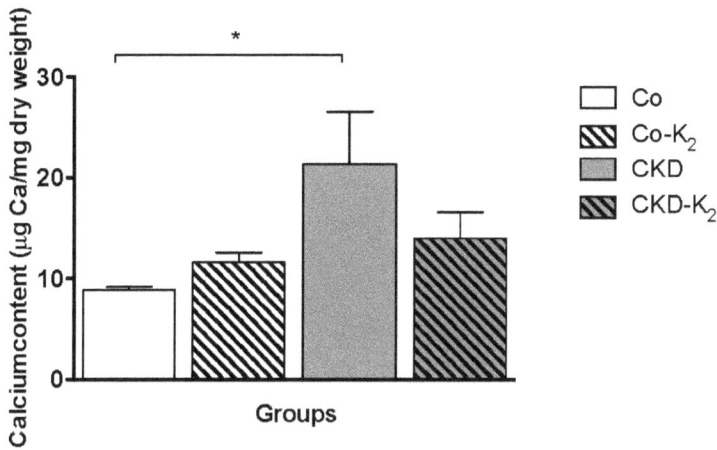

Figure 4. Myocardial calcium content. Measurement of myocardial calcium content using atomic absorption spectrometry in µg Ca/mg dry weight tissue. CKD animals display a significantly increased myocardial calcium content compared to Co animals. Co = control group; Co-K_2 = MK-7 supplemented control group; CKD = 5/6 nephrectomized group; CKD-K_2 = MK-7 supplemented 5/6 nephrectomized group; mg = milligrams; µg = micrograms. Significant differences: * $p < 0.05$.

Kidney: In renal tissues of CKD and CKD-K_2 animals we detected tubular calcification easily visible on von Kossa histology (Figures 5 and 6). Quantitative analysis detected no effect of MK-7 supplementation on renal calcification.

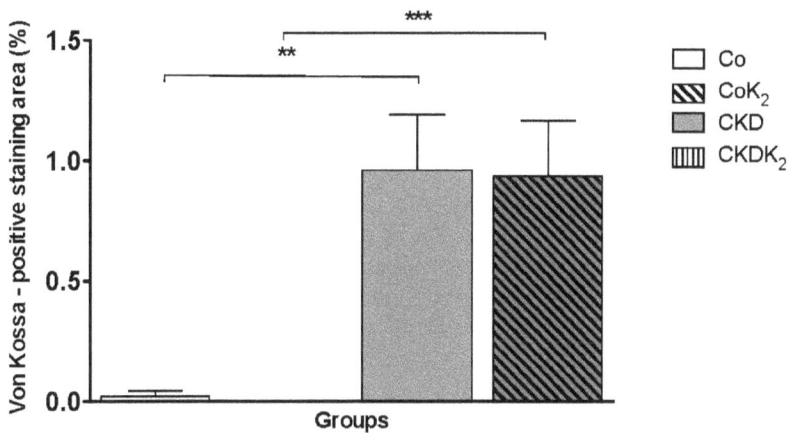

Figure 5. Renal calcification. Von Kossa positive staining area expressed as percentage of tissue area. In 5/6 nephrectomized animals significantly more von Kossa positivity was measured as compared to the control groups. No differences were seen between CKD and CKD-K_2 treated groups. Co = control group; Co-K_2 = MK-7 supplemented control group; CKD = 5/6 nephrectomized group; CKD-K_2 = MK-7 supplemented 5/6 nephrectomized group. Significant differences: ** $p < 0.01$, *** $p < 0.001$.

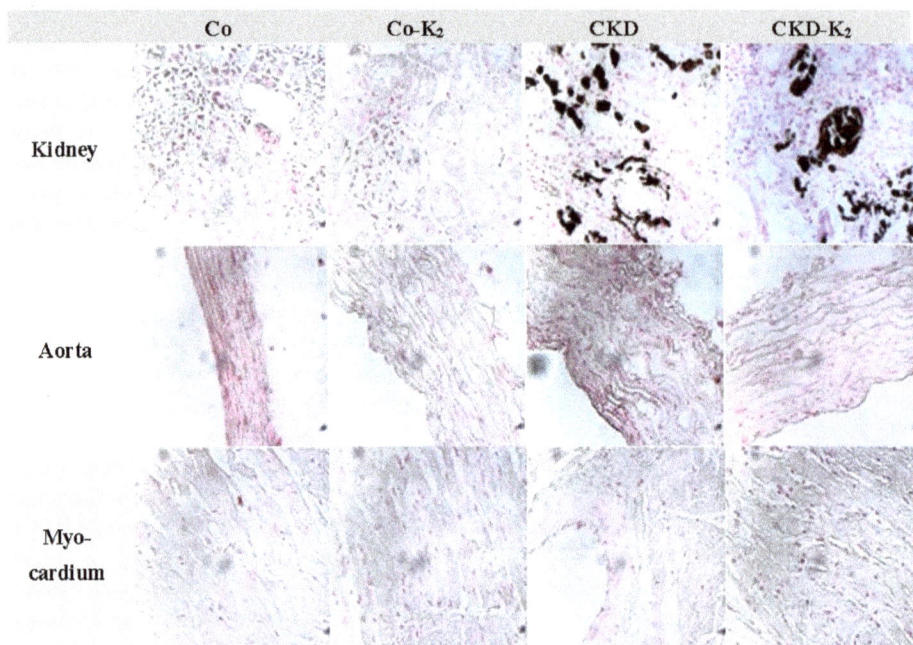

Figure 6. Representative sections of von Kossa stained tissue samples. Microscopically visible von Kossa positive staining was only detected in kidney tissue samples of CKD and CDK-K_2 animals. Magnification 40×; Counterstain: nuclear fast red; Co = control group; Co-K_2 = MK-7 supplemented control group; CKD = 5/6 nephrectomized group; CKD-K_2 = MK-7 supplemented 5/6 nephrectomized group.

3.3. Structural Alterations in Experimental CKD

Fiber breaking points: In order to evaluate the structural alterations induced by 5/6 nephrectomy and a high phosphate diet, we performed Elastica van Gieson staining of the aorta to illustrate elastic fiber breaking points. Both interventional groups (CKD, CKD-K_2) displayed significantly more elastic fiber breaking points compared to the control groups (CKD *vs.* Co, $p < 0.001$) (Figure 7). MK-7 supplementation had no effect on fiber breaking points in controls or CKD rats, respectively.

Proliferative response: Immunofluorescence staining of Ki67/DAPI revealed markedly increased cell proliferation in CKD and CKD-K_2 animals compared to controls (CKD *vs.* Co, $p < 0.001$). MK-7 supplementation did not alter the proliferative response to the CKD stimulus (Figure 8).

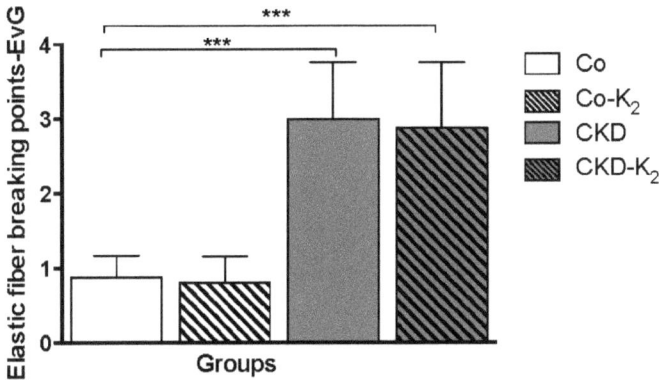

Figure 7. Elastic fiber breaking points. Elastica van Gieson (EvG) staining of aortic tissue samples with focus on elastic fiber breaking points. CKD animals display significantly more elastic fiber breaking points compared to Co animals. Co = control group; Co-K_2 = MK-7 supplemented control group; CKD = 5/6 nephrectomized group; CKD-K_2 = MK-7 supplemented 5/6 nephrectomized group. Significant differences: *** $p < 0.001$.

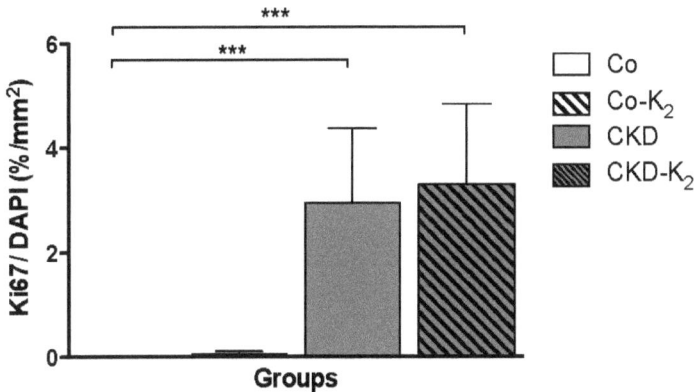

Figure 8. Proliferative response. Ratio of positive staining area for Ki67 per DAPI positive staining area in % per mm^2. DAPI values do not differ significantly between groups. CKD animals display significantly more Ki67 positive staining area per DAPI positive staining area compared to Co animals. Co = control group; Co-K_2 = MK-7 supplemented control group; CKD = 5/6 nephrectomized group; CKD-K_2 = MK-7 supplemented 5/6 nephrectomized group; mm = millimeters. Significant differences: *** $p < 0.001$.

3.4. Cardiovascular Function

Blood pressure: CKD and CKD-K_2 animals developed arterial hypertension (Figure 9). After 12 weeks, systolic as well as diastolic blood pressure values were elevated by 15–20 mmHg in CKD rats compared to controls (CKD-K_2 *vs.* Co-K_2, $p < 0.01$). MK-7 supplementation did not affect blood pressure (Figure 9).

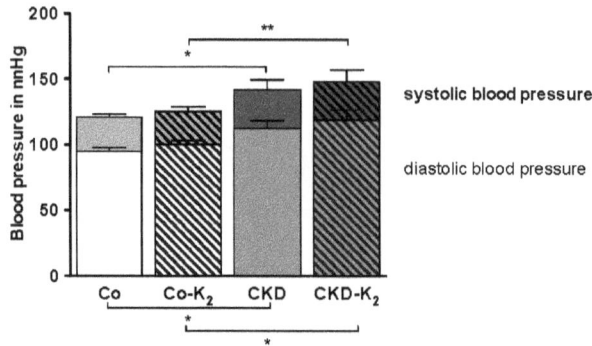

Figure 9. Systolic and diastolic blood pressure. Systolic and diastolic blood pressure after 12 weeks of treatment. CKD animals developed significantly increased systolic and diastolic blood pressure values compared to controls. Co = control group; Co-K_2 = MK-7 supplemented control group; CKD = 5/6 nephrectomized group; CKD-K_2 = MK-7 supplemented 5/6 nephrectomized group; mmHg = millimeters of mercury. Significant differences: * $p < 0.05$, ** $p < 0.01$.

Echocardiography: To quantify the impact of CKD and arterial hypertension on cardiovascular function we analyzed hypertrophy, contractility, and valvular function in the various treatment groups. CKD and CKD-K_2 animals exhibited significant myocardial hypertrophy, as depicted by increased diameters of the interventricular septum (by about 50%; CKD *vs.* Co, $p < 0.01$) (Figure 10). Myocardial contractility, as detected by fractional shortening, remained normal in all the animals studied. No relevant valvular disease or overt signs of valvular calcification were detected throughout the experiments (data not shown).

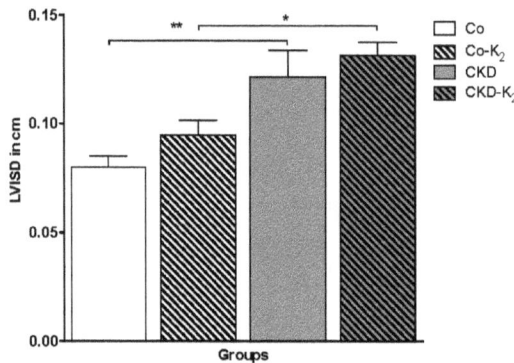

Figure 10. Echocardiography of diastolic interventricular septum diameter (LVISD) in cm. Echocardiography was performed in all animals after 12 weeks of study protocol. CKD animals developed significantly increased LVISD compared to controls. Co = control group; Co-K_2 = MK-7 supplemented control group; CKD = 5/6 nephrectomized group; CKD-K_2 = MK-7 supplemented 5/6 nephrectomized group; cm = centimeters. Significant differences: * $p < 0.05$, ** $p < 0.01$.

3.5. Aortic mRNA Expression

We analyzed regulation of relevant activators and inhibitors of VC in aortic tissue samples by quantitative real-time PCR. In a stepwise analysis, we investigated separately the effect of CKD (Figure 11a), MK-7 supplementation (Figure 11b), and finally the effect of MK-7 supplementation in CKD rats (Figure 11c), each compared to controls. For more clarity, pro-calcific changes are depicted by red columns while alterations associated with potential calcification inhibition are assigned with blue columns.

CKD compared to controls: The induction of CKD was associated with pro-calcific mRNA alterations within the aortas of the animals. MGP and SM22α gene expression was markedly decreased in CKD animals, while periostin and BMP-2 gene expression was increased compared to controls (Figure 11a).

MK-7 supplementation compared to controls: MK-7 supplementation revealed a significant induction of aortic MGP mRNA while procalcifing periostin mRNA levels were found to be significantly reduced (Figure 11b).

MK-7 supplementation and CKD compared to controls: MK-7 supplementation in CKD was associated with a calcification inhibitory effect in the aortic mRNA repertoire. Of note, we detected a significant induction of MGP mRNA levels. Moreover, the CKD-mediated reduction of SM22α mRNA was abolished, as depicted by a trend towards increased SM22α mRNA (Figure 11c).

4. Discussion

In this study we demonstrate that high-dose MK-7 supplementation inhibits calcification in a murine model of CKD-induced cardiovascular calcification. The effect of MK-7 is—at least in part—mediated via MGP and subsequent inhibition of ectopic calcification.

4.1. CKD and High Phosphate Diet

In our study we used a murine model of 5/6 nephrectomy and high phosphate diet to induce CKD-related cardiovascular damage. Shobeiri *et al.* compared different experimental CKD models for the induction of VC [38]. They observed a 2.2-fold increased serum creatinine concentration in 5/6 nephrectomized rats eight weeks after surgery, with corresponding values for BUN and creatinine clearance [38]. Our findings are similar with respect to serum creatinine and BUN levels and creatinine clearance but differ in severity of kidney injury. We observed moderate kidney injury, whereas others report severe kidney injury after 5/6 nephrectomy. This difference might arise from the technique we used to perform the 5/6 nephrectomy. We used unilateral nephrectomy, followed by ligation of the poles of the remaining kidney, whereas most studies describe surgical resection of the kidney poles or embolization of the pole-supplying arteries to induce renal impairment [38,39]. As expected, animals from CKD and CKD-K$_2$ groups gained less weight as compared to control animals, which is in accordance with previous studies [39]. Moreover, CKD and CKD-K$_2$ animals did not developed anemia. This finding is consistent with moderate kidney injury, since anemia is most frequently seen in patients with severe renal impairment [40].

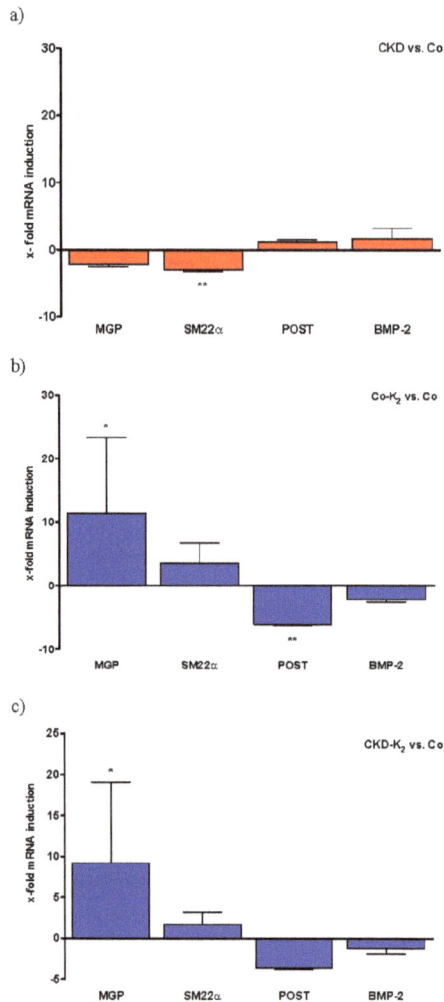

Figure 11. Aortic gene expression. The effect of CKD and MK-7 supplementation on aortic gene expression of calcification modifiers as x-fold induction compared to control group. Red columns depict pro-calcific changes, while alterations associated with potential calcification inhibition are assigned with blue columns. (**a**) In CKD animals SM22α expression is significantly decreased, whereas MGP expression is non-significantly decreased as compared to Co animals. (**b**) In Co-K$_2$ animals MGP mRNA concentration is significantly increased, whereas POST mRNA concentration is significantly decreased compared to Co animals. (**c**) In CKD-K$_2$ animals MGP mRNA concentration is significantly and SM22α mRNA concentration is tendentially increased compared to Co animals. Co = control group; Co-K$_2$ = MK-7 supplemented control group; CKD = 5/6 nephrectomized group; CKD-K$_2$ = MK-7 supplemented 5/6 nephrectomized group; MGP = matrix Gla-protein; POST = periostin; BMP-2 = bone morphogenetic protein 2. Significant differences: * $p < 0.05$, ** $p < 0.01$.

4.2. Cardiovascular Calcification

Animals in the CKD groups exhibited modest VCs with concomitant alkaline phosphatase presence. ALP may serve as a marker for osteoblastic activity [41]. However, increased deposits of ALP in the vasculature of animals in the CKD groups are also associated with the transdifferentiation of VSMCs towards osteochondrogenic-like cells [42]. These data are supported by the significantly decreased expression of SM22α, a protein specific for VSMCs. Our data are in line with previous observations that SM22α mRNA levels are decreased in a murine model of VC [43,44]. Moreover, we detected increased expression levels of periostin and BMP-2. Periostin is associated with increased extracellular matrix turnover, as seen in diseases like CKD [45,46]. Additionally, periostin is inversely correlated with decreased kidney function [47], which is in line with our results. BMP-2 expression is increased in atherosclerotic plaques [48] and in *in vitro* models of VC [49], supporting our data of CKD-induced VC.

MGP is a vitamin K-dependent protein known to inhibit VC. Functionality of MGP is dependent on vitamin K. We demonstrate that MGP expression is decreased in CKD animals as compared to controls. It has been described that MGP synthesis increases in response to VC [18,49]. Diabetes and CKD have an inhibitory effect on the protective upregulation of MGP expression, which is a possible pathomechanism for CKD-induced VC [50].

For the first time, we demonstrate that vitamin K (MK-7) affects MGP mRNA expression (>10-fold induction in controls and CKD rats) within the vascular wall. Earlier studies [17] showed that only locally expressed MGP in the arterial wall—and not systemic MGP over-expression—inhibits VC. Our results point to protective effects of MK-7 supplementation against imminent VC at the transcriptional level. There is evidence that MK-4 mediates MGP mRNA expression via activation of the SXR (steroid and xenobiotic receptor) nuclear receptor [51]. MK-4 has been shown to activate SXR in a dose-dependent manner [51]. Further studies are required to examine whether this observation can be replicated by MK-7. It is well known that vitamin K is a cofactor for the posttranslational carboxylation of MGP [16]. In our study we did not measure uncarboxylated and carboxylated MGP status.

MK-7 supplementation increased SM22α expression, whereas periostin and BMP-2 expression decreased, indicating that MK-7 affects VSMC phenotypic switching. This corroborates recent findings that the vitamin K-dependent Gla-rich protein (GRP) affects VC via VSMC phenotype modulation [52]. Thus, the impact of CKD on cardiovascular calcification might be counteracted by MK-7 supplementation via regulation of MGP expression and activity, and VSMC phenotypic switching.

Animals in both CKD and CKD-K_2 (MK-7 supplemented) groups significantly developed renal calcium deposits, particularly in the tubules. The significant amount of calcium deposits may be explained by the increased phosphate clearance by the remaining nephrons in combination with the high phosphate diet [53]. Phosphate levels in CKD play an important role in the development of cardiovascular calcification [54,55].

Interestingly, MK-7 supplementation normalized CKD-induced increased serum phosphate concentrations. More importantly, MK-7 supplementation inhibited both vascular and myocardial calcification in CKD animals on a high phosphate diet. Our results demonstrate a protective effect of MK-7 supplementation on early stages of cardiovascular calcification. Our results support previous data from our group, showing that both VK_1 and MK-4 supplementation reverses vitamin K antagonist-induced VC in rats [34]. To our best knowledge, this is the first study demonstrating a protective effect of MK-7 supplementation in a murine model of 5/6 nephrectomy-induced CKD. Compared to commonly applied models to induce VC (adenine diet, gene knockout animals, high-dose warfarin treatment), the VC calcification model applied in the current manuscript with mild CKD and phosphate loading more closely resembles the clinical situation of early CKD. As a matter of fact, cardiovascular mortality is already profoundly increased at early stages of CKD (e.g., below 60 mL/min GFR), rendering this model an attractive option to study the pathophysiological processes of imminent calcification and potential treatment options related to early CKD. Our results support the rationale for prophylactic supplementation of MK-7 in patients at risk for development of cardiovascular calcification. It has been shown that MK-7 supplementation is safe and has no side effects, both in experimental animals and humans [31,32,56]. Patients with CKD have been shown to be subclinically vitamin K deficient [21,22,57]. In an observational study in hemodialysis patients it was reported that a low circulating concentration of MK-4 was a predictor of aortic calcification [58], but this claim remains to be confirmed or refuted. Our group showed that MK-7 supplementation reduces levels of inactive MGP, osteocalcin, and PIVKA-II in hemodialysis patients [27]. It is tempting to speculate whether these results can be transferred to patients, a hypothesis that is currently being investigated in several studies [59].

4.3. Structural and Functional Alterations

In our model, CKD and a high phosphate diet induced increased systolic and diastolic blood pressure with cardiac hypertrophy. It is known that CKD and VC are associated with arterial hypertension [54] and reduced vascular compliance, with subsequent increased systolic and decreased diastolic blood pressure values [60]. Hypertension is most likely a consequence of kidney disease since blood pressure values were similarly elevated in both CKD and CKD-K$_2$ animals. CKD and hypertension are associated with vascular remodeling and increased cell proliferation [61,62]. VSMC proliferation increased in CKD and CKD-K$_2$ groups but was not affected by MK-7 treatment. Additionally, we detected increased elastic fiber breaking points in the tunica media, indicative of loss of vascular integrity in animals of the CKD and CKD-K$_2$ groups [63].

Importantly, we observed an inhibition of calcification of damaged tissues by MK-7 supplementation, whereas MK-7 was not able to continuously block the overwhelming harmful milieu of CKD and a high phosphate diet.

5. Conclusions

Our data provide evidence for a protective effect of high-dose MK-7 supplementation on cardiovascular calcification. MK-7 supplementation could not prevent CKD-associated hypertension and hypertrophy but prevented calcification of affected tissues. Since vitamin K has no reported side effects, it seems a promising therapeutic agent [59]. The effect of MK-7 is likely to act via vitamin K-dependent proteins such as MGP and it is tempting to speculate whether these results can be transferred to CKD patients.

Acknowledgments: This work was supported by: The Forschungskommission of the Medical Faculty, University Düsseldorf, Germany and the Susanne-Brunnenberg-Stiftung at Duesseldorf Heart Center.

Author Contributions: Ralf Westenfeld and Leon J. Schurgers conceived and designed the experiments. Verena Veulemans and Daniel Scheiber performed the experiments. Ralf Westenfeld, Verena Veulemans, and Daniel Scheiber analyzed the data. Patrick Horn, Marijn L. Chatrou, Sebastian Potthoff, and Malte Kelm contributed reagents, materials, and analysis tools. Ralf Westenfeld, Leon J. Schurgers, and Daniel Scheiber wrote the paper.

Conflicts of Interest: The authors declare no conflict of interest.

References

1. Allison, M.A.; Criqui, M.H.; Wright, C.M. Patterns and risk factors for systemic calcified atherosclerosis. *Arterioscler. Thromb. Vasc. Biol.* **2004**, *24*, 331–336. [CrossRef] [PubMed]
2. Giachelli, C.M. The emerging role of phosphate in vascular calcification. *Kidney Int.* **2009**, *75*, 890–897. [CrossRef] [PubMed]
3. Schurgin, S.; Rich, S.; Mazzone, T. Increased prevalence of significant coronary artery calcification in patients with diabetes. *Diabetes Care* **2001**, *24*, 335–338. [CrossRef] [PubMed]
4. Vliegenthart, R.; Oudkerk, M.; Hofman, A.; Oei, H.H.; van Dijck, W.; van Rooij, F.J.; Witteman, J.C. Coronary calcification improves cardiovascular risk prediction in the elderly. *Circulation* **2005**, *112*, 572–577. [CrossRef] [PubMed]

5. Ketteler, M.; Schlieper, G.; Floege, J. Calcification and cardiovascular health—New insights into an old phenomenon. *Hypertension* **2006**, *47*, 1027–1034. [CrossRef] [PubMed]
6. Wu, M.; Rementer, C.; Giachelli, C.M. Vascular calcification: An update on mechanisms and challenges in treatment. *Calcif. Tissue Int.* **2013**, *93*, 365–373. [CrossRef] [PubMed]
7. Moe, S.M.; O'Neill, K.D.; Duan, D.; Ahmed, S.; Chen, N.X.; Leapman, S.B.; Fineberg, N.; Kopecky, K. Medial artery calcification in esrd patients is associated with deposition of bone matrix proteins. *Kidney Int.* **2002**, *61*, 638–647. [CrossRef] [PubMed]
8. Demer, L.L.; Tintut, Y. Vascular calcification: Pathobiology of a multifaceted disease. *Circulation* **2008**, *117*, 2938–2948. [CrossRef] [PubMed]
9. Chatrou, M.L.; Winckers, K.; Hackeng, T.M.; Reutelingsperger, C.P.; Schurgers, L.J. Vascular calcification: The price to pay for anticoagulation therapy with vitamin K-antagonists. *Blood Rev.* **2012**, *26*, 155–166. [CrossRef] [PubMed]
10. Reaven, P.D.; Sacks, J. Coronary artery and abdominal aortic calcification are associated with cardiovascular disease in type 2 diabetes. *Diabetologia* **2005**, *48*, 379–385. [CrossRef] [PubMed]
11. Okuno, S.; Ishimura, E.; Kitatani, K.; Fujino, Y.; Kohno, K.; Maeno, Y.; Maekawa, K.; Yamakawa, T.; Imanishi, Y.; Inaba, M.; *et al.* Presence of abdominal aortic calcification is significantly associated with all-cause and cardiovascular mortality in maintenance hemodialysis. *Am. J. Kidney Dis.* **2007**, *49*, 417–425. [CrossRef] [PubMed]
12. Schurgers, L.J.; Cranenburg, E.C.M.; Vermeer, C. Matrix gla-protein: The calcification inhibitor in need of vitamin k. *Thromb. Haemost.* **2008**. [CrossRef]
13. Price, P.A.; Urist, M.R.; Otawara, Y. Matrix gla protein, a new gamma-carboxyglutamic acid-containing protein which is associated with the organic matrix of bone. *Biochem. Biophys. Res. Commun.* **1983**, *117*, 765–771. [CrossRef]
14. Luo, G.; Ducy, P.; McKee, M.D.; Pinero, G.J.; Loyer, E.; Behringer, R.R.; Karsenty, G. Spontaneous calcification of arteries and cartilage in mice lacking matrix gla protein. *Nature* **1997**, *386*, 78–81. [CrossRef] [PubMed]
15. Munroe, P.B.; Olgunturk, R.O.; Fryns, J.P.; van Maldergem, L.; Ziereisen, F.; Yuksel, B.; Gardiner, R.M.; Chung, E. Mutations in the gene encoding the human matrix gla protein cause keutel syndrome. *Nat. Genet.* **1999**, *21*, 142–144. [CrossRef] [PubMed]
16. Schurgers, L.J.; Uitto, J.; Reutelingsperger, C.P. Vitamin k-dependent carboxylation of matrix gla-protein: A crucial switch to control ectopic mineralization. *Trends Mol. Med.* **2013**, *19*, 217–226. [CrossRef] [PubMed]
17. Murshed, M.; Schinke, T.; McKee, M.D.; Karsenty, G. Extracellular matrix mineralization is regulated locally; different roles of two gla-containing proteins. *J. Cell Biol.* **2004**, *165*, 625–630. [CrossRef] [PubMed]
18. Schurgers, L.J.; Teunissen, K.J.; Knapen, M.H.; Kwaijtaal, M.; van Diest, R.; Appels, A.; Reutelingsperger, C.P.; Cleutjens, J.P.; Vermeer, C. Novel conformation-specific antibodies against matrix gamma-carboxyglutamic acid (gla) protein: Undercarboxylated matrix gla protein as marker for vascular calcification. *Arterioscler. Thromb. Vasc. Biol.* **2005**, *25*, 1629–1633. [CrossRef] [PubMed]
19. Berkner, K.L.; Runge, K.W. The physiology of vitamin k nutriture and vitamin k-dependent protein function in atherosclerosis. *J. Thromb. Haemost.* **2004**, *2*, 2118–2132. [CrossRef] [PubMed]
20. Rennenberg, R.J.M.W.; van Varik, B.J.; Schurgers, L.J.; Hamulyak, K.; ten Cate, H.; Leiner, T.; Vermeer, C.; de Leeuw, P.W.; Kroon, A.A. Chronic coumarin treatment is associated with increased extracoronary arterial calcification in humans. *Blood* **2010**, *115*, 5121–5123. [CrossRef] [PubMed]
21. Pilkey, R.M.; Morton, A.R.; Boffa, M.B.; Noordhof, C.; Day, A.G.; Su, Y.H.; Miller, L.M.; Koschinsky, M.L.; Booth, S.L. Subclinical vitamin k deficiency in hemodialysis patients. *Am. J. Kidney Dis.* **2007**, *49*, 432–439. [CrossRef] [PubMed]
22. Schurgers, L.J.; Barreto, D.V.; Barreto, F.C.; Liabeuf, S.; Renard, C.; Magdeleyns, E.J.; Vermeer, C.; Choukroun, G.; Massy, Z.A. The circulating inactive form of matrix gla protein is a surrogate marker for vascular calcification in chronic kidney disease: A preliminary report. *Clin. J. Am. Soc. Nephrol.* **2010**, *5*, 568–575. [CrossRef] [PubMed]
23. Shea, M.K.; O'Donnell, C.J.; Vermeer, C.; Magdeleyns, E.J.P.; Crosier, M.D.; Gundberg, C.M.; Ordovas, J.M.; Kritchevsky, S.B.; Booth, S.L. Circulating uncarboxylated matrix gla protein is associated with vitamin k nutritional status, but not coronary artery calcium, in older adults. *J. Nutr.* **2011**, *141*, 1529–1534. [CrossRef] [PubMed]

24. Ueland, T.; Gullestad, L.; Dahl, C.P.; Aukrust, P.; Aakhus, S.; Solberg, O.G.; Vermeer, C.; Schurgers, L.J. Undercarboxylated matrix gla protein is associated with indices of heart failure and mortality in symptomatic aortic stenosis. *J. Intern. Med.* **2010**, *268*, 483–492. [CrossRef] [PubMed]

25. Ueland, T.; Dahl, C.P.; Gullestad, L.; Aakhus, S.; Broch, K.; Skardal, R.; Vermeer, C.; Aukrust, P.; Schurgers, L.J. Circulating levels of non-phosphorylated undercarboxylated matrix gla protein are associated with disease severity in patients with chronic heart failure. *Clin. Sci.* **2011**, *121*, 119–127. [CrossRef] [PubMed]

26. Cranenburg, E.C.; Koos, R.; Schurgers, L.J.; Magdeleyns, E.J.; Schoonbrood, T.H.; Landewe, R.B.; Brandenburg, V.M.; Bekers, O.; Vermeer, C. Characterisation and potential diagnostic value of circulating matrix gla protein (mgp) species. *Thromb. Haemost.* **2010**, *104*, 811–822. [PubMed]

27. Westenfeld, R.; Krueger, T.; Schlieper, G.; Cranenburg, E.C.; Magdeleyns, E.J.; Heidenreich, S.; Holzmann, S.; Vermeer, C.; Jahnen-Dechent, W.; Ketteler, M.; *et al.* Effect of vitamin k2 supplementation on functional vitamin k deficiency in hemodialysis patients: A randomized trial. *Am. J. Kidney Dis.* **2012**, *59*, 186–195. [CrossRef] [PubMed]

28. Gonnet, M.; Lethuaut, L.; Boury, F. New trends in encapsulation of liposoluble vitamins. *J. Control. Release* **2010**, *146*, 276–290. [CrossRef] [PubMed]

29. Gijsbers, B.L.; Jie, K.S.; Vermeer, C. Effect of food composition on vitamin k absorption in human volunteers. *Br. J. Nutr.* **1996**, *76*, 223–229. [CrossRef] [PubMed]

30. Schurgers, L.J.; Vermeer, C. Determination of phylloquinone and menaquinones in food. Effect of food matrix on circulating vitamin k concentrations. *Haemostasis* **2000**, *30*, 298–307. [PubMed]

31. Beulens, J.W.J.; Bots, M.L.; Atsma, F.; Bartelink, M.L.E.L.; Prokop, M.; Geleijnse, J.M.; Witteman, J.C.M.; Grobbee, D.E.; van der Schouw, Y.T. High dietary menaquinone intake is associated with reduced coronary calcification. *Atherosclerosis* **2009**, *203*, 489–493. [CrossRef] [PubMed]

32. Geleijnse, J.M.; Vermeer, C.; Grobbee, D.E.; Schurgers, L.J.; Knapen, M.H.; van der Meer, I.M.; Hofman, A.; Witteman, J.C. Dietary intake of menaquinone is associated with a reduced risk of coronary heart disease: The rotterdam study. *J. Nutr.* **2004**, *134*, 3100–3105. [PubMed]

33. Kruger, T.; Oelenberg, S.; Kaesler, N.; Schurgers, L.J.; van de Sandt, A.M.; Boor, P.; Schlieper, G.; Brandenburg, V.M.; Fekete, B.C.; Veulemans, V.; *et al.* Warfarin induces cardiovascular damage in mice. *Arterioscler. Thromb. Vasc. Biol.* **2013**, *33*, 2618–2624. [CrossRef] [PubMed]

34. Schurgers, L.J.; Spronk, H.M.; Soute, B.A.; Schiffers, P.M.; DeMey, J.G.; Vermeer, C. Regression of warfarin-induced medial elastocalcinosis by high intake of vitamin k in rats. *Blood* **2007**, *109*, 2823–2831. [CrossRef] [PubMed]

35. Spronk, H.M.; Soute, B.A.; Schurgers, L.J.; Thijssen, H.H.; de Mey, J.G.; Vermeer, C. Tissue-specific utilization of menaquinone-4 results in the prevention of arterial calcification in warfarin-treated rats. *J. Vasc. Res.* **2003**, *40*, 531–537. [CrossRef] [PubMed]

36. Perez-Ruiz, L.; Ros-Lopez, S.; Cardus, A.; Fernandez, E.; Valdivielso, J.M. A forgotten method to induce experimental chronic renal failure in the rat by ligation of the renal parenchyma. *Nephron. Exp. Nephrol.* **2006**, *103*, e126–e130. [CrossRef] [PubMed]

37. Ng, K.; Hildreth, C.M.; Phillips, J.K.; Avolio, A.P. Aortic stiffness is associated with vascular calcification and remodeling in a chronic kidney disease rat model. *Am. J. Physiol. Renal Physiol.* **2011**, *300*, F1431–F1436. [CrossRef] [PubMed]

38. Shobeiri, N.; Adams, M.A.; Holden, R.M. Vascular calcification in animal models of ckd: A review. *Am. J. Nephrol.* **2010**, *31*, 471–481. [CrossRef] [PubMed]

39. Fleck, C.; Appenroth, D.; Jonas, P.; Koch, M.; Kundt, G.; Nizze, H.; Stein, G. Suitability of 5/6 nephrectomy (5/6nx) for the induction of interstitial renal fibrosis in rats—Influence of sex, strain, and surgical procedure. *Exp. Toxicol. Pathol.* **2006**, *57*, 195–205. [CrossRef] [PubMed]

40. El-Achkar, T.M.; Ohmit, S.E.; McCullough, P.A.; Crook, E.D.; Brown, W.W.; Grimm, R.; Bakris, G.L.; Keane, W.F.; Flack, J.M. Higher prevalence of anemia with diabetes mellitus in moderate kidney insufficiency: The kidney early evaluation program. *Kidney Int.* **2005**, *67*, 1483–1488. [CrossRef] [PubMed]

41. Shioi, A.; Katagi, M.; Okuno, Y.; Mori, K.; Jono, S.; Koyama, H.; Nishizawa, Y. Induction of bone-type alkaline phosphatase in human vascular smooth muscle cells: Roles of tumor necrosis factor-alpha and oncostatin m derived from macrophages. *Circ. Res.* **2002**, *91*, 9–16. [CrossRef]

42. Kendrick, J.; Chonchol, M. The role of phosphorus in the development and progression of vascular calcification. *Am. J. Kidney Dis.* **2011**, *58*, 826–834. [CrossRef] [PubMed]

43. El-Abbadi, M.M.; Pai, A.S.; Leaf, E.M.; Yang, H.Y.; Bartley, B.A.; Quan, K.K.; Ingalls, C.M.; Liao, H.W.; Giachelli, C.M. Phosphate feeding induces arterial medial calcification in uremic mice: Role of serum phosphorus, fibroblast growth factor-23, and osteopontin. *Kidney Int.* **2009**, *75*, 1297–1307. [CrossRef] [PubMed]

44. Steitz, S.A.; Speer, M.Y.; Curinga, G.; Yang, H.Y.; Haynes, P.; Aebersold, R.; Schinke, T.; Karsenty, G.; Giachelli, C.M. Smooth muscle cell phenotypic transition associated with calcification: Upregulation of cbfa1 and downregulation of smooth muscle lineage markers. *Circ. Res.* **2001**, *89*, 1147–1154. [CrossRef] [PubMed]

45. Hakuno, D.; Kimura, N.; Yoshioka, M.; Mukai, M.; Kimura, T.; Okada, Y.; Yozu, R.; Shukunami, C.; Hiraki, Y.; Kudo, A.; *et al.* Periostin advances atherosclerotic and rheumatic cardiac valve degeneration by inducing angiogenesis and mmp production in humans and rodents. *J. Clin. Invest.* **2010**, *120*, 2292–2306. [CrossRef] [PubMed]

46. Hixson, J.E.; Shimmin, L.C.; Montasser, M.E.; Kim, D.K.; Zhong, Y.; Ibarguen, H.; Follis, J.; Malcom, G.; Strong, J.; Howard, T.; *et al.* Common variants in the periostin gene influence development of atherosclerosis in young persons. *Arterioscler. Thromb. Vasc. Biol.* **2011**, *31*, 1661–1667. [CrossRef] [PubMed]

47. Sen, K.; Lindenmeyer, M.T.; Gaspert, A.; Eichinger, F.; Neusser, M.A.; Kretzler, M.; Segerer, S.; Cohen, C.D. Periostin is induced in glomerular injury and expressed de novo in interstitial renal fibrosis. *Am. J. Pathol.* **2011**, *179*, 1756–1767. [CrossRef] [PubMed]

48. Bostrom, K.; Watson, K.E.; Horn, S.; Wortham, C.; Herman, I.M.; Demer, L.L. Bone morphogenetic protein expression in human atherosclerotic lesions. *J. Clin. Invest.* **1993**, *91*, 1800–1809. [CrossRef] [PubMed]

49. Ciceri, P.; Elli, F.; Brenna, I.; Volpi, E.; Romagnoli, S.; Tosi, D.; Braidotti, P.; Brancaccio, D.; Cozzolino, M. Lanthanum prevents high phosphate-induced vascular calcification by preserving vascular smooth muscle lineage markers. *Calcif. Tissue Int.* **2013**, *92*, 521–530. [CrossRef] [PubMed]

50. Kaesler, N.; Magdeleyns, E.; Herfs, M.; Schettgen, T.; Brandenburg, V.; Fliser, D.; Vermeer, C.; Floege, J.; Schlieper, G.; Kruger, T. Impaired vitamin k recycling in uremia is rescued by vitamin k supplementation. *Kidney Int.* **2014**, *86*, 286–293. [CrossRef] [PubMed]

51. Tabb, M.M.; Sun, A.; Zhou, C.; Grun, F.; Errandi, J.; Romero, K.; Pham, H.; Inoue, S.; Mallick, S.; Lin, M.; *et al.* Vitamin k2 regulation of bone homeostasis is mediated by the steroid and xenobiotic receptor sxr. *J. Biol. Chem.* **2003**, *278*, 43919–43927. [CrossRef] [PubMed]

52. Viegas, C.S.; Rafael, M.S.; Enriquez, J.L.; Teixeira, A.; Vitorino, R.; Luis, I.M.; Costa, R.M.; Santos, S.; Cavaco, S.; Neves, J.; *et al.* Gla-rich protein acts as a calcification inhibitor in the human cardiovascular system. *Arterioscler. Thromb. Vasc. Biol.* **2015**, *35*, 399–408. [CrossRef]

53. Tsuchiya, N.; Matsushima, S.; Takasu, N.; Kyokawa, Y.; Torii, M. Glomerular calcification induced by bolus injection with dibasic sodium phosphate solution in sprague-dawley rats. *Toxicol. Pathol.* **2004**, *32*, 408–412. [CrossRef] [PubMed]

54. Eknoyan, G.; Levin, N.W. K/doqi clinical practice guidelines for chronic kidney disease: Evaluation, classification, and stratification. *Am. J. Kidney Dis.* **2002**, *39*, S14–S266.

55. McCarty, M.F.; DiNicolantonio, J.J. Bioavailable dietary phosphate, a mediator of cardiovascular disease, may be decreased with plant-based diets, phosphate binders, niacin, and avoidance of phosphate additives. *Nutrition* **2014**, *30*, 739–747. [CrossRef] [PubMed]

56. Pucaj, K.; Rasmussen, H.; Moller, M.; Preston, T. Safety and toxicological evaluation of a synthetic vitamin k2, menaquinone-7. *Toxicol. Mech. Methods* **2011**, *21*, 520–532. [CrossRef] [PubMed]

57. Holden, R.M.; Morton, A.R.; Garland, J.S.; Pavlov, A.; Day, A.G.; Booth, S.L. Vitamins k and d status in stages 3–5 chronic kidney disease. *Clin. J. Am. Soc. Nephrol.* **2010**, *5*, 590–597. [CrossRef] [PubMed]

58. Fusaro, M.; Noale, M.; Viola, V.; Galli, F.; Tripepi, G.; Vajente, N.; Plebani, M.; Zaninotto, M.; Guglielmi, G.; Miotto, D.; *et al.* Vitamin k, vertebral fractures, vascular calcifications, and mortality: Vitamin k italian (viki) dialysis study. *J. Bone Miner. Res.* **2012**, *27*, 2271–2278. [CrossRef] [PubMed]

59. Brandenburg, V.M.; Schurgers, L.J.; Kaesler, N.; Pusche, K.; van Gorp, R.H.; Leftheriotis, G.; Reinartz, S.; Koos, R.; Kruger, T. Prevention of vasculopathy by vitamin k supplementation: Can we turn fiction into fact? *Atherosclerosis* **2015**, *240*, 10–16. [CrossRef] [PubMed]

60. Taddei, S.; Nami, R.; Bruno, R.M.; Quatrini, I.; Nuti, R. Hypertension, left ventricular hypertrophy and chronic kidney disease. *Heart Fail. Rev.* **2011**, *16*, 615–620. [CrossRef] [PubMed]

61. Feihl, F.; Liaudet, L.; Levy, B.I.; Waeber, B. Hypertension and microvascular remodelling. *Cardiovasc. Res.* **2008**, *78*, 274–285. [CrossRef] [PubMed]

62. Li, S.; Wang, X.; Li, Y.; Kost, C.K., Jr.; Martin, D.S. Bortezomib, a proteasome inhibitor, attenuates angiotensin ii-induced hypertension and aortic remodeling in rats. *PLoS One* **2013**, *8*, e78564. [CrossRef] [PubMed]
63. Ro, A.; Kageyama, N. Pathomorphometry of ruptured intracranial vertebral arterial dissection: Adventitial rupture, dilated lesion, intimal tear, and medial defect. *J. Neurosurg.* **2013**, *119*, 221–227. [CrossRef] [PubMed]

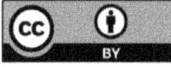

nutrients

MDPI

Article

Total and Differential Phylloquinone (Vitamin K₁) Intakes of Preterm Infants from All Sources during the Neonatal Period

Paul Clarke [1,*], Simon J. Mitchell [2] and Martin J. Shearer [3]

[1]   Neonatal Unit, Norfolk and Norwich University Hospitals NHS Foundation Trust, Colney Lane, Norwich, Norfolk NR4 7UY, UK

[2]   Newborn Intensive Care, St Mary's Hospital, Oxford Road, Manchester M13 9WL, UK; simon.mitchell@cmft.nhs.uk

[3]   The Centre for Haemostasis and Thrombosis, St. Thomas' Hospital, Westminster Bridge Road, London SE1 7EH, UK; martin.shearer@gstt.nhs.uk

*   Correspondence: paul.clarke@nnuh.nhs.uk; Tel.: +44-1603-286-337; Fax: +44-1603-287-584

Received: 26 July 2015 ; Accepted: 16 September 2015 ; Published: 25 September 2015

Abstract: All newborns require phylloquinone after birth to prevent vitamin K deficiency bleeding. Babies born prematurely may be at particular risk of deficiency without adequate supplementation during infancy. The main sources of phylloquinone in preterm babies during the neonatal period are the prophylactic dose of phylloquinone given at birth, and that derived from parenteral and/or enteral feeding. This observational study formed part of a prospective, multicentre, randomised, controlled trial that examined the vitamin K status of preterm infants after random allocation to one of three phylloquinone prophylactic regimens at birth (0.5 or 0.2 mg intramuscularly or 0.2 mg intravenously). In this nutritional sub-study we quantified the proportional and total phylloquinone intakes of preterm infants within the neonatal period from all sources. Almost all infants had average daily phylloquinone intakes that were in excess of the currently recommended amounts. In infants who did not receive parenteral nutrition, the bolus dose of phylloquinone given at birth was the major source of phylloquinone intake, whereas in infants who received parenteral nutrition, the intake from the parenteral preparation exceeded that from the bolus dose by a ratio of approximately 3:1. Our study supports the concern of others that preterm infants who receive current parenteral nutrition formulations may be receiving excessive vitamin K.

Keywords: phylloquinone; prophylaxis; prematurity; deficiency; bleeding; dietary; micronutrients; supplement; nutrition

1. Introduction

Vitamin K-dependent coagulation factors are synthesised exclusively in the liver and so the maintenance of adequate hepatic vitamin K reserves is essential for normal haemostasis. Preterm as well as term babies are born with extremely low hepatic stores of vitamin K [1,2]. Unlike in adults, the major hepatic form of vitamin K in neonates is phylloquinone (vitamin K₁) which is also the major form of the vitamin in human breast milk. After birth, the combination of low hepatic reserves and relatively low concentrations of phylloquinone in breast milk (compared to formula milks) places the breast-fed infant at increased risk of developing vitamin K deficiency. They are consequently dependent upon adequate intakes of vitamin K postnatally and during early infancy to keep them healthy. Supplementary vitamin K prophylaxis is offered at birth to protect against vitamin K deficiency bleeding (VKDB), a now rare but still potentially lethal disorder which may cause devastating brain injury and lifelong impairment in survivors [3–5]. Preterm infants may be at higher risk of developing VKDB without adequate ongoing phylloquinone intakes following birth [6], so a baseline understanding of their current typical intakes from various sources during the neonatal period is clearly important.

In both term and preterm infants the very large bolus dose of phylloquinone given prophylactically at birth is considered to be the major source of phylloquinone in early infancy [7,8], and, therefore, to provide the mainstay of protection provided against VKDB during early infancy. Preterm neonates receive an on-going supply of phylloquinone from dietary sources, including from enteral and often parenteral feeding. No previous study has reported in detail the total phylloquinone intakes of preterm infants from all the various sources during their first weeks of life. The aims of this study were: (i) to quantify phylloquinone intake by preterm infants from all sources during the first postnatal weeks of life; and (ii) to assess the relative contribution of the various sources to the total phylloquinone intake of preterm infants during the neonatal period.

2. Experimental Section

2.1. Study Design

This observational study was done as part of a prospective, multicentre, randomised controlled trial that examined the vitamin K status of preterm infants after random allocation to one of three phylloquinone prophylactic regimens at birth [9]. The setting was three neonatal intensive care units (NICUs) in the United Kingdom (UK). The present study reports the detailed phylloquinone intakes of these infants during the first weeks after birth. Data on the functional outcome measures of phylloquinone status and metabolism in this cohort, including undercarboxylated prothrombin (PIVKA-II), prothrombin time, and factor II concentrations, were reported previously [9]. Assessment of other vitamin-K dependent proteins (such as osteocalcin and matrix Gla protein) was beyond the scope of the study.

2.2. Subjects

Infants eligible for inclusion were born at a gestational age of <32 completed weeks and admitted to one of the three participating NICUs. Exclusion criteria included fetal intracranial haemorrhage suspected antenatally, history of maternal antiplatelet antibodies or alloimmune thrombocytopenia, maternal drug treatment with known vitamin K antagonists, life-threatening congenital abnormality, and marked bruising present from birth. Infants with bowel diseases (such as necrotising enterocolitis) or other expected complications of prematurity were not excluded or discontinued from the study. Written parental consent was obtained for inclusion, and the period of recruitment was between November 2001 and February 2003.

2.3. Sources of Vitamin K Intake

There are only three prospective sources of phylloquinone intake by preterm infants during the neonatal period: (i) the prophylactic bolus dose received soon after birth and any extra bolus doses given while in the NICU; (ii) enteral milk feeds and human milk fortifiers (HMFs); and (iii) parenteral nutrition (PN).

2.3.1. Prophylactic Phylloquinone Formulation and Dose

The phylloquinone preparation provided for prophylaxis and for any subsequent bolus dose for infants in this study was Konakion® Neonatal Ampoules (Roche Ltd, Basel, Switzerland). This formulation contained phytomenadione 2 mg/mL and had Cremophor EL (BASF AG, Ludwigshafen, Germany) as the solubilising excipient. Although unlicensed for use in preterm infants, this vitamin K formulation was at the time the commonest preparation used for prophylaxis in the UK [10].

For the main study [2,9], infants were randomly allocated to receive one of three vitamin K prophylaxis regimens within a few hours of birth: phylloquinone 0.5 mg intramuscularly (IM), 0.2 mg IM, or 0.2 mg intravenously (IV). As a safety provision, the study protocol provided that a 0.2 mg IM additional bolus dose of phylloquinone would be given during the study period to any infant with abnormal coagulation values or clinical bleeding in case these findings represented vitamin K deficiency.

2.3.2. Enteral Feeding and Human Milk Fortifiers

The introduction and grading of enteral feeds proceeded in line with standard practices. In general, small "trophic" volumes (totalling ~20 mL/kg/day) of colostrum/human milk and/or a preterm milk formula were commenced within the first few days postnatal. Maternal expression of breast milk was actively encouraged, and expressed breast milk (EBM) was the preferred milk feed for preterm infants at all participating neonatal units. Bolus aliquots of milk were given via a nasogastric tube, initially on an hourly basis. Any increment in the feed volume was a decision of the clinical ward round and would depend upon an infant's stability and any recent history of feed tolerance. Infants were considered to have established full enteral feeds when they were tolerating a volume of at least 150 mL/kg/day of milk and no longer on PN. An infant who tolerated the gradual feed increase without event or setback would potentially establish full feeds by 7–10 days postnatal.

It was standard clinical practice at all three participating NICUs to add HMF routinely to breast milk once the full enteral feed volume of 150 mL/kg/day was attained. Three commercially-available HMFs were available in the UK during the study period. Infants at the participating units all received Eoprotin HMF (Nutricia Ltd., Trowbridge, UK). Coincidentally, a new formulation of Eoprotin with a higher phylloquinone content was introduced nationally in the UK during the study period. Initially one scoop was given per 100 mL of breast milk, and this was graded up to three scoops (old Eoprotin formulation) or four scoops (new Eoprotin formulation) on successive days as tolerated. Infants discharged to neonatal centres outside of the three trial centres prior to study completion who subsequently received a different HMF had their phylloquinone intake calculated according to the actual fortifier received.

2.3.3. Parenteral Nutrition

Administration of PN solution was routine for the sickest neonates in the participating NICUs. It was generally reserved for all very preterm infants (less than ~29 weeks' gestation), extremely low birth weight infants (ELBW; <1000 g), and also any other neonate that was considered unlikely to achieve full enteral feeding by 7–10 days postnatal. It was expected that many of the more mature and heavier preterm infants in the study group would not require PN.

PN was usually commenced within the first three days of life. The daily volume of lipid infused was routinely graded up over the first three days to minimise fat intolerance and hyperlipidaemia. The phylloquinone-containing components of the PN solution were 20% Intralipid®, an intravenous fat emulsion, and Vitlipid N Infant®, a fat-soluble vitamin emulsion (Fresenius Kabi Ltd, Runcorn, Cheshire, UK). Nursing charts recorded the dates when PN began and ended, and also the exact daily volumes of the respective PN solutions delivered to each infant.

2.4. Assessment of Phylloquinone Intake

Phylloquinone intakes from all sources were calculated between birth and the date that the infant had tolerated full enteral feeds (*i.e.*, ⩾150 mL/kg/day of milk) for a continuous full 2-week period, the latter date being considered the date of "study completion". The total vitamin intake was thus calculated for each enrolled infant between birth and the date that full enteral feeds had been tolerated for two weeks.

Each infant's absolute phylloquinone intake between birth and study completion was calculated from the sum amounts received from: (i) allocated prophylactic phylloquinone dose and any extra bolus phylloquinone doses given during the study period, obtained from review of the prescription charts; (ii) daily enteral feed volumes and HMF, obtained from the daily nursing charts; and (iii) PN intake, with daily volumes of Intralipid and Vitlipid received being obtained from the PN prescription charts and the nursing infusion administration charts.

An average daily phylloquinone intake was calculated for each infant from its total phylloquinone intake (expressed in µg/kg, using the infant's weight at completion of the study) divided by the number of days from birth to study completion. The phylloquinone intake from enteral feeds was calculated from the actual milk types and volumes fed to each infant between birth and study completion, as recorded on the neonatal nursing charts.

2.4.1. Phylloquinone Content of Milk Feeds and Fortifier

Table 1 shows the phylloquinone content of human preterm breast milk, and of the preterm artificial milk formulae that were available in the UK during the study period. The values for phylloquinone content of term infant human breast milk and term infant milk formulae are also provided for comparison purposes. Milk formulae phylloquinone contents are compiled from the various manufacturers' contemporaneous data sheets. Values for the phylloquinone content of HMF-fortified preterm breast milk are also provided; these are based upon the manufacturer-published phylloquinone content of the various HMFs that were commercially-available during the study period, and upon the mean phylloquinone concentration value reported for preterm EBM. The value for mean phylloquinone concentration of human preterm EBM (3.0 µg/L) derives from a study of human milk obtained on postnatal one day from mothers of preterm infants prior to maternal phylloquinone supplementation [11]. To date this study of Bolisetty *et al.* [11] remains the only known study in which breast milk phylloquinone concentrations have been measured in mothers of preterm infants. Nevertheless, this mean value compares well to the mean concentration of phylloquinone in mature human breast milk (2.1 µg/L) from mothers of term infants reported by Haroon *et al.* [12], and to the mean value (2.5 µg/L) that was used in the calculation of the Adequate Intake (AI) by the Food and Nutrition Board [7]. Addition of HMF to EBM provided a total phylloquinone concentration of 5–66 µg/L depending on brand used (Table 1). Artificial preterm milk formulae provided 40–66 µg/L of phylloquinone depending on brand. These values were used to calculate exact phylloquinone intakes from the enteral feeds for all study individuals up to completion of the study.

Table 1. Phylloquinone content of human milk, commercial milk formulae, and fortifiers.

Nutrient	Phylloquinone Content (µg/100 mL)	Phylloquinone Content (µg/L)
Human Milk		
Term colostrum [a]	0.23	2.3
Term mature EBM [a]	0.21	2.1
Preterm colostrum/EBM [b]	0.30	3.0
Formula Milks		
PreAptamil	6.6	66
Aptamil	4.0	40
Nutriprem 1	6.6	66
Nutriprem 2	5.9	59
SMA Low Birth Weight	8.0	80
SMA Gold	6.7	67
C + G Premium	5.1	51
C + G Plus	5.0	50

Table 1. *Cont.*

Nutrient	Phylloquinone Content (µg/100 mL)	Phylloquinone Content (µg/L)
Human Milk Fortifiers		
Eoprotin (old formulation)	0.2 per 3 scoops (3 g powder) [c]	2
Eoprotin (new formulation)	6.3 per 4 scoops (4.2 g powder) [c]	63
Nutriprem HMF	6.2 per 2 sachets (4.2 g powder) [c]	62
SMA Breast Milk Fortifier	11.0 per 2 sachets (4 g powder) [c]	110
Fortified EBM [d]		
Eoprotin old formulation	0.5	5
Eoprotin new formulation	6.6	66
Nutriprem HMF	6.5	65
SMA HMF	11.3	113

EBM, expressed breast milk; HMF, human milk fortifier. [a] Analysis of colostrum and breast milk obtained within five days *post-partum*, from Haroon *et al.* [12]; [b] Mean preterm EBM concentration on the first postnatal day in unsupplemented mothers, from Bolisetty *et al.* [11]; [c] Quantities recommended by manufacturers for addition to each 100 mL of human milk; [d] Values listed refer to content of fortified human milk after adding the recommended amount of HMF according to manufacturers' instructions

2.4.2. Phylloquinone Content of Parenteral Nutrition Solution

The phylloquinone content of Vitlipid N Infant (fat soluble vitamin emulsion) was 20 mg/L. That of 20% Intralipid IV fat emulsion varied between batches, and ranged from 0.50 to 0.77 mg/L [13]; for calculation purposes a figure of 0.6 mg/L was used. Infants on PN received 4 mL/kg of Vitlipid and 5–15 mL/kg of 20% Intralipid per day, providing daily phylloquinone supplementation of 80 µg/kg and 3–9 µg/kg respectively.

2.4.3. Calculation of Total and Proportional Phylloquinone Intake from All Sources

The average daily phylloquinone intake was calculated for each infant from the total phylloquinone intake (expressed as µg/kg body weight at study completion) divided by number of days between birth and study completion. The proportional intake of phylloquinone from each route was also assessed: for each infant the contribution to overall total intake from each phylloquinone source was expressed as a percentage of total intake. In addition to calculating the proportional intake for all infants who completed the study (because not all preterm infants required or received PN feeding) the proportional intake was calculated separately for infants who received PN and for infants who did not receive any PN.

2.4.4. Statistical Analysis

Infants who died before study completion were excluded from analysis. Data for all randomised infants who completed the study were analysed using StatsDirect statistical software (www.statsdirect.com) version 2.4.5. The Mann-Whitney U test was used to compare phylloquinone intakes between the three randomisation cohorts, and a *p*-value of <0.05 was considered statistically significant.

2.5. Ethics Approvals

The study received prior ethical review board approval from Salford and Trafford Local Research Ethics Committee on 5 November 2001 (Project No. 01198). Further Research Ethics Committee approvals were given on 10 July 2002 and on 10 December 2002 for extension of the study to two additional sites.

3. Results

3.1. Baseline Characteristics

Of 98 infants randomised to the main trial [2,9], 15 died before study completion and three infants with incomplete data were excluded from the analysis. All deaths were related to the common complications of prematurity and no infant in the study had vitamin K deficiency bleeding [9]. A total of 80 infants completed the study. Table 2 shows their baseline characteristics, including feeding characteristics, overall and subgrouped according to initial allocated dose of phylloquinone prophylaxis. There were no significant differences between subgroups for any of these baseline characteristics. As already reported, all infants had satisfactory vitamin K status at study completion and there were no significant differences in any functional outcome measures of phylloquinone status and metabolism between the subgroups in this cohort [9]. No infant suffered any suspected adverse event or reaction in relation to phylloquinone dosage or its route of administration. There were no differences between sub-groups in incidence of significant intraventricular haemorrhage ($n = 6$ infants overall, $p = 0.9$), other significant bleeding, such as gastro-intestinal or pulmonary ($n = 7$ infants overall, $p = 0.2$), or numbers transfused with fresh frozen plasma during the study ($n = 7$ infants overall, $p = 0.7$).

Table 2. Baseline characteristics of the $n = 80$ infants who completed the study and subgroups according to initial phylloquinone prophylaxis regimen.

Characteristic	All Infants ($n = 80$)	0.5 mg IM ($n = 28$)	0.2 mg IM ($n = 26$)	0.2 mg IV ($n = 26$)
Gestational Age, weeks	29.4 (22.4–31.9)	29.0 (24.1–31.9)	29.9 (24.0–31.7)	29.6 (22.4–31.4)
Birth Weight, g	1092 (454–1910)	1033 (454–1910)	1143 (534–1910)	1203 (575–1892)
Male gender, *n*	36 (45%)	10 (36%)	13 (50%)	13 (50%)
Received any PN, *n*	56 (70%)	18 (64%)	17 (65%)	21 (81%)
Duration of PN [a], days median (range) (IQR)	10 (3–78) (7–17)	9 (4–78) (7–13)	10 (5–29) (9–21)	9 (3–48) (5–18)
Postnatal age reached full enteral feeds, days	10 (4–80)	9 (4–80)	12 (4–43)	11 (4–49)
Postnatal age at study completion, days	25 (17–90)	24 (19–90)	26 (19–58)	26 (17–64)
Weight at study completion, g	1495 (600–2710)	1281 (605–2650)	1595 (600–2270)	1572 (612–2710)

Data are median (range) unless indicated. IM, intramuscular; IV, intravenous; PN, parenteral nutrition; IQR, inter-quartile range. [a] Data shown here include only babies who received any period of PN. There were no statistically significant differences between any subgroups for any of the baseline characteristics shown.

3.2. Total Phylloquinone Intakes

Table 3 shows total phylloquinone intakes from all sources between birth and study completion overall and for the subgroups. There were no significant differences in absolute phylloquinone intakes from all sources between the three study groups at study completion. However, after correcting for birth weight and days to study completion, the average daily intake of phylloquinone adjusted for birth weight was significantly lower for infants who had received 0.2 mg boluses at birth ($p < 0.05$).

Table 3. Phylloquinone intakes from all sources between birth and study completion (adapted from Clarke *et al.* [9], with permission).

Phylloquinone Intake (µg)	All infants (*n* = 80)	0.5 mg IM (*n* = 28)	0.2 mg IM (*n* = 26)	0.2 mg IV (*n* = 26)
Via bolus doses				
Mean (SD)	378 (256)	629 (264)	238 (80) *	246 (130) *
Median (range)	200 (200–1500)	500 (500–1500)	200 (200–400) *	200 (200–800)
From PN [†]				
Mean (SD)	784 (939)	610 (972)	754 (768)	1001 (1045)
Median (range)	542 (0–5071)	440 (0–5071)	674 (0–2441)	713 (0–3895)
Via enteral feeds				
Mean (SD)	124 (90)	118 (85)	125 (97)	131 (91)
Median (range)	133 (2–340)	116 (2–340)	122 (6–304)	145 (8–300)
Total phylloquinone intake µg				
Mean (SD)	1286 (1025)	1357 (1133)	1118 (775)	1378 (1136)
Median (range)	1011 (214–6574)	1038 (507–6574)	958 (332–2730)	1020 (214–4822)
µg/kg				
Mean (SD)	914 (597)	1070 (633)	808 (591)	853 (548)
Median (range)	775 (141–2594)	1048 (408–2594)	699 (173–2057)	704 (141–2343)
µg/kg/day				
Mean (SD)	30 (15)	37 (15)	26 (15) [‡]	27 (11) [‡]
Median (range)	28 (7–75)	39 (18–75)	27 (8–55) [‡]	27 (7–65) [‡]

SD, standard deviation. [†] Includes infants who received any period of PN as well as those who did not receive PN; * *Versus* 0.5 mg IM group, $p < 0.001$; [‡] *Versus* 0.5 mg IM group, $p < 0.05$.

3.2.1. Phylloquinone Intakes According to Parenteral Nutrition Administration

Table 4 shows the total phylloquinone intake from all sources in study infants who received any period of PN and completed the study (*n* = 56). PN-derived phylloquinone intake in these 56 infants was comparable in the 0.5 mg IM (*n* = 18) and 0.2 mg IV (*n* = 21) groups, and slightly higher in the 0.2 mg IM group (*n* = 17).

Table 5 shows total phylloquinone intakes by route confined to study infants who did not receive any PN (*n* = 24).

Table 4. Relative intakes of phylloquinone from all sources together with total intakes at study completion in infants who received parenteral nutrition.

Phylloquinone Intake (µg)	All Infants Given PN (n = 56)	0.5 mg IM (n = 18)	0.2 mg IM (n = 17)	0.2 mg IV (n = 21)
Via bolus doses				
Mean (SD)	391 (277)	672 (303)	259 (94) *	275 (143) *
Median (range)	200 (200–1500)	500 (500–1500)	200 (200–400) *	200 (200–800) *
From PN				
Mean (SD)	1120 (940)	950 (1077)	1153 (658) [†]	1240 (1027)
Median (range)	759 (305–5071)	589 (350–5071)	767 (515–2441) [†]	946 (305–3895)
Via enteral feeds				
Mean (SD)	101 (80)	97 (63)	80 (82)	120 (89)
Median (range)	94 (2–304)	105 (2–198)	79 (6–304)	142 (8–300)
Total phylloquinone intake µg				
Mean (SD)	1612 (1066)	1719 (1280)	1492 (714)	1617 (1140)
Median (range)	1234 (596–6574)	1423 (956–6574)	1189 (771–2730)	1240 (596–4822)
µg/kg				
Mean (SD)	1168 (535)	1410 (540)	1119 (498)	1000 (506) [‡]
Median (range)	1136 (438–2594)	1269 (721–2594)	971 (529–2057)	813 (438–2343) [‡]
µg/kg/day				
Mean (SD)	37 (13)	46 (12)	34 (11) [‡]	30 (10) *
Median (range)	33 (18–75)	44 (28–75)	33 (19–55) [‡]	29 (18–65) *

Statistically-significant comparisons (using Mann-Whitney U test) are shown thus: * *versus* 0.5 mg IM group, *p* < 0.0001; [†] *Versus* 0.5 mg IM group, *p* < 0.05; [‡] *Versus* 0.5 mg IM group, *p* < 0.01.

Table 5. Relative intakes of phylloquinone from bolus doses and enteral feeds together with total intakes at study completion for infants who did not receive parenteral nutrition.

Phylloquinone Intake (µg)	All Infants Not Given PN (n = 24)	0.5 mg IM (n = 10)	0.2 mg IM (n = 9)	0.2 mg IV (n = 5)
Via bolus doses				
Mean (SD)	346 (202)	550 (158)	200 (NA) *	200 (NA) [†]
Median (range)	200 (200–1000)	500 (500–1000)	200 (NA) *	200 (NA) [†]
Via enteral feeds				
Mean (SD)	181 (88)	156 (107)	212 (55)	176 (94)
Median (range)	195 (7–340)	149 (7–340)	214 (132–292)	208 (14–254)
Total phylloquinone intake µg				
Mean (SD)	527 (187)	706 (145)	412 (55) *	376 (94) [†]
Median (range)	466 (214–1016)	690 (507–1016)	414 (332–492) *	408 (214–454) [†]
µg/kg				
Mean (SD)	322 (124)	458 (48)	220 (27) *	233 (54) [†]
Median (range)	251 (141–562)	439 (408–562)	215 (173–249) *	249 (141–284) [†]
µg/kg/day				
Mean (SD)	15 (6)	22 (3)	10 (1) *	12 (4) [†]
Median (range)	13 (7–25)	21 (18–25)	10 (8–12) *	13 (7–17) [†]

NA, not applicable because all infants received 0.2 mg dose. Statistically-significant comparisons (using Mann-Whitney U test) are shown thus: * *versus* 0.5 mg IM group, *p* < 0.0001; [†] *Versus* 0.5 mg IM group, *p* < 0.001.

3.2.2. Proportional Contribution of Various Sources to Overall Phylloquinone Intakes

Table 6 shows the proportional intake of phylloquinone from each route as a percentage of the total intake, for all infants and for the subgroups. Analysis of the proportional intake of phylloquinone from the various routes shows that for the infants receiving 0.5 mg phylloquinone after delivery and who received PN, the bolus dose comprised ~40% of total phylloquinone intake over the study period, while PN comprised ~50% of intake, and enteral feeding <10% of intake. In contrast for the 0.2 mg groups, only ~20% of the total phylloquinone intake in the study period came from the bolus prophylaxis dose, whereas 70% came from PN, and <10% came from enteral feeding.

Table 6. Proportional intake of phylloquinone from each route from birth until study completion as a percentage of the total intake.

Proportional Phylloquinone Intake	All Infants	0.5 mg IM	0.2 mg IM	0.2 mg IV
All Infants	*n* = 80	*n* = 28	*n* = 26	*n* = 26
% Via bolus doses				
Mean (SD)	38 (23)	56 (21)	30 (16) *	27 (19) *
Median (range)	33 (5–99)	52 (23–99)	22 (7–60) *	20 (5–94) *
% From PN				
Mean (SD)	46 (33)	32 (26)	49 (37) [†]	57 (31) *
Median (range)	56 (0–92)	37 (0–77)	69 (0–89) [†]	68 (0–92) *
% Via enteral feeds				
Mean (SD)	17 (18)	12 (11)	21 (23)	16 (17)
Median (range)	8 (0–59)	8 (0–41)	10 (0–59)	8 (0–56)
Infants given PN	*n* = 56	*n* = 18	*n* = 17	*n* = 21
% Via bolus doses				
Mean (SD)	27 (14)	43 (11)	20 (8) *	19 (8) *
Median (range)	23 (5–64)	45 (23–64)	19 (7–42) *	17 (5–34) *
% From PN				
Mean (SD)	65 (16)	50 (13)	75 (10) *	71 (13) *
Median (range)	68 (28–92)	50 (28–77)	78 (54–89) *	74 (43–92) *
% Via enteral feeds				
Mean (SD)	8 (7)	7 (5)	6 (6)	10 (9)
Median (range)	6 (0–28)	7 (0–16)	3 (0–21)	8 (0–28)

Table 6. *Cont.*

Infants not given PN	n = 24	n = 10	n = 9	n = 5
% Via bolus doses				
Mean (SD)	63 (18)	78 (13)	49 (7) *	57 (21) [†]
Median (range)	58 (41–99)	77 (60–99)	48 (41–60) *	49 (44–94) [†]
% Via enteral feds				
Mean (SD)	37 (18)	22 (13)	51 (7) *	43 (21) [†]
Median (range)	42 (1–59)	23 (1–41)	52 (40–59) *	51 (7–56) [†]

Statistically-significant comparisons (using Mann-Whitney U test) are shown thus: * *versus* 0.5 mg IM group, $p <$ 0.0001; [†] *Versus* 0.5 mg IM group, $p <$ 0.05.

Considering infants who had not received any period of PN, the bolus dose for those receiving 0.5 mg phylloquinone after delivery represented ~80% of the total study intake (with enteral feeding ~20% of the total intake), whereas for the 0.2 mg groups the bolus dose and enteral feeding each comprised ~50% of the total phylloquinone intake.

4. Discussion

This is the first study to describe in detail the absolute phylloquinone intake by preterm infants from all sources during their first weeks of postnatal life. We quantified the relative proportional intake of phylloquinone from the various nutritional routes for infants who received PN and for those who did not receive PN. We found no differences in overall intakes between the three study groups that had been randomly allocated different phylloquinone regimens at birth. However after correcting for birth weight and days to study completion, the average daily intake of phylloquinone adjusted for birth weight was significantly lower for infants who had received the lower dose prophylactic bolus dose of 0.2 mg phylloquinone. We had speculated that the initial bolus doses of phylloquinone given for prophylaxis at birth would assume less importance as a source of the vitamin contributing to the overall intake at study completion, due to the increasing respective contributions to overall phylloquinone intake derived from other nutritional (dietary) sources. In infants who did not receive any PN, the bolus dose given at birth represented approximately 50% of the overall phylloquinone intake at study completion, compared to only approximately 20% in infants who had received PN.

Preterm infants represent a neglected group with respect to current knowledge of their phylloquinone intakes and recommendations for their nutritional requirements. As pointed out by Kumar *et al.* [14], published recommendations for vitamin K intakes and/or supplementation are specific for all ages except for preterm infants. As a result, recommendations for preterm infants are arbitrary and historically have ranged from 5 to 10 μg/kg/day in 1993 [15] and as high as 100 μg/kg/day in 1988 [16]. In this context it is important to note that the principles and knowledge base of dietary recommendations have changed over time. For example, the recommendations of 5–10 μg/kg/day for preterm infants in 1993 [15] came out during the lifespan of the 10th Edition of the US Food and Nutrition Board guidelines published in 1989, at which time they took the form of Recommended Daily Allowances (RDA) instead of the current Dietary Reference Intakes (DRI). At that time the RDA for term infants over the first six months was 5 μg/day, which in turn was based on the adult RDA of 1 μg/kg/day [17]. This means that the 5–10 μg/kg/day recommendation for preterm infants by Greer *et al.* [15] was 5–10 fold greater than the intake recommendations for term infants at that time. More recent guidelines published in 2005 recommended a phylloquinone intake of 8–10 μg/kg/day as an AI for preterm infants [18], representing the top end of the 1993 recommendations [15].

There is an inevitable degree of arbitrariness of recommendations even for healthy term infants. In the current United States recommendations published in 2001, the AI for healthy term infants is based on an average daily milk intake of 0.78 L and an average phylloquinone concentration in human milk of 2.5 μg/L [7]. This gave an AI of 2.0 μg/day after rounding [7]. The weak link in this calculation as a precise AI value lies with the fairly wide variations in the reported concentrations of phylloquinone in breast milk which taking the lower and upper values would result in estimated phylloquinone intakes of ~0.5 μg/day and 2.5 μg/day respectively [8].

Another weakness of current recommendations is that they are based solely on the phylloquinone content of breast milk. Although phylloquinone is the major vitamer of vitamin K in breast milk, it also contains a member of the menaquinone series, namely menaquinone-4 (MK-4) at concentrations that are about half that of phylloquinone [19,20]. There is also evidence that this MK-4 in breast milk is derived from dietary phylloquinone [20]. Future neonatal AI recommendations should also consider the contribution to intakes made by MK-4 as well as its potential contribution to neonatal vitamin K status.

Whether the dietary guidelines have been in the form of an RDA or AI, a common underlying assumption is that the infant is also given a prophylactic dose at birth in amounts recommended by the relevant paediatric societies [7,17]. For any individual infant, the optimal daily ongoing phylloquinone required from feeding will depend in part upon what prophylactic dose was given at birth and any postnatal supplementation received from PN. However there is also likely to be inter-individual variation in storage and metabolism.

For the purposes of discussion we have taken the most recent recommendation of 8–10 μg/kg/day [18] as a benchmark against which the phylloquinone intakes in this study can be compared. The median phylloquinone intake for infants who completed this study was approximately three-fold this recommended amount, and up to five to seven-fold more in some infants (Table 3).

For infants who received PN, there was little difference between allocation groups. The median of the average phylloquinone intake was three to four times the recommended amount, and all had an average phylloquinone intake that ranged between ~20–70 µg/kg/day, *i.e.*, two to seven times the daily recommendation (Table 4). For infants who did not receive any PN, the median average daily intake received by 0.5 mg IM group infants was approximately twice that currently recommended, whereas for infants in the 0.2 mg IM and 0.2 mg IV bolus groups the medians and ranges of average daily intakes were remarkably close to the currently recommended intakes of 8–10 µg/kg/day (Table 5).

For infants who did not receive any PN, the bolus dose(s) of phylloquinone constituted the major source of phylloquinone intake in the study period. In contrast, for infants who had received a period of PN by far their major intake source was, somewhat surprisingly, that delivered by the PN solution. For comparison, the ratio of median phylloquinone intake from PN to that from bolus doses was ~3:1.

In infants given PN, the median overall phylloquinone intake from enteral feeds was 6% (range: 0%–28%) of the total intake. In contrast in the infants not given PN the proportional intake from enteral feeds was significantly higher, and comprised 23% of overall intake for infants receiving a 0.5 mg bolus dose of phylloquinone after delivery, and 50% of overall intake for infants who received a 0.2 mg dose. Thus the contribution towards overall phylloquinone intake made by enteral feeding is small, but becomes more important in infants not given PN and particularly so for infants who receive lower bolus prophylactic doses (0.2 mg) and who do not receive PN.

These data show that in almost all infants, the average daily phylloquinone intake was in excess of the currently recommended amounts. The intakes were particularly high at three to four times the recommended amounts in all who received PN (irrespective of prophylactic dose), and were approximately twice the recommended amounts in infants given 0.5 mg prophylactic doses who did not receive PN. Only infants who received the 0.2 mg dose and who did not receive PN had an intake which approximated well to the current recommended daily phylloquinone intake of 8–10 µg/kg/day. Our data provide further evidence that the amounts of phylloquinone currently added to manufactured PN multivitamin solutions are excessive for the needs of preterm infants and should be reviewed.

Although there are no known clinical manifestations of toxicity from phylloquinone prophylaxis in neonates, nor indeed any known toxic effects in adults consuming high amounts of vitamin K [7], we previously found evidence of hepatic overload in a sub-group of preterm infants from our main study who had received the 0.5 mg rather than the 0.2 mg dose for prophylaxis [9]. The larger dose was more likely to be associated with elevated serum phylloquinone 2,3-epoxide concentrations, and suggested overload of the hepatic vitamin K 2,3-epoxide reductase enzyme in some preterm infants [2,9]. Furthermore, in a separate study we previously obtained evidence of metabolic overload in a subgroup of preterm infants who predominantly excreted the less extensively metabolised urinary 7C-side chain metabolite of vitamin K instead of the usual 5C-side chain metabolite [21]. This subgroup also had the highest serum concentrations of phylloquinone together with raised blood concentrations of phylloquinone 2,3-epoxide that is normally undetectable. This combination of increased excretion of the 7C-metabolite, high serum phylloquinone and raised phylloquinone 2,3-epoxide is indicative of a metabolic overload of both vitamin K recycling and catabolic pathways [21]. None of the infants in these studies who had biochemical evidence of overload showed any clinical manifestations of an overload status.

Because of their special nutritional requirements preterm babies are often provided with multivitamin supplements—including the fat-soluble vitamins A, D, and E—at the time of discharge home from the neonatal unit; these are usually continued throughout infancy. However post-discharge phylloquinone supplements are rarely provided to this group at present. Yet without adequate ongoing supplementation preterm infants may be at increased risk of developing vitamin K deficiency in early infancy, particularly if they continue to be exclusively breast fed. National surveillance studies of VKDB continue to report sporadic cases in preterm infants [6]. The most recent study in the United Kingdom and the Irish Republic reported a case of probable VKDB in a 24-week gestation infant

Nutrients **2015**, *7*, 8308–8320

who had received 0.4 mg/kg IM at birth [22]. This infant was primarily human milk fed and had no liver disease but suffered gastro-intestinal bleeding aged three months postnatal. Further study is required to assess whether phylloquinone supplements should be given routinely to preterm infants on discharge home from the neonatal unit.

5. Conclusions

In conclusion, this study of phylloquinone intake in the first weeks of life shows that all preterm infants received at least the minimum daily recommended intake of phylloquinone, but that most received an excessive intake. These data support the calls for the amount of phylloquinone added to standard PN multivitamin solutions to be reduced [14,23,24], and also support lower initial phylloquinone bolus doses being used for prophylaxis at birth [6]. For all infants studied, a bolus prophylactic phylloquinone dose of 0.2 mg (or ~0.3 mg/kg) was more appropriate than 0.5 mg because it resulted in an average daily intake over the study period closer to the currently recommended intake amounts. Also, average daily intakes were remarkably close to the currently recommended intake values in infants given 0.2 mg prophylaxis who did not receive any PN. In infants who do not receive PN, a 0.2 mg or 0.5 mg bolus dose given at birth represents a significant proportion of overall phylloquinone intake.

Future research in preterm infants should focus on their post-discharge vitamin K status and address the question whether additional supplementation with phylloquinone during infancy should also be routine.

Acknowledgments: This study was supported by the Hope Neonatal Unit Research Endowment Fund. We thank the staff of the Human Nutristasis Unit at Guy's and St Thomas's Hospital, London, and the respective biochemistry and haematology departments of the participating hospitals. We thank the paediatricians who allowed us to gather follow-up data on back-transferred infants. P.C. wishes to sincerely thank Mark Turner and Suresh Victor for very helpful constructive critical review of this and the other studies that comprised his doctoral thesis. Above all we sincerely thank all the parents who kindly allowed their infants to participate.

Author Contributions: The authors thank the American Academy of Pediatrics for kindly granting us permission to use and adapt the data presented in Table 3 from *Pediatrics* vol. 118, page e1663 [9], Copyright © 2006 by the AAP.

Author Contributions: S.J.M. conceived the idea for this study. P.C. collected the data, performed the statistical analyses, and wrote the first manuscript draft. All authors contributed to manuscript revisions, provided intellectual input in data interpretation, and approve of the final version. P.C. is guarantor.

Conflicts of Interest: Conflicts of Interest: P.C. gratefully received a small travel bursary from Roche (UK) that assisted presentation of this work in abstract form at the Pediatric Academic Societies annual scientific meeting, San Francisco, 2004. Roche had no input into the design, conduct or funding of this study, or the interpretation of data or decision to publish.

References

1. Shearer, M.J. Vitamin K metabolism and nutriture. *Blood Rev.* **1992**, *6*, 92–104. [CrossRef]
2. Clarke, P. A Comparison of Vitamin K Status in Preterm Infants Following Intravenous or Intramuscular Prophylaxis and the Effects of Feeding with Preterm Formula or Fortified Human Milk. Ph.D. Thesis, University of Manchester, Manchester, UK, 2008.
3. Lane, P.A.; Hathaway, W.E. Vitamin K in infancy. *J. Pediatr.* **1985**, *106*, 351–359. [CrossRef]
4. Sutor, A.H.; von Kries, R.; Cornelissen, E.A.; McNinch, A.W.; Andrew, M. Vitamin K deficiency bleeding (VKDB) in infancy. ISTH Pediatric/Perinatal Subcommittee. International Society on Thrombosis and Haemostasis. *Thromb. Haemost.* **1999**, *81*, 456–461. [PubMed]
5. Shearer, M.J. Vitamin K deficiency bleeding (VKDB) in early infancy. *Blood Rev.* **2009**, *23*, 49–59. [CrossRef] [PubMed]
6. Clarke, P. Vitamin K prophylaxis for preterm infants. *Early Hum. Dev.* **2010**, *86* (Suppl. 1), 17–20. [CrossRef] [PubMed]

7. Food and Nutrition Board, Institute of Medicine. *Dietary Reference Intakes for Vitamin A, Vitamin K, Arsenic, Boron, Chromium, Copper, Iodine, Iron, Manganese, Molybdenum, Nickel, Silicon, Vanadium, and Zinc*; National Academy Press: Washington, DC, USA, 2001.
8. Shearer, M.J.; Fu, X.; Booth, S.L. Vitamin K nutrition, metabolism, and requirements: Current concepts and future research. *Adv. Nutr.* **2012**, *3*, 182–195. [CrossRef] [PubMed]
9. Clarke, P.; Mitchell, S.J.; Wynn, R.; Sundaram, S.; Speed, V.; Gardener, E.; Roeves, D.; Shearer, M.J. Vitamin K prophylaxis for preterm infants: A randomized, controlled trial of 3 regimens. *Pediatrics* **2006**, *118*, e1657–e1666. [CrossRef] [PubMed]
10. Clarke, P.; Mitchell, S. Vitamin K prophylaxis in preterm infants: Current practices. *J. Thromb. Haemost.* **2003**, *1*, 384–386. [CrossRef] [PubMed]
11. Bolisetty, S.; Gupta, J.M.; Graham, G.G.; Salonikas, C.; Naidoo, D. Vitamin K in preterm breastmilk with maternal supplementation. *Acta Paediatr.* **1998**, *87*, 960–962. [CrossRef] [PubMed]
12. Haroon, Y.; Shearer, M.J.; Rahim, S.; Gunn, W.G.; McEnery, G.; Barkhan, P. The content of phylloquinone (vitamin K_1) in human milk, cows' milk and infant formula foods determined by high-performance liquid chromatography. *J. Nutr.* **1982**, *112*, 1105–1117. [PubMed]
13. Smith, R.J. (Fresenius Kabi Ltd, Runcorn, UK). Personal communication, 2004.
14. Kumar, D.; Greer, F.R.; Super, D.M.; Suttie, J.W.; Moore, J.J. Vitamin K status of premature infants: Implications for current recommendations. *Pediatrics* **2001**, *108*, 1117–1122. [CrossRef] [PubMed]
15. Greer, F. Vitamin K. In *Nutritional Needs of the Preterm Infant: Scientific Basis and Practical Guidelines*; Tsang, R.C., Lucas, A., Eds.; Williams & Wilkins: Baltimore, MD, USA, 1993; pp. 111–119.
16. Greene, H.L.; Hambidge, K.M.; Schanler, R.; Tsang, R.C. Guidelines for the use of vitamins, trace elements, calcium, magnesium, and phosphorus in infants and children receiving total parenteral nutrition: Report of the subcommittee on pediatric parenteral nutrient requirements from the committee on clinical practice issues of the American Society for Clinical Nutrition. *Am. J. Clin. Nutr.* **1988**, *48*, 1324–1342. [PubMed]
17. Food and Nutrition Board Commission on Life Sciences; National Research Council. *Recommended Dietary Allowances*, 10th ed.; National Academy Press: Washington, DC, USA, 1989.
18. Tsang, R.C. *Nutrition of the Preterm Infant: Scientific Basis and Practical Guidelines*, 2nd ed.; Digital Educational Publishing: Cincinnati, OH, USA, 2005.
19. Indyk, H.E.; Woollard, D.C. Vitamin K in milk and infant formulas: Determination and distribution of phylloquinone and menaquinone-4. *Analyst* **1997**, *122*, 465–469. [CrossRef] [PubMed]
20. Thijssen, H.H.; Drittij, M.J.; Vermeer, C.; Schoffelen, E. Menaquinone-4 in breast milk is derived from dietary phylloquinone. *Br. J. Nutr.* **2002**, *87*, 219–226. [CrossRef] [PubMed]
21. Harrington, D.J.; Clarke, P.; Card, D.J.; Mitchell, S.J.; Shearer, M.J. Urinary excretion of vitamin K metabolites in term and preterm infants: Relationship to vitamin K status and prophylaxis. *Pediatr. Res.* **2010**, *68*, 508–512. [CrossRef] [PubMed]
22. Busfield, A.; Samuel, R.; McNinch, A.; Tripp, J.H. Vitamin K deficiency bleeding after NICE guidance and withdrawal of Konakion Neonatal: British Paediatric Surveillance Unit study, 2006–2008. *Arch. Dis. Child.* **2013**, *98*, 41–47. [CrossRef] [PubMed]
23. Costakos, D.T.; Greer, F.R.; Love, L.A.; Dahlen, L.R.; Suttie, J.W. Vitamin K prophylaxis for premature infants: 1 mg *versus* 0.5 mg. *Am. J. Perinatol.* **2003**, *20*, 485–490. [PubMed]
24. Costakos, D.T.; Porte, M. Did "controversies concerning vitamin K and the newborn" cover all the controversies? *Pediatrics* **2004**, *113*, 1466–1467. [CrossRef] [PubMed]

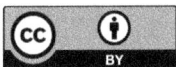

nutrients

MDPI

Article

Prevalence and Predictors of Functional Vitamin K Insufficiency in Mothers and Newborns in Uganda

Data Santorino [1,*], Mark J. Siedner [2], Juliet Mwanga-Amumpaire [1], Martin J. Shearer [3], Dominic J. Harrington [3] and Unni Wariyar [1]

1   Department of Pediatrics and Child Health, Mbarara University of Science and Technology,
     Plot 8-18 Mbarara–Kabale Road, P.O. Box 1410, Mbarara, Uganda; jmwanga@must.ac.ug (J.M.-A.);
     wariyarunniwariyar@gmail.com (U.W.)
2   Department of Medicine and Infectious Diseases, Massachusetts General Hospital and Harvard
     Medical School, 125 Nashua Street, Boston, MA 02114, USA; MSIEDNER@mgh.harvard.edu
3   Centre for Haemostasis and Thrombosis, St. Thomas' Hospital, Westminster Bridge Road, London SE1 7EH,
     UK; Martin.Shearer@gstt.nhs.uk (M.J.S.); Dominic.Harrington@viapath.co.uk (D.J.H.)
*   Correspondence: boymukedata@gmail.com; Tel.: +256-71221-4456; Fax: +256-4852-0782

Received: 10 July 2015 ; Accepted: 28 September 2015 ; Published: 16 October 2015

Abstract: Vitamin K deficiency bleeding (VKDB) in infancy is a serious but preventable cause of mortality or permanent disability. Lack of epidemiologic data for VKDB in sub-Saharan Africa hinders development and implementation of effective prevention strategies. We used convenience sampling to consecutively enroll mothers delivering in a southwestern Uganda Hospital. We collected socio-demographic and dietary information, and paired samples of maternal venous and neonatal cord blood for the immunoassay of undercarboxylated prothrombin (PIVKA-II), a sensitive marker of functional vitamin K (VK) insufficiency. We used univariable and multivariable logistic regression models to identify predictors of VK insufficiency. We detected PIVKA-II of $\geqslant$0.2 AU (Arbitrary Units per mL)/mL (indicative of VK insufficiency) in 33.3% (47/141) of mothers and 66% (93/141) of newborns. Importantly, 22% of babies had PIVKA-II concentrations $\geqslant$5.0 AU/mL, likely to be associated with abnormal coagulation indices. We found no significant predictors of newborn VK insufficiency, including infant weight (AOR (adjusted odds ratio) 1.85, 95% CI (confidence interval) 0.15–22.49), gender (AOR 0.54, 95% CI 0.26–1.11), term birth (AOR 0.72, 95% CI 0.20–2.62), maternal VK-rich diet (AOR 1.13, 95% CI 0.55–2.35) or maternal VK insufficiency (AOR 0.99, 95% CI 0.47–2.10). VK insufficiency is common among mothers and newborn babies in southwestern Uganda, which in one fifth of babies nears overt deficiency. Lack of identifiable predictors of newborn VK insufficiency support strategies for universal VK prophylaxis to newborns to prevent VKDB.

Keywords: vitamin K; undercarboxylated prothrombin; deficiency; insufficiency; newborn; bleeding; haemorrhage; prophylaxis

1. Introduction

Vitamin K Deficiency Bleeding (VKDB) in infancy is a rare but potentially serious worldwide problem with a high risk of mortality or permanent disability, primarily due to the high incidence of intracranial haemorrhage (ICH) of the later onset syndrome [1–5]. It is a disease of breastfeeding infants [1,6–9] and can be prevented by administration of vitamin K (VK) to newborns shortly after birth [1,9–12]. VKDB is classified according to the age of presentation as early, classical and late [1]. Early VKDB occurs in the first 24 h after birth, it is generally rare and often associated with maternal anticoagulant and or anticonvulsant usage during pregnancy. Classical and late VKDB occur between days 2 to 7, and days 8 to 6 months of life, respectively [9]. In classical VKDB, bleeding typically occurs from the gastrointestinal tract, umbilicus, skin, nose or after circumcision [1,9,10] while in late VKDB, bleeding predominantly occurs within the brain with prevalence rates of ICH as high as 60%–80% [2,3]. Reported incidence rates of classical and late VKDB over the last 50 years in infants who have not been given VK prophylaxis vary widely across different countries.

Apart from reflecting the lack of standardization for case definitions [4,10], there is evidence that the incidence of VKDB reflects economic and nutritional status [6,8,9], social customs such as male circumcision [6,13], and probably genetic variations such as those known to influence the metabolism and intracellular recycling of VK [14]. For classical VKDB, the extremely high incidence rates of 1.7% in Cincinnati, USA in the 1960s [6] and 0.8% in Addis Ababa, Ethiopia from 1982–1991 [8] are noteworthy for the economic deprivation of the populations studied. Incidence rates were strongly influenced by male circumcision in the Cincinnati study [6] but not in the Addis Ababa study where circumcision occurred after 7 days of age and outside the window of classical VKDB [8]. In contrast, the incidence of classical and late VKDB from national surveys in two European countries (Germany and the British Isles) in the late 1980s reveal a markedly lower incidence of 4–7 cases per 10^5 births in infants given no VK prophylaxis [9,10,15]. A much higher prevalence of late VKDB has been reported in countries of South East Asia (e.g., Japan, Thailand, Malaysia, Vietnam and China) with incidence rates ranging from 11 to 116 cases per 10^5 births [3,4,9,16]. There is no data for the prevalence of late VKDB in sub-Saharan Africa. Apart from exclusive breastfeeding [1,6–9], other known risk factors for classical and late VKDB are diarrhea, prolonged antibiotic use and the presence of underlying diseases (e.g., biliary atresia, alpha-1-antitrypsin deficiency, cystic fibrosis) causing malabsorption of VK [1,5,17,18]. Feeding infants with milk formulas (both unsupplemented and supplemented) offers a high protection against VKDB owing to their higher VK content compared to breast milk [19,20] resulting in a greatly superior VK status of formula-fed infants [21].

The lack of data about the epidemiology of VKDB in sub-Saharan Africa has limited the development and implementation of guidelines for prevention of VKDB. As such, VK is not typically listed as a priority drug for children by programmatic organizations such as in the World Health Organization's Model Medicines list for children [13]. To estimate the incidence of neonatal haemorrhage in Uganda, we performed a retrospective chart review from June–August 2010 at Mbarara Regional Referral Hospital (MRRH) in Southwestern Uganda where VK prophylaxis is not routinely administered to newborns at birth. We found a 6.6% incidence of haemorrhage among all neonatal admissions to the Hospital during the observation period (unpublished data). This was higher than the neonatal haemorrhage prevalence previously reported by Lulseged in Ethiopia [8]. Based on this high prevalence of newborn haemorrhage, we conducted a study to determine the epidemiology and predictors of functional VK insufficiency among mothers and their newborns at MRRH. We define "functional VK insufficiency" as a nutritional state in which the hepatic stores of vitamin K are insufficient to ensure full gamma-glutamyl carboxylation of the VK-dependent procoagulant proteins, factors II (prothrombin), VII, IX and X. In states of VK insufficiency, functionally defective undercarboxylated species of factors such as prothrombin are released into the bloodstream where they can be measured [9,22]. Historically the collective name for these undercarboxylated species is PIVKA (Proteins Induced by vitamin K Absence or Antagonism). In the present study functional VK insufficiency was assessed by the measurement of undercarboxylated prothrombin (PIVKA-II) which has been shown to be a highly sensitive and selective functional marker of VK status with respect to its coagulation function [9,22]. Our choice of PIVKA-II has several advantages over traditional biomarkers of VK status. First, global coagulation tests such as the prothrombin time (PT) or activated partial thromboplastin time (APTT) are insufficiently sensitive to detect early VK insufficiency. As reviewed by Suttie [23], a 1–2 second increase in the PT only occurs when the percent of active (carboxylated) prothrombin has dropped to below 50% of normal whereas immunoassays of PIVKA-II can readily detect undercarboxylated species of prothrombin when there are no observable changes in the PT. For example, even when the concentration of active prothrombin is as high as 90% there is a 20-fold increase in the concentrations of PIVKA-II as measured by an immunoassay such as that used in our study [23]. Second, a prolonged PT lacks specificity for VK insufficiency: for example in a VK supplementation trial carried out in 98 preterm infants, 21 infants who had a significantly prolonged PT were shown to have satisfactory VK status as assessed by serum PIVKA-II and phylloquinone measurements [24]. Thus while a prolonged PT (and APTT) are expected findings in advanced vitamin K deficiency, they have important limitations as early biomarkers of VK insufficiency.

2. Experimental Section

2.1. Enrollment and Study Procedures

We consecutively enrolled mothers delivering during daytime hours on the peripartum ward at MRRH. Women in active labour were consented before the onset of second stage of labor and were followed until delivery for blood collection at birth. Women with self-reported liver disease, visible jaundice or taking warfarin were excluded [25,26]. We used interviewer administered structured questionnaires to collect socio-demographic data. We also recorded gestational age, newborn weight, and newborn gender. We assessed maternal diet using a 22-item non-validated, and non-quantitative food frequency questionnaire to determine intake frequency of VK rich food [27]. Participants stated daily, weekly and monthly frequency with which they ate VK-rich foods using an interviewer administered food frequency questionnaire. We defined a frequent VK rich food intake as five or more servings per week of green vegetables and or peas.

2.2. Blood Collection and Laboratory Procedures

Maternal venous blood from the brachial vein and newborn cord blood were collected immediately at birth in the delivery room. Serum was separated and stored at negative 70 degrees Celsius. At the conclusion of study procedures, samples were transported by courier on dry ice to the Centre for Haemostasis and Thrombosis, Guy's and St. Thomas' Hospital Foundation Trust in London for analysis. We measured undercarboxylated prothrombin (factor II) also known as Protein Induced by vitamin K Absence-II (PIVKA-II) serum concentrations using a conformation-specific PIVKA-II monoclonal antibody with a sandwich ELISA [22,28–30]. Concentrations of PIVKA-II were expressed as Arbitrary Units per mL (AU/mL) with 1 AU/mL being equivalent to 1 µg of multiple species of uncarboxylated or partially carboxylated prothrombin purified by electrophoresis [22,28–30]. Using this same immunoassay, PIVKA-II concentrations in healthy VK replete adults and infants are <0.20 AU/mL. Newborn babies with PIVKA-II values ≥0.20 AU/mL are defined as having vitamin K insufficiency with values ≥5.0 AU/mL approaching a state of overt VK deficiency that are likely to be associated with abnormal coagulation indices and which are clinically relevant to bleeding risk [22]. However, it was not possible to perform any coagulation tests (e.g., prothrombin time) in our study.

2.3. Statistical Analyses

Our primary outcome was VK insufficiency at birth as defined by PIVKA-II of greater than or equal to 0.2 AU/mL. Exposures of interest were newborn weight, gender, gestational age [31] and maternal intake of VK rich foods [25]. We fitted univariable and multivariable logistic regression models to estimate associations between the primary outcome of interest (raised PIVKA-II) and exposures of interest. All variables for which we had a priori reason to consider as potential confounders or correlates of vitamin K insufficiency were maintained in the multivariable model. A *p*-value of less than or equal to 0.05 was considered statistically significant [32]. Data analysis was performed with Stata Version 12 (Statcorp, College Station, TX, USA).

2.4. Ethics Statement

All participants gave signed informed consent. All babies received intramuscular prophylactic VK after blood sample collection. The study procedures were reviewed and approved by Mbarara University Faculty of Medicine Research and Ethics committee, the Institutional Review Committee at the Mbarara University of Science and Technology and the Uganda National Council for Science and Technology.

3. Results

We enrolled 141 mother-baby pairs over a period of 4 months (June–September). The median maternal age was 25 years (Interquartile range: 21–29 years). All mothers approached to participate in the study, gave their written consent. All samples analyzed yielded useable laboratory values. Sixty six percent (93/141) of mothers came from town/urban settings mainly from Mbarara town where MRRH is located. Ninety six (136/141) of the women were married, 57.5% had no secondary education, and 33.3% were primigravidae. Sixty four percent of babies (90/141) were male, 9% (13/141) were preterm (born before 37 completed weeks of amenorrhea) and 3% (4/141) had low birth weight (<2.5 kg). The median birth weight was 3.2 kg (IQR: 2.9–3.8 kg). Spontaneous vaginal delivery accounted for 75% (107/141) of deliveries, caesarian section, 23.4% (33/141) and only one baby was delivered by vacuum extraction. VK insufficiency defined by a detectable PIVKA-II of ⩾0.2 AU/mL was present in 33% (47/141) of mothers and 66% (93/141) of babies as shown in Table 1. Six sets of twins were enrolled in the study, there was no PIVKA-II value-category difference between twin siblings, therefore, for the purposes of this study, the PIVKA-II value of the first-born twin were used for analysis. Highly elevated, concentrations of PIVKA-II (⩾5.0 AU/mL) indicative of likely abnormal coagulation [22] were found in 22% (31/141) of newborns but in none of their mothers. No newborn babies had detectable postpartum bleeding before hospital discharge. However, all newborn babies received intramuscular vitamin K within one hour of delivery during the period of the study irrespective of study enrolment status.

Table 1. Maternal dietary habits and newborn characteristics at birth for the total cohort and by presence of vitamin K (VK) insufficiency.

Variable	Total Cohort (n = 282)	PIVKA-II ⩾ 0.2 AU/mL [ℓ] (n = 140)	PIVKA-II < 0.2 AU/mL [π] (n = 142)	p-Value
Mothers, % (n)	100 (141)	33 (47)	67 (94)	
Newborn babies, % (n)	100 (141)	66 (93)	34 (48)	
Female newborn, % (n)	36 (51)	57 (29)	43 (22)	0.086
Low birth weight (<2.5 kg), % (n)	3 (4)	75 (3)	25 (1)	0.699
Preterm, % (n)	9 (13)	62 (8)	38 (5)	0.724
Maternal VK-rich intake *, % (n)	40 (56)	32 (18)	68 (38)	0.808

* Vitamin K-rich intake as defined by intake of greens and or peas five or more times a week; [ℓ] PIVKA-II: Protein induced in vitamin K absence, with a level ⩾ 0.2 Arbitrary Units indicative of vitamin K insufficiency; [π] PIVKA-II level < 0.20 AU/mL indicative of normal vitamin K status. AU/mL: Arbitrary Units per mL.

We found no significant predictors of newborn VK insufficiency among newborn or maternal characteristics including: infant weight (AOR (adjusted odds ratio) 1.85, 95% CI (confidence interval) 0.15–22.49), gender (AOR 0.54, 95% CI 0.26–1.11), term birth (AOR 0.72, 95% CI 0.20–2.62), maternal VK-rich diet (AOR 1.13, 95% CI 0.55–2.35) and maternal VK insufficiency (AOR 0.99, 95% CI 0.47–2.10) as shown in Table 2.

Table 2. Univariate and multivariate logistic regression models of correlates of vitamin K (VK) insufficiency in newborns, as defined by a PIVKA II concentration $\geqslant 0.2$ AU/mL.

Characteristic	Univariable Logistic Regression		Multivariable Logistic Regression	
	AOR (95% CI)	*p*-Value	AOR (95% CI)	*p*-Value
Female newborn	0.54 (0.26–1.09)	0.088	0.54 (0.26–1.11)	0.093
Low birth weight (<2,500 g)	1.57 (0.16–15.48)	0.701	1.85 (0.15–22.49)	0.630
Preterm (<37 weeks of gestation)	0.81 (0.25–2.62)	0.725	0.72 (0.20–2.62)	0.619
Maternal VK insufficiency	1.00 (0.48–2.09)	1.000	0.99 (0.47–2.10)	0.983
Maternal VK-rich intake *	0.915 (045–1.88)	0.808	1.13 (0.55–2.35)	0.737

* Vitamin K rich intake as defined by intake of greens and or peas five or more times a week; PIVKA-II: Protein induced in vitamin K absence, with a level $\geqslant 0.2$ Arbitrary Units indicative of vitamin K insufficiency. AOR: adjusted odds ratio; CI: confidence interval.

Up to 61.5% (8/13) of all premature babies had detectable PIVKA-II and 23% (3/13) had highly elevated PIVKA-II values ($\geqslant 5$ AU/mL).

4. Discussion

Among mothers delivering at a publicly-operated referral hospital in rural southwestern Uganda, VK insufficiency is very common in both mothers (33%) and their newborns (66%). Our study is the first to characterize the prevalence of VK insufficiency in a Sub-Saharan Africa setting using the gold standard measurement (PIVKA-II assay) for functional VK insufficiency with respect to its coagulation function. We found no maternal or infant clinical or dietary predictors of VK insufficiency, implying that routine, prophylactic VK administration should continue to be the standard of care for prevention of VKDB in newborns. Given the high prevalence of VK insufficiency and potential devastating effects of VKDB, availability of VK should be prioritized in resource-limited settings, and especially in health facilities that perform perinatal care.

The 33% prevalence of functional VK insufficiency among mothers in our study is notable and higher than other previous reports. For example, using the same PIVKA-II assay, Chuansumrit *et al.*, found a prevalence of VK insufficiency of 12% among mothers delivering at Ramathibodi hospital in Thailand [22], a country in which the incidence of VKDB was estimated to be 72 cases per 10^5 births before universal prophylaxis was introduced [3]. Lower dietary intakes of VK by Ugandan mothers compared to Thai mothers may explain the high prevalence of VK insufficiency in our study population. However, the two studies used different methods to measure VK intake, limiting direct comparability.

Similarly, the prevalence of detectable PIVKA-II of 66% in newborn babies in our study was much higher than the 16% prevalence in the Thai study [22] or the 23% prevalence in a study of preterm infants in England [29], all done with the same PIVKA-II assay. Another notable difference between this Ugandan and the Thai study was that 22.0% (31/141) of Ugandan babies had clinically significant PIVKA-II concentrations ($\geqslant 5.0$ AU/mL) compared to 1.5% (10/683) of Thai babies despite the fact that both cohorts were comparable in their birth characteristics. PIVKA-II concentrations greater than 5 AU/mL are likely associated with abnormal coagulopathy and an increased risk for spontaneous bleeding [22].

We found no consistent correlation between the presence or absence of detectable PIVKA-II in cord blood with its presence or absence in the respective paired sample from the mother. In other words, the concentration of PIVKA-II in the mother was not predictive of the concentration in her newborn baby. We should emphasize however that while highly raised PIVKA-II concentrations ($\geqslant 5.0$ AU/mL) were found in 22% of newborns, none of their mothers showed evidence of such a similarly severe degree of VK insufficiency. In addition, the frequency of intakes of VK-rich foods in mothers was not predictive of the functional VK status of their newborns. This lack of correlation between maternal and newborn vitamin K status has been reported previously in a much smaller European study of PIVKA-II measurements in 22 infant-mother pairs [33], but the reasons for this disparity remain unexplained. Certainly, case reports have linked severe maternal dietary VK deficiency to intracranial bleeding in fetal life showing the importance of maintaining adequate maternal intakes of vitamin K during pregnancy [34,35]. Importantly, the lack of clear predictors or correlates of VKD in women or their babies reinforce the need for routine VK administration to newborn babies independent of maternal or newborn factors to help prevent VKDB.

We acknowledge limitations to our study, most importantly the use of a non-standardized dietary questionnaire for determination of VK intake. It should also be noted that our sample size and confidence intervals did not exclude the possibility of a type II error. For example, our estimated adjusted odds of VK insufficiency for each kilogram of birth weight was 1.85 (95% CI 0.15–22.49), suggesting that a significant effect of birth weight on VK insufficiency might have been detected with a larger sample size. To address these shortcomings and further explore these relationships, we intend to conduct a multicenter clinical study to measure VK intakes using a more accurate dietary assessment method (e.g., weighed dietary records) and the prevalence of VK insufficiency in pregnant women and their newborn babies in Sub-Saharan Africa. This additional data will broaden our understanding of the epidemiology of VK intake and deficiency, and help guide recommendations for VK requirements and administration in the region. The study also is characterized by a convenience sampling method in a regional referral Hospital located in an urban area in southwestern Uganda, which might affect generalizability to mothers in rural areas or those without means to reach a referral hospital.

5. Conclusions

Functional VK insufficiency evidenced by raised PIVKA-II is common among mothers and newborn babies in southwestern Uganda. Worryingly, 22% of babies had highly elevated PIVKA-II concentrations that are likely to be associated with an increased risk of bleeding. We found no predictors of newborn VK insufficiency, supporting a strategy of universal administration of newborn vitamin K prophylaxis to prevent VKDB.

Acknowledgments: We would like to thank Mbarara University of Science and Technology, The German Academic Exchange Service and the Centre for Haemostasis and Thrombosis, St. Thomas' Hospital, London for funding different aspects of this study either directly or indirectly. Additionally, we wish to thank Kieran Voong of the Centre for Haemostasis and Thrombosis, St Thomas' Hospital for performing the PIVKA-II assays.

Author Contributions: Santorino Data: Data took the lead in study conception and design, data and sample collection and analysis, led data analysis, wrote the first draft of the manuscript, and participated in editing of subsequent drafts. Unni Wariyar: Wariyar assisted in study conception, editing of manuscript drafts and approved the final version for submission. Martin Shearer: Shearer advised on study methodology, supervised analysis and interpretation of PIVKA-II measurements, edited manuscript drafts and approved the final version for submission. Juliet Mwanga-Amumpaire: Mwanga-Amumpaire helped in supervision and quality control during data collection, edited manuscript drafts and approved the final version for submission. Mark Siedner: Siedner assisted in data analysis, interpretation, edited manuscript drafts and approved the final version for submission. Dominic Harrington: Harrington assisted in sample analysis, edited manuscript drafts and approved the final version for submission.

Conflicts of Interest: The authors declare no conflict of interest.

References

1. Lane, P.A.; Hathaway, W.E. Vitamin K in infancy. *J. Pediatr.* **1985**, *106*, 351–359. [CrossRef]
2. Loughnan, P.M.; McDougall, P.N. Epidemiology of late onset haemorrhagic disease: A pooled data analysis. *J. Paediatr. Child Health* **1993**, *29*, 177–181. [CrossRef] [PubMed]
3. Chuansumrit, A.; Isarangkura, P.; Hathirat, P. Vitamin K deficiency bleeding in Thailand: A 32-year history. *Southeast Asian J. Trop. Med. Public Health* **1998**, *29*, 649–654. [PubMed]
4. Danielsson, N.; Hoa, D.P.; Thang, N.V.; Vos, T.; Loughnan, P.M. Intracranial haemorrhage due to late onset vitamin K deficiency bleeding in Hanoi province, Vietnam. *Arch. Dis. Child Fetal Neonatal Ed.* **2004**, *89*, F546–F550. [CrossRef] [PubMed]

5. Elalfy, M.; Elagouza, I.; Ibrahim, F.; Abdelmessieh, S.; Gadallah, M. Intracranial haemorrhage is linked to late onset vitamin K deficiency in infants aged 2–24 weeks. *Acta Paediatr.* **2014**, *17*, 12598. [CrossRef] [PubMed]
6. Sutherland, J.M.; Glueck, H.I.; Gleser, G. Hemorrhagic disease of the newborn: Breast feeding as a necessary factor in the pathogenesis. *Am. J. Dis. Child* **1967**, *113*, 524–533. [CrossRef] [PubMed]
7. Greer, F.R. Vitamin K status of lactating mothers and their infants. *Acta Paediatr. Suppl.* **1999**, *88*, 95–103. [CrossRef] [PubMed]
8. Lulseged, S. Haemorrhagic disease of the newborn: A review of 127 cases. *Ann. Trop. Paediatr.* **1993**, *13*, 331–336. [PubMed]
9. Shearer, M.J. Vitamin K deficiency bleeding (VKDB) in early infancy. *Blood Rev.* **2009**, *23*, 49–59. [CrossRef] [PubMed]
10. Von Kries, R.; Hanawa, Y. Neonatal vitamin K prophylaxis. Report of Scientific and Standardization Subcommittee on Perinatal Haemostasis. *Thromb. Haemost.* **1993**, *69*, 293–295. [PubMed]
11. Martin-Lopez, J.E.; Carlos-Gil, A.M.; Rodriguez-Lopez, R.; Villegas-Portero, R.; Luque-Romero, L.; Flores-Moreno, S. Prophylactic vitamin K for vitamin K deficiency bleeding of the newborn. *Farm Hosp.* **2011**, *35*, 148–155. [CrossRef] [PubMed]
12. Watson, R.R.; Grimble, G.; Preedy, V.R.; Zibaldi, S. *Nutrition in Infancy*; Springer Science: New York, NY, USA, 2013.
13. Plank, R.M.; Steinmetz, T.; Sokal, D.C.; Shearer, M.J.; Data, S. Vitamin K deficiency bleeding and early infant male circumcision in Africa. *Obstet. Gynecol.* **2013**, *122*, 503–505. [CrossRef] [PubMed]
14. Shearer, M.J.; Fu, X.; Booth, S.L. Vitamin K nutrition, metabolism, and requirements: Current concepts and future research. *Adv. Nutr.* **2012**, *3*, 182–195. [CrossRef] [PubMed]
15. McNinch, A.W.; Tripp, J.H. Haemorrhagic disease of the newborn in the British Isles: Two year prospective study. *BMJ* **1991**, *303*, 1105–1109. [CrossRef] [PubMed]
16. Choo, K.E.; Tan, K.K.; Chuah, S.P.; Ariffin, W.A.; Gururaj, A. Haemorrhagic disease in newborn and older infants: A study in hospitalized children in Kelantan, Malaysia. *Ann. Trop. Paediatr.* **1994**, *14*, 231–237. [PubMed]
17. Van Hasselt, P.M.; Kok, K.; Vorselaars, A.D.; van Vlerken, L.; Nieuwenhuys, E.; de Koning, T.J.; de Vries, R.A.; Houwen, R.H. Vitamin K deficiency bleeding in cholestatic infants with alpha-1-antitrypsin deficiency. *Arch. Dis. Child Fetal Neonatal Ed.* **2009**, *94*, 3. [CrossRef] [PubMed]
18. Miyao, M.; Abiru, H.; Ozeki, M.; Kotani, H.; Tsuruyama, T.; Kobayashi, N.; Omae, T.; Osamura, T.; Tamaki, K. Subdural hemorrhage: A unique case involving secondary vitamin K deficiency bleeding due to biliary atresia. *Forensic Sci. Int.* **2012**, *221*, 16. [CrossRef] [PubMed]
19. Haroon, Y.; Shearer, M.J.; Rahim, S.; Gunn, W.G.; McEnery, G.; Barkhan, P. The content of phylloquinone (vitamin K1) in human milk, cows' milk and infant formula foods determined by high-performance liquid chromatography. *J. Nutr.* **1982**, *112*, 1105–1117. [PubMed]
20. Von Kries, R.; Shearer, M.; McCarthy, P.T.; Haug, M.; Harzer, G.; Gobel, U. Vitamin K1 content of maternal milk: Influence of the stage of lactation, lipid composition, and vitamin K1 supplements given to the mother. *Pediatr. Res.* **1987**, *22*, 513–517. [CrossRef] [PubMed]
21. Greer, F.R.; Marshall, S.; Cherry, J.; Suttie, J.W. Vitamin K status of lactating mothers, human milk, and breast-feeding infants. *Pediatrics* **1991**, *88*, 751–756. [PubMed]
22. Chuansumrit, A.; Plueksacheeva, T.; Hanpinitsak, S.; Sangwarn, S.; Chatvutinun, S.; Suthutvoravut, U.; Herabutya, Y.; Shearer, M.J. Prevalence of subclinical vitamin K deficiency in Thai newborns: Relationship to maternal phylloquinone intakes and delivery risk. *Arch. Dis. Child Fetal Neonatal Ed.* **2010**, *95*, 11. [CrossRef] [PubMed]
23. Suttie, J.W. Vitamin K and human nutrition. *J. Am. Diet. Assoc.* **1992**, *92*, 585–590. [PubMed]
24. Clarke, P.; Mitchell, S.J.; Sundaram, S.; Sharma, V.; Wynn, R.; Shearer, M.J. Vitamin K status of preterm infants with a prolonged prothrombin time. *Acta Paediatr.* **2005**, *94*, 1822–1824. [CrossRef] [PubMed]
25. Booth, S.L.; Centurelli, M.A. Vitamin K: A practical guide to the dietary management of patients on warfarin. *Nutr. Rev.* **1999**, *57*, 288–296. [CrossRef] [PubMed]
26. Mager, D.R.; McGee, P.L.; Furuya, K.N.; Roberts, E.A. Prevalence of vitamin K deficiency in children with mild to moderate chronic liver disease. *J. Pediatr. Gastroenterol. Nutr.* **2006**, *42*, 71–76. [CrossRef] [PubMed]

27. Kowalkowska, J.; Slowinska, M.A.; Slowinski, D.; Dlugosz, A.; Niedzwiedzka, E.; Wadolowska, L. Comparison of a full food-frequency questionnaire with the three-day unweighted food records in young Polish adult women: Implications for dietary assessment. *Nutrients* **2013**, *5*, 2747–2776. [CrossRef] [PubMed]

28. Belle, M.; Brebant, R.; Guinet, R.; Leclercq, M. Production of a new monoclonal antibody specific to human des-gamma-carboxyprothrombin in the presence of calcium ions. Application to the development of a sensitive ELISA-test. *J. Immunoass.* **1995**, *16*, 213–229. [CrossRef]

29. Clarke, P.; Mitchell, S.J.; Wynn, R.; Sundaram, S.; Speed, V.; Gardener, E.; Roeves, D.; Shearer, M.J. Vitamin K prophylaxis for preterm infants: A randomized, controlled trial of 3 regimens. *Pediatrics* **2006**, *118*, 13. [CrossRef] [PubMed]

30. O'Shaughnessy, D.; Allen, C.; Woodcock, T.; Pearce, K.; Harvey, J.; Shearer, M. Echis time, under-carboxylated prothrombin and vitamin K status in intensive care patients. *Clin. Lab. Haematol.* **2003**, *25*, 397–404. [CrossRef] [PubMed]

31. Salonvaara, M.; Riikonen, P.; Kekomaki, R.; Vahtera, E.; Mahlamaki, E.; Kiekara, O.; Heinonen, K. Intraventricular haemorrhage in very-low-birthweight preterm infants: Association with low prothrombin activity at birth. *Acta Paediatr.* **2005**, *94*, 807–811. [CrossRef] [PubMed]

32. Hosmer, D.W.; Lemeshow, S. *Applied Logistic Regression*; Wiley: New York, NY, USA, 1989.

33. Von Kries, R.; Shearer, M.J.; Widdershoven, J.; Motohara, K.; Umbach, G.; Gobel, U. Des-gamma-carboxyprothrombin (PIVKA II) and plasma vitamin K1 in newborns and their mothers. *Thromb. Haemost.* **1992**, *68*, 383–387. [PubMed]

34. Kawamura, Y.; Kawamata, K.; Shinya, M.; Higashi, M.; Niiro, M.; Douchi, T. Vitamin K deficiency in hyperemesis gravidarum as a potential cause of fetal intracranial hemorrhage and hydrocephalus. *Prenat. Diagn.* **2008**, *28*, 59–61. [CrossRef] [PubMed]

35. Eventov-Friedman, S.; Klinger, G.; Shinwell, E.S. Third trimester fetal intracranial hemorrhage owing to vitamin K deficiency associated with hyperemesis gravidarum. *J. Pediatr. Hematol. Oncol.* **2009**, *31*, 985–988. [CrossRef] [PubMed]

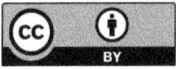

nutrients

MDPI

Article

Menaquinone-7 Supplementation to Reduce Vascular Calcification in Patients with Coronary Artery Disease: Rationale and Study Protocol (VitaK-CAC Trial)

Liv M. Vossen [1,2,*], Leon J. Schurgers [3], Bernard J. van Varik [1], Bas L. J. H. Kietselaer [4], Cees Vermeer [5], Johannes G. Meeder [6], Braim M. Rahel [6], Yvonne J. M. van Cauteren [6], Ge A. Hoffland [7], Roger J. M. W. Rennenberg [1], Koen D. Reesink [3], Peter W. de Leeuw [1,2,3] and Abraham A. Kroon [1,3]

[1] Department of Internal Medicine, Maastricht University Medical Centre (MUMC+), Maastricht 6229HX, The Netherlands; b.vanvarik@maastrichtuniversity.nl (B.J.V.); r.rennenberg@mumc.nl (R.J.M.W.R.); p.deleeuw@maastrichtuniversity.nl (P.W.L.); aa.kroon@mumc.nl (A.A.K.)
[2] Department of Internal Medicine, Zuyderland Medical Centre, Sittard 6162BG, The Netherlands
[3] Department of Biochemistry, Cardiovascular Research Institute Maastricht (CARIM), University of Maastricht, Maastricht 6229ER, The Netherlands; l.schurgers@maastrichtuniversity.nl (L.J.S.); k.reesink@maastrichtuniversity.nl (K.D.R.)
[4] Departments of Cardiology and Radiology, Maastricht University Medical Centre (MUMC+), Maastricht 6229HX, The Netherlands; b.kietselaer@mumc.nl
[5] R&D Group VitaK, Maastricht University, Maastricht 6229EV, The Netherlands; c.vermeer@vitak.com
[6] Department of Cardiology, VieCuri Medical Centre, Venlo 5912 BL, The Netherlands; jmeeder@viecuri.nl (J.G.M.); brahel@viecuri.nl (B.M.R.); yvonne.cauteren@mumc.nl (Y.J.M.C.)
[7] Department of Radiology, VieCuri Medical Centre, Venlo 5912BL, The Netherlands; ghoffland@viecuri.nl
* Correspondence: liv.vossen@mumc.nl; Tel.: +31-43-3877366; Fax: +31-43-3875642

Received: 5 August 2015 ; Accepted: 10 October 2015 ; Published: 28 October 2015

Abstract: Coronary artery calcification (CAC) develops early in the pathogenesis of atherosclerosis and is a strong and independent predictor of cardiovascular disease (CVD). Arterial calcification is caused by an imbalance in calcification regulatory mechanisms. An important inhibitor of calcification is vitamin K-dependent matrix Gla protein (MGP). Both preclinical and clinical studies have shown that inhibition of the vitamin K-cycle by vitamin K antagonists (VKA) results in elevated uncarboxylated MGP (ucMGP) and subsequently in extensive arterial calcification. This led us to hypothesize that vitamin K supplementation may slow down the progression of calcification. To test this, we designed the VitaK-CAC trial which analyses effects of menaquinone-7 (MK-7) supplementation on progression of CAC. The trial is a double-blind, randomized, placebo-controlled trial including patients with coronary artery disease (CAD). Patients with a baseline Agatston CAC-score between 50 and 400 will be randomized to an intervention-group (360 microgram MK-7) or a placebo group. Treatment duration will be 24 months. The primary endpoint is the difference in CAC-score progression between both groups. Secondary endpoints include changes in arterial structure and function, and associations with biomarkers. We hypothesize that treatment with MK-7 will slow down or arrest the progression of CAC and that this trial may lead to a treatment option for vascular calcification and subsequent CVD.

Keywords: vascular calcification; coronary artery calcification; matrix gla protein; vitamin K2; menaquinone-7

Nutrients **2015**, *7*, 8905–8915

1. Introduction and Rationale

Coronary artery calcification (CAC) develops early in the pathogenesis of atherosclerosis [1] and is a strong and independent risk marker of cardiovascular complications [2,3]. Moreover, annual changes in CAC-score are thought to reflect changes in atherosclerotic plaque burden [1,3]. Vascular calcification is not merely a passive phenomenon but rather, is caused by an imbalance between the mechanisms that promote and inhibit the deposition of calcium in the vascular wall. In this regard the vitamin K dependent Matrix Gla protein (MGP) plays an important role [3–7] as an inhibitor of soft tissue calcification, as was first shown in MGP-deficient mice [4]. Inhibition of the vitamin-K-cycle by vitamin K antagonists (VKA) results in the accumulation of uncarboxylated MGP which is biologically inactive. This is associated with extensive arterial calcification in experimental animals [5,8]. In line with the experimental data, humans on VKA treatment also tend to have more aortic and valve calcification in comparison to patients not on anticoagulant therapy [9]. Furthermore, observational studies show that long-term use of VKA is associated with both increased extra-coronary vascular calcification [10] and increased coronary calcification [11]. Because VKA induce vascular calcification, vitamin K supplementation presents an attractive treatment option to reduce vascular calcifications [9,12,13]. Indeed, in rats, dietary supplementation with high doses of either phylloquinone (vitamin K1) or menaquinone-4 (vitamin K2) resulted in the regression of post-warfarin-induced arterial calcifications [14,15]. In mice, co-administration of low-dose MK-4 in the concurrent warfarin plus phylloquinone model of vascular calcification reduced the development of calcification [16]. Note that in this animal model of warfarin-induced vascular calcification, the concurrent administration of phylloquinone is needed to support hepatic synthesis of coagulation factors but does not itself prevent vascular calcification while warfarin is still being administered. Observational studies in humans show an inverse relationship between menaquinone intake and CAC in healthy elderly [17,18]. However, phylloquinone supplementation itself was shown to slow the progression of CAC and had a beneficial effect on vascular stiffness in healthy adults with coronary artery calcification after 3 years of follow-up [19–21]. Dalmeijer *et al.* performed a randomized, double blind, placebo controlled trial to investigate the effect of menaquinone-7 (MK-7) supplementation on MGP species and found a dose-dependent decrease of dephospho-uncarboxylated MGP (dp-ucMGP) concentrations [22]. Furthermore, MK-7 improves arterial stiffness and elastic properties of the carotid artery [23]. Altogether, this data suggests that vitamin K administration may have beneficial effects on the vasculature. So far, however, the effect of MK-7 supplementation on CAC and its long-term progression has not been studied in humans in a randomized clinical trial (RCT). Therefore, we designed the VitaK-CAC trial to analyze the effect of MK-7 supplementation in comparison to placebo on the annual progression of CAC. We hypothesize that treatment with MK-7 will slow down or arrest the progression of CAC in comparison to placebo and that MK-7 supplementation may lead to a treatment option for vascular calcification and cardiovascular disease.

Our proposed RCT has several highly innovative features. First it will be the first RCT to study the effect of nutritional supplementation with MK-7 on the progression of arterial calcification using state of the art techniques for the quantification of calcification in atherosclerotic lesions in patients with pre-existing CAC. The mainstay of the assessment of CAC progression will be multi-slice computed tomography in addition to measurements of arterial stiffness used in previous studies of MK-7 [23]. The only other comparable RCT using Computed Tomography (CT) scans showed that daily supplementation with 500 μg phylloquinone (high dietary range) reduced the progression of CAC in older people by 6% [19]. From the animal and human studies outlined above [12,16–18,24] we hypothesize that MK-7 should be more effective than phylloquinone in ameliorating the progression of CAC. One likely reason for the greater effectiveness of MK-7 is that its rate of clearance from the human circulatory system is much longer than that for phylloquinone and enhances the degree of gamma-carboxylation of Gla proteins in extrahepatic tissues such as bone and arteries [12]. Finally we should emphasize that the proposed daily amounts of 360 μg MK-7 are within the nutritional range of certain diets. For example the MK-7 content of Japanese fermented food natto is approximately

1000 μg/100 g in a highly bioactive form for gamma-carboxylation of hepatic and extrahepatic Gla proteins [12,25].

2. The Vitamin K—Coronary Artery Calcification (VitaK-CAC) Study

2.1. Trial Objectives

The primary objective of our trial is to assess whether oral MK-7 supplementation will slow down the rate of CAC progression after 12 and 24 months in patients with pre-existing CAC in comparison to treatment with placebo. Secondary endpoints include CT angiographically defined plaque composition alterations, and changes in parameters of arterial stiffness, extra-coronary atherosclerosis and biomarkers (Table 1).

Table 1. Secondary endpoints.

Changes in plaque morphology of existing atherosclerotic lesions
Incidence of new calcified atherosclerotic lesions
Changes in arterial structure and function
Carotid-femoral pulse wave velocity (cfPWV)
Pulse-waveform and central aortic blood pressure (CABP)
Common carotid artery intima media thickness (cIMT)
Common carotid artery distensibility coefficient (DC)
Biochemical associations between CAC progression
Circulating matrix Gla protein (MGP) species with different phosphorylation and carboxylation forms
Osteocalcin (OC)
Lipid profile (Total cholesterol, Low-Density Lipoprotein-cholesterol (LDL), High-Density Lipoprotein-cholesterol (HDL) and Triglycerides)
Glucose status (Fasting glucose)
Calcium metabolism (Calcium, Albumine, Phosphate and Parathyroid Hormone)
Kidney function (Creatinine)
Prothrombin time-International normalized ratio (PT-INR)

2.2. Patient Recruitment

The VitaK-CAC trial is a double-blind, randomized, placebo-controlled trial in two centers. Eligible patients suspected of having coronary artery disease (CAD) and who are scanned by 128-slice multiple detector CT (MDCT) to assess the presence of coronary atherosclerotic plaques and CAC will be identified from the outpatient clinic of the departments of Cardiology. Patients with a baseline Agatston CAC-score between 50 and 400 will be recruited and randomized into two groups. This Agatston score corresponds with a moderately increased risk of cardiovascular events or death [2].

The study has been approved by the Medical Ethics Committee (MEC) of the Maastricht University Medical Center, Maastricht, the Netherlands. The study complies with the Declaration of Helsinki. All patients have to give written informed consent.

The VitaK-CAC trial is registered at clinicaltrials.gov as NCT01002157.

2.3. Inclusion and Exclusion Criteria

We include all patients older than 18 years with a baseline CAC-score (Agatston) between 50 and 400. Patients who meet any of the exclusion criteria (Table 2) will be excluded. Specifically, patients with chronic kidney disease (CKD) will be excluded because of differences in pathophysiology of vascular calcification and higher prevalence of cardiovascular death [26]. Disorders of calcium and phosphate metabolism and a high prevalence of subclinical vitamin K deficiency in this population contribute to the higher rate of vascular calcification and mortality [14].

Table 2. Exclusion criteria.

Baseline-scan of insufficient quality (due to the presence of motion artefacts, breathing artefacts or high noise-levels)
Heart rate greater than 70 beats per min during first scan because of impaired scan quality
Chronic or paroxysmal atrial fibrillation
Presence or scheduled bypass-grafting in more than one coronary artery
Presence or scheduled coronary revascularization procedure (stent-placement > 1 coronary artery)
History of myocardial infarction or stroke < 6 months before coronary Coronary Tomography (CT)
Presence of diabetes mellitus type 1
Known kidney disease or an estimated Glomerular Filtration Rate (eGFR) < 60 mL/min/1.73 m^2, calculated by the MDRD-formula
Malignant disease (exception: treated basal-cell or squamous cell carcinoma)
Use of Vitamin K antagonists
A life-expectancy < 2 years
Pregnancy or wish to become pregnant in the near future

2.4. Measurements

2.4.1. Interviewing, Physical Examination and Blood-Pressure Measurement

At baseline, information on medical history, lifestyle factors (smoking, alcohol consumption, physical activity and dietary habits) and use of medication will be assessed. Furthermore, height, weight and waist-hip circumference will be measured. Arterial blood pressures (systolic, diastolic and mean) will be measured on both arms with a validated electronic (oscillometric) blood-pressure measurement device (Datascope Accutorr Plus, Soma Technology, Paramus, NJ, USA). Before measurement, subject will be seated for at least 5 min. At every study visit, drug adherence and any co-medication will be recorded.

2.4.2. Multi-Slice Computed Tomography

Scans will be performed using a dual-source CT-scanner (Somatom Definition Flash, Siemens Medical Solutions, Forchheim, Germany). In line with routine clinical procedures, patients can be premedicated with beta blocking agents to achieve a stable heart rate and/or sublingual nitrates to ensure vasodilatation. First, a native scan is performed using 120 kV and 3 mm slice thickness to determine the calcium score according to the Agatston method [27]. Subsequently, a 20 mL contrast test bolus will be injected to assess the time to peak in the ascending aorta. Coronary computed tomography angiography (CCTA) will be performed using 80–100 mL of contrast agent (Ultravist 300; Bayer Pharma AG, Berlin, Germany), which is injected into an antecubital vein at a rate of 5.2–7.4 mL/s followed by 60 mL intravenous saline (6.0 mL/s) using a dual-head power injector (Medrad Inc., Pittsburgh, PA, USA). A prospectively gated high pitch spiral "flash" protocol will be used in patients with a stable heart rate <60 beats per minute (bpm). In patients with a stable heart rate between 60 and 90 bpm, a prospectively gated axial "adaptive sequence" protocol is used. In patients with a heart rate > 90 bpm or in case of an irregular heart rhythm (because of new diagnosed atrial fibrillation or ventricular extrasystoles), a retrospectively gated "helical" protocol with dose modulation will be used. Data acquisition parameters are $2 \times 128 \times 0.6$ mm slice collimation, a gantry rotation time of 280 millisecond (ms) and a tube voltage of 100 or 120 kV depending on patients' height and weight.

The assessment will be performed using the source images on the provided software (Syngo CT 2010A, Siemens, Forchheim, Germany). The coronary artery tree will be analyzed for the presence and severity of CAD, according to the classification of the American Heart Association 16-segment model [28]. Coronary plaques are defined as visible structures within or adjacent to the coronary artery lumen, which can be clearly distinguished from the vessel lumen and the surrounding pericardial tissue. Quantification of coronary plaque components is done via semi-automated analysis as has been described before [29]. Scans are analyzed independently by a cardiologist and a radiologist, both experienced in the assessment of CCTA. In case of disagreement, consensus is reached by discussion.

2.4.3. Measurement of the Central Aortic Blood Pressure (CABP)

Measurement of the CABP is based on pulse wave analysis using a Sphygmocor device (SphygmoCor, Atcor Medical, Sydney, Australia). The waveform is recorded using a pen-shaped transducer that is placed on the skin of the patient's wrist overlying the radial artery (application tonometry). Using brachial mean arterial pressure and diastolic blood pressure for calibration and a transfer function, the CABP is estimated by the Sphygmocor internal algorithms.

2.4.4. Measurement of Pulse Wave Velocity (PWV)

The carotid-to-femoral and carotid-to-radial pulse wave velocities (cfPWV and crPWV) will be determined according to recent guidelines by using tonometry (Complior, Artech Medical, Patin, France) [30]. With the participant in supine position, sensors will be placed on the skin over the right common carotid artery, right radial artery, and right femoral artery. After obtaining simultaneous waveforms of sufficient quality, two consecutive series of 10 to 15 waveforms will be recorded for derivation of transit times. The transit time will be determined using the intersecting tangent algorithm. The distances between the sensors will be measured to calculate the cfPWV and crPWV. The median of two consecutive cfPWV and crPWV recordings will be used in the analysis.

2.4.5. Measurement of the Carotid Intima Media Thickness (cIMT)

The carotid Intima Media Thickness is measured using a vascular ultrasound scanner equipped with the ArtLab wall-track system (Esaote/Pie Medical, Maastricht, the Netherlands). With the participant lying supine, both rights and left Common Carotid Arteries (CCA) are identified on a longitudinal ultra-sonographic image. During ultrasound measurements, a double line pattern on both walls of the CCA is detected in real-time, consisting of the echoes of the lumen-intima transition and media-adventitia transition (automated radiofrequency-based IMT). The cIMT measurement will be done 10 mm proximal to the carotid bulb and is determined on the far wall of the CCA as the distance between these two lines in micrometers (spatial average). Images will be taken at four different angles (90°, 120°, 150° and 180° for the right carotid artery, and 180°, 210°, 240° and 270° for the left carotid artery). The median diameter and IMT of the measurements will be used in the analysis. The cIMT measurements will we performed by certified operators. Because of the radiofrequency-based IMT measurement we don't expect interobserver nor intra-observer variability [31]. The reproducibility will be calculated.

2.4.6. Measurement of the Common Carotid Artery Distensibility Coefficient (DC)

The CCA distensibility coefficient (DC) is measured using a vascular ultrasound scanner equipped with an ArtLab wall-track system (Esaote Europe, Maastricht, the Netherlands). The DC is calculated as follows: $DC = \frac{2\Delta D \times D + \Delta D^2}{PP \times D^2}$, in ($10^{-3} \cdot kPa^{-1}$), where D is the arterial (diastolic) diameter, ΔD is the distension, and PP is the brachial pulse pressure (calculated as systolic minus diastolic blood pressure). The median DC of two measurements will be used in the analysis.

2.4.7. Laboratory Assessment

Fasting blood samples will be obtained for routine biochemical and hematological measurements and specific laboratory variables (see Table 3). In addition, 7 mL of blood will be stored for future research. MGP will be quantified using an automated method available on the market (supplied by IDS, Boldon, UK). OCN will be measured using Gla-OC and Glu-OC ELISAs from Takara (Shiga, Japan).

Table 3. Laboratory assessment.

Routine Laboratory Variables	Specific Laboratory Variables
Total cholesterol	
LDL-cholesterol	
HDL-cholesterol	
Triglycerides	
Creatinine	MGP
Glucose	OCN
Albumin	
Calcium	
Phosphate	
Coagulation function (PT-INR)	

2.5. Treatment Schedule

Treatment of both groups will last for 24 months. During this time participants will visit our research unit five times, at 6-month intervals (Figure 1). At every study visit we will perform an interview and blood pressure measurements. During the first visit, at 12, and at 24 months of follow-up, measurements of CABP, cfPWV, crPWV, cIMT and DC are scheduled. In addition, fasting blood-samples will be drawn at 0, 12, and 24 months. We will repeat CT-scans of the heart and coronary arteries at 12 and 24 months of follow-up. At 12 months only a non-contrast CT scan will be performed to obtain a calcium score. At 24 months a CT-angiography will be performed, using the same acquisition protocol and reconstruction techniques as the initial CT scan (See Figure 1).

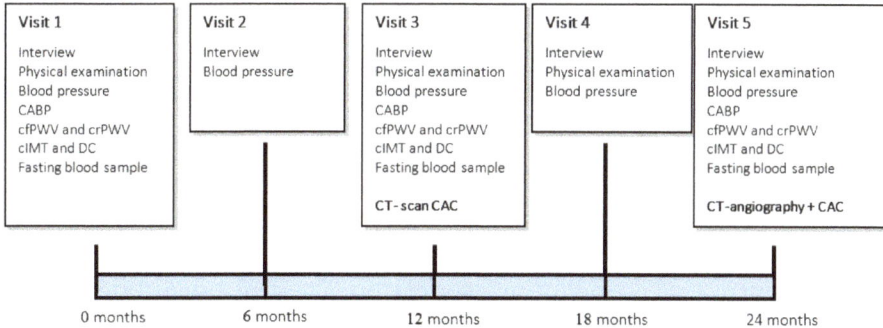

Figure 1. Trial design.

2.6. Vitamin K Product

Subjects in the intervention group will receive a once-daily oral tablet of 360 micrograms of MK-7. In our study we use a pure synthetic MK-7 provided by NattoPharma ASA (Hovik, Norway). The choice for MK-7 as K-vitamer is based on the longer half-life and extra-hepatic tissue distribution as compared to other vitamin K-forms [12,24]. The chosen dose in this trial was established in a dose-finding study, in which the effect of increasing doses of MK-7 on OCN and MGP-carboxylation was monitored. A daily dose of 360 µg MK-7 most effectively reduced the amount of non-functional MGP [22,32].

MK-7 is well tolerated and does not cause a hypercoagulable state [33]. There are no reported adverse effects associated with the use of MK-7.

2.7. Randomization Procedure

If the patient is eligible and willing to participate in the study, the patient will be randomly assigned to the MK-7 or placebo group. Subjects will be randomized after stratification for age, sex, BMI, statin- and bisphosphonate-use using the minimization technique [34]. An independent investigator who is not involved in the coordination or analysis of this study, will randomize consecutive patients using custom-made computer software. The randomization-list will be stored in a secure location and will not be accessible to the investigators during the study.

2.8. Statistical Analysis

The main outcome parameters (CAC-score) and CAC-score progression will be presented as continuous variables. In addition, the amount of CAC-score progression (in both Agatston-score and Mass-score) will be dichotomized (rapid progression and slow progression) using a cut-off of an annual progression of 15% [33].

Data will be analyzed based on the intention-to-treat principle. To adjust for potential confounders (age, gender, BMI, blood-pressure, smoking, cholesterol, glucose and medication use), multiple analysis of variance will be performed. For continuous variables, multivariable linear regression will be applied. For longitudinal data analysis (*i.e.*, progression between baseline, 12 months, and 24 months of follow-up) Generalized Estimating Equations (GEE) analysis will be applied to adjust for multiple testing. Additional statistical analyses will be performed as appropriate (e.g., Hazzard ratio calculation). All statistical analysis will be performed using the statistical package SPSS 22 (IBM Corp, Armonk, New York, USA). The statistical tests will be performed using a two-sided significance level of 5%.

2.9. Sample Size

The mean annual CAC-progression reported in literature ranges from 24% to 51% and has a large inter-individual variation depending on many factors such as the baseline CAC-score, medical history, medication-use, body-mass index, scanner type and manufacturer. The standard deviation in CAC-score progression in a population comparable to our intended population is reported to range from 21% to 36% [33]. Since we use strict inclusion and exclusion criteria and use a 128-slice MDCT with better reproducibility of measurements, we estimate the standard deviation of CAC-progression to be 25%. We consider an absolute difference of 15% in CAC-progression between the two treatment groups a significant effect [33]. To test this difference with a statistical power of 90% (alpha 0.05) we require 59 patients per group. Based on analysis of available data from our center, we estimate a patient drop-out of approximately 35%. This drop-out may have various reasons such as patients requiring coronary artery stenting over the course of the study, occurrence of cardiovascular events such as myocardial infarction requiring percutaneous coronary intervention (PCI) or death, development of exclusion criteria, or subjects no longer willing to participate in the study. Therefore, to obtain sufficient statistical power to demonstrate a possible treatment-effect, we require 90 patients per group for a total number of 180 patients.

2.10. Organization

2.10.1. Data Safety Monitoring Board (DSMB)

An independent DSMB will be established to perform ongoing safety surveillance and to perform interim analyses on the safety data. None of the DSMB-members are directly or indirectly involved in the coordination, execution or analysis of the proposed study.

The DSMB's primary task is to monitor the safety of participants. Interim analysis will be performed to assess whether a treatment-group has relatively more adverse events than the other. The DSMB will assess the number of cardiovascular events (myocardial infarction, coronary revascularization procedures, and cardiovascular deaths) and the number of adverse reactions/side effects as reported by the study-participants at every interim analysis.

Furthermore, the DSMB will calculate the rate of progression of vascular calcification in both groups. If there is a reason for concern, the DSMB can advise to interrupt the study for further analysis or terminate the study. This will be discussed in a meeting with the investigators and DSMB.

The investigator will inform the subjects and the reviewing accredited MEC if anything occurs, on the basis of which it appears that the disadvantages of participation may be significantly greater than was foreseen in the research proposal.

2.10.2. Adverse and Serious Adverse Events (AE and SAE)

Adverse events are defined as any undesirable experience occurring to a subject during a clinical trial, whether or not they are considered related to the investigational drug. All adverse events are recorded. An abnormal laboratory result will not be considered as an adverse event except where it is indicative of disease and/or organ toxicity. Details of all adverse events reported spontaneously by subjects or observed by the investigator or medical staff will be recorded. All SAEs will be reported to the accredited MEC that approved the protocol, according to the local requirements.

2.10.3. Suspected Unexpected Serious Adverse Reactions (SUSAR)

Adverse reactions are all untoward and unintended responses to an investigational product related to any dose administered. Unexpected adverse reactions are adverse reactions, of a nature or severity that is not consistent with the applicable product information. The investigator will report all SUSARs to the MEC. In case of a SUSAR, the randomization-code will be broken for the individual patient only so blinding of treatment allocation can be maintained for the remaining study subjects. The treatment allocation of that individual patient will be reported to the investigators.

2.10.4. Premature Termination of the Study

The study can be terminated prematurely if the number of SAEs or the rate of vascular calcification is significantly higher in the treatment group *versus* the placebo group.

The study will be terminated if a causal relation between MK-7 treatment and the adverse events or progression of vascular calcification is highly suspected. If the study is terminated prematurely, all subjects will be informed about their results and the reason why the study is terminated.

2.10.5. Withdrawal of Individual Subjects

Subjects can leave the study at any time for any reason if they wish to do so, without any consequences. The investigator can decide to withdraw a subject from the study for urgent medical reasons or in case of demonstrable poor adherence to the study medication. This is assessed by interview and pill-count. If subjects are required to take vitamin-K antagonists (coumarins) during the course of the study (for example due to Deep-Venous Thrombosis or Pulmonary Embolism) they will be withdrawn from the study.

2.10.6. Participating Centers

The Maastricht University Medical Centre (MUMC) is the initiating center of the VitaK-CAC trial and the VieCuri Medical Centre is participating. The principal investigator is Abraham A. Kroon, internist at the MUMC.

3. Concluding Remarks

In conclusion, the VitaK-CAC trial will study the effect of menaquinone-7 supplementation on progression of CAC in a randomized, placebo-controlled trial. We hypothesize that MK-7 supplementation will slow down the progression of CAC in patients with CAD. So far, no treatment options are available for vascular calcification, and this trial may lead to a treatment option for vascular calcification and cardiovascular disease.

Nutrients **2015**, *7*, 8905–8915

The result of this study will be expected at the end of 2017.

Acknowledgments: The study is supported by a grant from the Netherlands Heart Foundation (NHS 2010 B161). The study-tablets are provided for free of charge by NattoPharma ASA (Hovik, Norway).

Author Contributions: Abraham A. Kroon, Leon J. Schurgers, Peter W. de Leeuw, Roger J.M.W. Rennenberg and Bernard J. van Varik conceived and designed the study. Bas L.J.H. Kietselaer contributed information about the Coronary computed tomography angiography (CCTA) and will analyze the scans with his colleagues. Koen D. Reesink contributed information about the Measurement of the Common Carotid Artery Distensibility Coefficient (DC). Liv M. Vossen and Bernard J. van Varik will perform the experiments in Maastricht, Yvonne J.M. van Cauteren will perform the experiments in the VieCuri Medical Centre. Johannes G. Meeder, Braim M. Rahel and Ge A. Hoffland will analyze the baseline CCTA of the patient of the VieCuri Medical Centre with their colleagues. Cees Vermeer will monitor the quality and concentration of the Menaquinone-7 tablets. Leon J. Schurgers, Abraham A. Kroon, Peter W. de Leeuw, Bernard J. van Varik and Liv M. Vossen wrote the paper.

Conflicts of Interest: The authors declare no conflict of interest.

References

1. Henein, M.Y.; Koulaouzidis, G.; Granåsen, G.; Wiklund, U.; Guerci, A.; Schmermund, A. The natural history of coronary calcification: A meta-analysis from St Francis and EBEAT trials. *Int. J. Cardiol.* **2013**, *168*, 3944–3948. [PubMed]
2. Budoff, M.J.; Shaw, L.J.; Liu, S.T.; Weinstein, S.R.; Mosler, T.P.; Tseng, P.H.; Flores, F.R.; Callister, T.Q.; Raggi, P.; Berman, D.S. Long-term prognosis associated with coronary calcification: Observations from a registry of 25,253 patients. *J. Am. Coll. Cardiol.* **2007**, *49*, 1860–1870. [PubMed]
3. Madhavan, M.V.; Tarigopula, M.; Mintz, G.S.; Maehara, A.; Stone, G.W.; Généreux, P. Coronary artery calcification: Pathogenesis and prognostic implications. *J. Am. Coll. Cardiol.* **2014**, *63*, 1703–1714. [PubMed]
4. Luo, G.; Ducy, P.; McKee, M.D.; Pinero, G.J.; Loyer, E.; Behringer, R.R.; Karsenty, G. Spontaneous calcification of arteries and cartilage in mice lacking matrix GLA protein. *Nature* **1997**, *386*, 78–81. [PubMed]
5. Schurgers, L.J.; Cranenburg, E.C.M.; Vermeer, C. Matrix Gla-protein: The calcification inhibitor in need of vitamin K. *Thromb. Haemost.* **2008**, *100*, 593–603. [PubMed]
6. Schurgers, L.J.; Uitto, J.; Reutelingsperger, C.P. Vitamin K-dependent carboxylation of matrix Gla-protein: A crucial switch to control ectopic mineralization. *Trends Mol. Med.* **2013**, *19*, 217–226. [PubMed]
7. Rennenberg, R.J.; Schurgers, L.J.; Kroon, A.A.; Stehouwer, C.D. Arterial calcifications. *J. Cell Mol. Med.* **2010**, *14*, 2203–2210. [PubMed]
8. Price, P.A.; Faus, S.A.; Williamson, M.K. Warfarin causes rapid calcification of the elastic lamellae in rat arteries and heart valves. *Arterioscler. Thromb. Vasc. Biol.* **1998**, *18*, 1400–1407. [PubMed]
9. Chatrou, M.L.L.; Winckers, K.; Hackeng, T.M.; Reutelingsperger, C.P.; Schurgers, L.J. Vascular calcification: The price to pay for anticoagulation therapy with vitamin K-antagonists. *Blood Rev.* **2012**, *26*, 155–166. [PubMed]
10. Rennenberg, R.J.; van Varik, B.J.; Schurgers, L.J.; Hamulyak, K.; ten Cate, H.; Leiner, T.; Vermeer, C.; de Leeuw, P.W.; Kroon, A.A. Chronic coumarin treatment is associated with increased extracoronary arterial calcification in humans. *Blood* **2010**, *115*, 5121–5123. [PubMed]
11. Weijs, B.; Blaauw, Y.; Rennenberg, R.J.M.W.; Schurgers, L.J.; Timmermans, C.C.M.M.; Pison, L.; Nieuwlaat, R.; Hofstra, L.; Kroon, A.A.; Wildberger, J.; *et al.* Patients using vitamin K antagonists show increased levels of coronary calcification: An observational study in low-risk atrial fibrillation patients. *Eur. Heart J.* **2011**, *32*, 2555–2562. [PubMed]
12. Schurgers, L.J.; Teunissen, K.J.F.; Hamulyák, K.; Knapen, M.H.J.; Vik, H.; Vermeer, C. Vitamin K-containing dietary supplements: Comparison of synthetic vitamin K1 and natto-derived menaquinone-7. *Blood* **2007**, *109*, 3279–3283. [PubMed]
13. Brandenburg, V.M.; Schurgers, L.J.; Kaesler, N.; Püsche, K.; van Gorp, R.H.; Leftheriotis, G.; Reinartz, S.; Koos, R.; Krüger, T. Prevention of vasculopathy by vitamin K supplementation: Can we turn fiction into fact? *Atherosclerosis* **2015**, *240*, 10–16. [PubMed]
14. McCabe, K.M.; Booth, S.L.; Fu, X.; Shobeiri, N.; Pang, J.J.; Adams, M.A.; Holden, R.M. Dietary vitamin K and therapeutic warfarin alter the susceptibility to vascular calcification in experimental chronic kidney disease. *Kidney Int.* **2013**, *83*, 835–844. [CrossRef] [PubMed]

15. Schurgers, L.J.; Spronk, H.M.H.; Soute, B.A.M.; Schiffers, P.M.; DeMey, J.G.R.; Vermeer, C. Regression of warfarin-induced medial elastocalcinosis by high intake of vitamin K in rats. *Blood* **2007**, *109*, 2823–2831. [CrossRef] [PubMed]

16. Krüger, T.; Oelenberg, S.; Kaesler, N.; Schurgers, L.J.; van de Sandt, A.M.; Boor, P.; Schlieper, G.; Brandenburg, V.M.; Fekete, B.C.; Veulemans, V.; *et al.* Warfarin induces cardiovascular damage in mice. *Arterioscler. Thromb. Vasc. Biol.* **2013**, *33*, 2618–2624. [CrossRef] [PubMed]

17. Beulens, J.W.J.; Bots, M.L.; Atsma, F.; Bartelink, M.-L.E.L.; Prokop, M.; Geleijnse, J.M.; Witteman, J.C.M.; Grobbee, D.E.; van der Schouw, Y.T. High dietary menaquinone intake is associated with reduced coronary calcification. *Atherosclerosis* **2009**, *203*, 489–493. [PubMed]

18. Geleijnse, J.M.; Vermeer, C.; Grobbee, D.E.; Schurgers, L.J.; Knapen, M.H.J.; van der Meer, I.M.; Hofman, A.; Witteman, J.C.M. Dietary intake of menaquinone is associated with a reduced risk of coronary heart disease: The Rotterdam study. *J. Nutr.* **2004**, *134*, 3100–3105. [PubMed]

19. Shea, M.K.; O'Donnell, C.J.; Hoffmann, U.; Dallal, G.E.; Dawson-Hughes, B.; Ordovas, J.M.; Price, P.A.; Williamson, M.K.; Booth, S.L. Vitamin K supplementation and progression of coronary artery calcium in older men and women. *Am. J. Clin. Nutr.* **2009**, *89*, 1799–1807. [CrossRef] [PubMed]

20. Braam, L.A.J.L.M.; Hoeks, A.P.G.; Brouns, F.; Hamulyák, K.; Gerichhausen, M.J.W.; Vermeer, C. Beneficial effects of vitamins D and K on the elastic properties of the vessel wall in postmenopausal women: A follow-up study. *Thromb. Haemost.* **2004**, *91*, 373–380. [CrossRef] [PubMed]

21. Shea, M.K.; Holden, R.M. Vitamin K status and vascular calcification: Evidence from observational and clinical studies. *Adv. Nutr.* **2012**, *3*, 158–165. [CrossRef] [PubMed]

22. Dalmeijer, G.W.; van der Schouw, Y.T.; Magdeleyns, E.; Ahmed, N.; Vermeer, C.; Beulens, J.W.J. The effect of menaquinone-7 supplementation on circulating species of matrix Gla protein. *Atherosclerosis* **2012**, *225*, 397–402. [CrossRef] [PubMed]

23. Knapen, M.H.J.; Braam, L.A.J.L.M.; Drummen, N.E.; Bekers, O.; Hoeks, A.P.G.; Vermeer, C. Menaquinone-7 supplementation improves arterial stiffness in healthy postmenopausal women. A double-blind randomised clinical trial. *Thromb. Haemost.* **2015**, *113*, 1135–1144. [CrossRef] [PubMed]

24. Gast, G.C.M.; de Roos, N.M.; Sluijs, I.; Bots, M.L.; Beulens, J.W.J.; Geleijnse, J.M.; Witteman, J.C.; Grobbee, D.E.; Peeters, P.H.M.; van der Schouw, Y.T. A high menaquinone intake reduces the incidence of coronary heart disease. *Nutr. Metab. Cardiovasc. Dis.* **2009**, *19*, 504–510. [CrossRef] [PubMed]

25. Schurgers, L.J.; Shearer, M.J.; Hamulyák, K.; Stöcklin, E.; Vermeer, C. Effect of vitamin K intake on the stability of oral anticoagulant treatment: Dose-response relationships in healthy subjects. *Blood* **2004**, *104*, 2682–2689. [CrossRef] [PubMed]

26. Schurgers, L.J. Vitamin K: Key vitamin in controlling vascular calcification in chronic kidney disease. *Kidney Int.* **2013**, *83*, 782–784. [CrossRef] [PubMed]

27. Agatston, A.S.; Janowitz, W.R.; Hildner, F.J.; Zusmer, N.R.; Viamonte, M.; Detrano, R. Quantification of coronary artery calcium using ultrafast computed tomography. *J. Am. Coll. Cardiol.* **1990**, *15*, 827–832. [CrossRef]

28. Austen, W.G.; Edwards, J.E.; Frye, R.L.; Gensini, G.G.; Gott, V.L.; Griffith, L.S.; McGoon, D.C.; Murphy, M.L.; Roe, B.B. A reporting system on patients evaluated for coronary artery disease. Report of the Ad Hoc Committee for Grading of Coronary Artery Disease, Council on Cardiovascular Surgery, American Heart Association. *Circulation* **1975**, *51*, 5–40. [CrossRef] [PubMed]

29. Versteylen, M.O.; Kietselaer, B.L.; Dagnelie, P.C.; Joosen, I.A.; Dedic, A.; Raaijmakers, R.H.; Wildberger, J.E.; Nieman, K.; Crijns, H.J.; Niessen, W.J.; *et al.* Additive value of semiautomated quantification of coronary artery disease using cardiac computed tomographic angiography to predict future acute coronary syndrome. *J. Am. Coll. Cardiol.* **2013**, *61*, 2296–2305. [CrossRef] [PubMed]

30. Van Bortel, L.M.; Laurent, S.; Boutouyrie, P.; Chowienczyk, P.; Cruickshank, J.K.; de Backer, T.; Filipovsky, J.; Huybrechts, S.; Mattace-Raso, F.U.S.; Protogerou, A.D.; *et al.* Expert consensus document on the measurement of aortic stiffness in daily practice using carotid-femoral pulse wave velocity. *J. Hypertens.* **2012**, *30*, 445–448. [CrossRef] [PubMed]

31. Willekes, C.; Brands, P.J.; Willigers, J.M.; Hoeks, A.P.G.; Reneman, R.S. Assessment of local differences in intima-media thickness in the human common carotid artery. *J. Vasc. Res.* **1999**, *36*, 222–228. [CrossRef] [PubMed]

32. Westenfeld, R.; Krueger, T.; Schlieper, G.; Cranenburg, E.C.M.; Magdeleyns, E.J.; Heidenreich, S.; Holzmann, S.; Vermeer, C.; Jahnen-Dechent, W.; Ketteler, M.; *et al.* Effect of vitamin K2 supplementation on functional vitamin K deficiency in hemodialysis patients: A randomized trial. *Am. J. Kidney Dis.* **2012**, *59*, 186–195. [CrossRef] [PubMed]

33. Theuwissen, E.; Cranenburg, E.C.; Knapen, M.H.; Magdeleyns, E.J.; Teunissen, K.J.; Schurgers, L.J.; Smit, E.; Vermeer, C. Low-dose menaquinone-7 supplementation improved extra-hepatic vitamin K status, but had no effect on thrombin generation in healthy subjects. *Br. J. Nutr.* **2012**, *108*, 1652–1657. [CrossRef] [PubMed]

34. Scott, N.W.; McPherson, G.C.; Ramsay, C.R.; Campbell, M.K. The method of minimization for allocation to clinical trials: A review. *Control. Clin. Trials* **2002**, *23*, 662–674. [CrossRef]

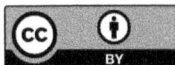

nutrients

MDPI

Review

New Insights into the Pros and Cons of the Clinical Use of Vitamin K Antagonists (VKAs) Versus Direct Oral Anticoagulants (DOACs)

Rick H. van Gorp [1,2] and Leon J. Schurgers [1,*]

[1] Department of Biochemistry, Cardiovascular Research Institute Maastricht, Maastricht University, PO Box 616, 6200 MD Maastricht, The Netherlands; rick.vangorp@maastrichtuniversity

[2] Nattopharma ASA, 1363 Høvik, Norway

* Correspondence: l.schurgers@maastrichtuniversity.nl; Tel.: +31-43-388-1680

Received: 15 May 2015 ; Accepted: 5 November 2015 ; Published: 17 November 2015

Abstract: Vitamin K-antagonists (VKA) are the most widely used anticoagulant drugs to treat patients at risk of arterial and venous thrombosis for the past 50 years. Due to unfavorable pharmacokinetics VKA have a small therapeutic window, require frequent monitoring, and are susceptible to drug and nutritional interactions. Additionally, the effect of VKA is not limited to coagulation, but affects all vitamin K-dependent proteins. As a consequence, VKA have detrimental side effects by enhancing medial and intimal calcification. These limitations stimulated the development of alternative anticoagulant drugs, resulting in direct oral anticoagulant (DOAC) drugs, which specifically target coagulation factor Xa and thrombin. DOACs also display non-hemostatic vascular effects via protease-activated receptors (PARs). As atherosclerosis is characterized by a hypercoagulable state indicating the involvement of activated coagulation factors in the genesis of atherosclerosis, anticoagulation could have beneficial effects on atherosclerosis. Additionally, accumulating evidence demonstrates vascular benefit from high vitamin K intake. This review gives an update on oral anticoagulant treatment on the vasculature with a special focus on calcification and vitamin K interaction.

Keywords: oral anticoagulants; vitamin K; vascular calcification; coumarin; DOACs

1. Arterial and Venous Thrombosis

In 1856 Rudolf Virchow, often regarded as the founder of modern pathology, delineated three major components that were responsible for the formation of emboli in the venous circulation. These three elements, now known as Virchow's triad, can be briefly summarized as: (1) changes in the composition of blood; (2) alterations in the vessel wall; and (3) disruption of the blood flow. Coagulation is a protective response after vascular injury to prevent bleeding [1] and can be initiated via either the so-called intrinsic or extrinsic pathways, which although simplistic, are still useful schematic models of the coagulation process (Figure 1a). Both pathways are characterized by a series of enzymatic events whereby the activation of members of a hierarchical chain of coagulation enzymes (called coagulation factors) are successively activated by the preceding factor in the chain. Although the initiation steps are different, both pathways converge and lead to activation of pro-thrombin (FII) to produce thrombin (FIIa). An important feature of this coagulation cascade is that it functions as a biochemical amplifier [2] in which the final product, thrombin catalyses the production of fibrin which forms a meshwork clot [3]. The coagulation events leading to the formation of a blood clot (thrombus) that adheres to the wall of a blood vessel and obstructs the flow of blood is termed thrombosis. Thrombosis can take place in both arteries and veins. Atherothrombosis is the term describing the occlusion of a blood vessel by a ruptured atherosclerotic plaque [4,5]. Arterial thrombosis can lead to stroke and myocardial infarction. In contrast to arterial thrombosis, venous thrombosis is associated with dysregulation of coagulation proteins and manifests in deep-vein thrombosis and pulmonary embolism [6]. Obesity and diabetes mellitus are risk factors for both arterial and venous thrombosis whereas other risk factors such as smoking, hypertension and hyperlipidemia increase only the risk for arterial thrombosis [6]. Oral anticoagulant drugs are prescribed to patients to reduce the risk and incidence of both arterial and venous thrombosis, although mainly for the latter.

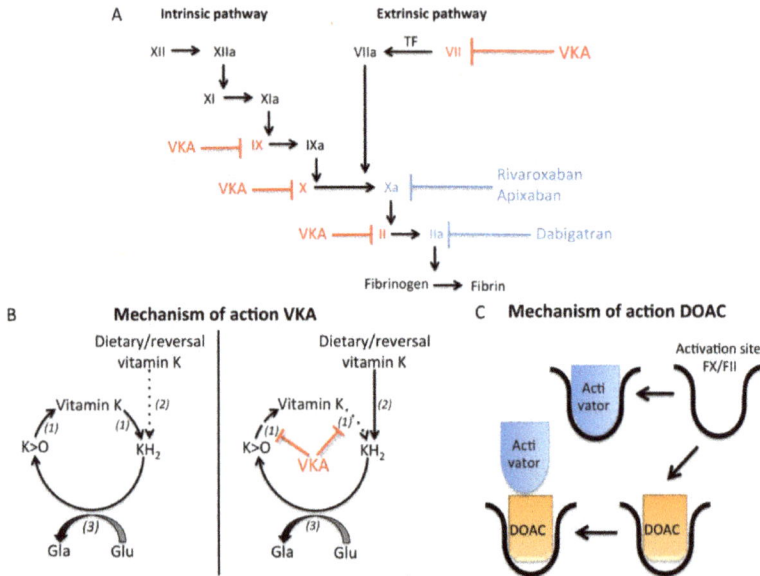

Figure 1. Effects of vitamin K antagonists and direct oral anticoagulants on coagulation. (**A**) The coagulation cascade can be activated by both the intrinsic and extrinsic pathway, which finally results in activation of thrombin and subsequently fibrin formation. Vitamin K antagonists (VKA) induce anticoagulation via inhibiting activation of the coagulation factors depicted in red (factors X, IX, VII, and II). Direct oral anticoagulants (DOACs) induce anticoagulation via blocking the activity of coagulation factors Xa (rivaroxaban and apixaban) and IIa (dabigatran) depicted in blue; (**B**) Vitamin K cycle is required to carboxylate, and thus activate, vitamin K dependent proteins. Vitamin K is converted to vitamin hydroquinone (KH_2), which is oxidized by γ-glutamylcarboxylase (3) to convert glutamate (Glu) residues in γ-carboxyglutamate (Gla) residues. This reaction results in vitamin K epoxide (K > O), which is recycled to vitamin K through vitamin K epoxide reductase (1). VKA disrupts the vitamin K cycle by inhibiting vitamin K epoxide reductase (VKOR) leading to depletion of vitamin K and uncarboxylated vitamin K dependent proteins. In the liver, the inhibition of warfarin can be circumvented via NAD(P)H quinone reductase (2), which can convert vitamin K into KH_2 even in the presence of VKA. In extra-hepatic tissues NAD(P)H quinone reductase activity is *ca.* 100 fold less, resulting in inactive vitamin K dependent proteins in the presence of VKA; (**C**) DOACs induce anticoagulation via inhibiting the activity of FXa and FIIa via binding to the activation site.

2. The Discovery of Oral Anticoagulant Drugs

The story of the discovery of vitamin K antagonists (VKA) began in the 1920s as a result of an often fatal bleeding disorder in cattle that manifested after the animals had been fed on the hay derived from sweet clover [7]. For this reason the haemorrhagic disease became known as "sweet clover disease". A crucial observation was the animals that bled had been fed on sweet clover hay that had become mouldy; those animals fed mould-free hay did not present with bleeding [7]. During the subsequent classical studies by Karl Link's group in Wisconsin it was first shown that bleeding was associated with a low plasma activity of prothrombin as measured by early coagulation assays that were the precursors of the modern day prothrombin time. Link's group then undertook the task of isolating the haemorrhagic component in spoiled sweet clover that was responsible for the prolonged prothrombin time. This proved a long and arduous process but finally resulted in the isolation and identification of the haemorrhagic agent that we now know as the compound dicoumarol and the first VKA [8]. Dicoumarol is a 4-hydroxycoumarin derivative and originated from microbial action on the compound coumarin which is rich in sweet clover.

After animal trials, dicoumarol was rapidly introduced into the clinic with considerable success. At that time, dicoumarol had also been tested in field trials as a potential rodenticide but it was concluded that the anticoagulant activity of dicoumarol in the rat was not high enough to make it practical for rodent control [8]. Therefore, Link's group synthesized a large number of different 4-hydroxycoumarin compounds to try and find a derivative with increased anticoagulant activity over dicoumarol. It turned out that a 4-hydroxycoumarin anticoagulant number 42 (out of 150 synthetic variants) was more potent than dicoumarol and had superior pharmacokinetics [8]. This coumarin derivative is today known as warfarin, the word originating from the combination of the Wisconsin Alumni Research Foundation (WARF) and "arin" from coum"arin". Warfarin revolutionized rodent control but clinicians were reluctant to use a rat poison in humans until an unforeseen event changed their minds. In 1951 an army conscript tried to commit suicide with warfarin. According to Link the slow onset time of warfarin gave him "too much time for thinking" enabling him to reconsider and admit himself to hospital where after receiving vitamin K supplementation he completely recovered. Clinical trials with warfarin in the 1950s confirmed its superiority over dicoumarol, being better absorbed and some 5–10 times more potent, although no head to head comparison was performed. Moreover, it became apparent that an overdose could easily be corrected by vitamin K supplementation [8,9]. Today, warfarin is the most prescribed oral anticoagulant world-wide [10].

2.1. Vitamin K and Vitamin K Antagonists

Vitamin K is a fat-soluble vitamin that exists in different forms (Table 1). All forms of vitamin K contain a 2-methyl-1,4-naphthoquinone ring structure, also known as menadione (vitamin K_3). Phylloquinone (vitamins K_1) and menaquinones (vitamin K_2) are classified according to the length and degree of saturation of the aliphatic side chain. Phylloquinone contains a phytyl side chain, and its main dietary sources are green leafy vegetables and certain vegetable oils. Menaquinones have an unsaturated aliphatic side chain comprising a varying number of prenyl units, abbreviated as MK-n (menaquinone with n representing the number of prenyl units). All menaquinones, except MK-4, are produced by bacteria and can be found in fermented foods such as cheese. Additionally, some bacteria in our intestines produce long-chain menaquinones (mainly MK-10 and MK-11) and although they make up the majority of human hepatic reserves their bioavailability for the synthesis of coagulation Gla proteins in the liver is debatable [11]. Both phylloquinone and menaquinones can participate in the γ-glutamylcarboxylation of both hepatic and extra-hepatic vitamin K-dependent proteins, although the longer residence times and better absorption of long chain menaquinones such as MK-7 and MK-9 in the circulation [12,13] makes them more effective for carboxylating both hepatic and extrahepatic vitamin K-dependent proteins [14]. Interestingly, menadione has been shown to act as a endogenous metabolite formed during the *in vivo* conversion of phylloquinone to MK-4 [15]. Furthermore, whereas phylloquinone and menaquinones can reverse VKA induced anticoagulation, menadione per se has no cofactor activity for γ-carboxylation and thus cannot reverse VKA-induced anticoagulation.

Table 1. Structural forms of vitamin K.

Drug	Characterization		Dietary Sources
Phylloquinone (vitamin K$_1$)	Phytyl side chain		Leafy green vegetables
Menaquinones (vitamin K$_2$)	Isoprenoid side chain	MK-4 MK-7 MK-9	Meat, eggs Natto, Cheese Cheese, curd, sauerkraut
Menadione (vitamin K$_3$)	2-methyl-1,4- naphthoquinone		Non-dietary metabolite. Precursor of MK-4

The molecular function of vitamin K is to serve as an essential cofactor to drive the γ-glutamyl carboxylation reaction (Figure 1b). In this vitamin K-dependent reaction, specific protein bound glutamate residues are modified to γ-glutamate residues, hence the name of the γ-carboxylated protein products as vitamin K-dependent proteins (VKDP). To achieve this protein modification vitamin K is first reduced to the active cofactor vitamin hydroquinone (KH$_2$) via quinone reductases. Next, the enzyme γ-glutamyl carboxylase (GGCX) oxidizes vitamin KH$_2$ with vitamin K epoxide (K > O) as the product. This oxidation reaction is intimately linked and essential to the γ-carboxylation modification of VKDP [16]. The metabolite K > O can be recycled by the microsomal enzyme vitamin K epoxide reductase (VKOR), first to vitamin K and then to KH$_2$. This cyclic pathway is called the "vitamin K-epoxide cycle" or simply the "vitamin K cycle" [17,18]. By this salvage mechanism, one molecule of vitamin K is able to carboxylate some 500 glutamate residues [17].

A deficiency of vitamin K can result from an insufficient dietary intake of vitamin K leading to depletion of local vitamin K tissue stores or via interference with the vitamin K cycle by VKA [18,19]. VKA exert their anticoagulant effect by inhibiting the VKOR enzyme resulting in reduced recycling of K > O, thereby limiting KH$_2$ production. As the cellular concentrations of KH$_2$ decline a stage is reached when the cofactor supply to the GGCX becomes insufficient to fully carboxylate the VKDP that are synthesized in a particular tissue. This in turn leads to the secretion of undercarboxylated species of VKDP in the circulation. The anticoagulant balance exerted by VKA can be said to be ultimately determined by the concentrations of γ-carboxylated coagulation proteins II, VII, IX and X that are secreted into the circulation. Changes in nutritional vitamin K intake interfere with VKA treatment by altering the size of the available pool of KH$_2$ cofactor because dietary vitamin K in its quinone state can be converted to KH$_2$ by a dehydrogenase enzyme not affected by VKA [18]. Remarkably, despite the long use of VKA the exact mechanism of inhibition of VKOR remains to be elucidated [18].

Owing to their unfavorable pharmacokinetics, VKA have a small therapeutic window, require frequent monitoring, and are susceptible to drug and nutritional interactions. A major disadvantage is that because of their indirect mechanism of action there is a lag phase of 2–3 days before a therapeutic anticoagulant effect is achieved. Therefore, considerable resources have been directed to the discovery of new anticoagulant agents that can directly target specific factors in the coagulation cascade. Several of these so-called direct oral anticoagulants (DOACs) have been approved for clinical use and can be subdivided into agents that either target coagulation factor IIa (FIIa, thrombin) or factor Xa (FXa).

2.2. Direct Thrombin Inhibitors

As with the discovery of VKA, the presence in nature of another anticoagulant (albeit in this case an anticoagulant without a lag phase) proved a catalyst to the future discovery of direct inhibitors of coagulation factors. Here it was the isolation of hirudin, a peptide present in the saliva of leeches as a direct inhibitor of thrombin, and long known to prevent coagulation [20,21]. For a detailed review on hirudin, see [22]. Hirudin binds to both the active and substrate recognition sites of thrombin. In addition, it is slowly reversible and excreted predominantly by the kidneys. In the 1990s, recombinant hirudin was shown to prevent postoperative venous thromboembolism [23]. However, a major concern was the increased bleeding tendency with hirudin treatment [21,24]. As with heparin another major disadvantage of hirudin is that it could only be administered by subcutaneous injection. Despite the specific concerns with hirudin, the theory behind designing a direct thrombin inhibitor as a clinical anticoagulant gained support and in the early 2000s a compound called ximelagatran became the first synthetic direct inhibitor of thrombin to be trialed as an oral anticoagulant. However, although initial human trials were promising, later trials led to concerns of hepatotoxicity, which ultimately prevented ximelagatran from being used in the clinical setting [25,26].

The second direct oral anticoagulant to undergo clinical trials was dabigatran etexilate, and this agent received approval for clinical use in 2008 (Table 2). Dabigatran etexilate is a prodrug that requires hydrolysis by carboxylesterases in the body to the active metabolite dabigatran [27]. Dabigatran binds with high specificity to the active site of thrombin thereby inhibiting both bound and free thrombin activity (Figure 1c). It takes two hours before dabigatran etexilate is metabolically active, which eliminates the need for parental anticoagulation. Dabigatran has a half-life of 12–17 h and is usually taken twice daily. Since 80% of dabigatran is excreted by the kidneys, patients with renal problems are not suited for this drug [25,28,29].

Table 2. Characteristics of VKA and DOACs.

	VKA [10]			Dabigatran Etexilate [24,27,28]	Rivaroxaban [30,31]	Apixaban [32]
	Warfarin	Acenocoumarol	Phenprocoumon			
Target	Vitamin K epoxide reductase	Vitamin K epoxide reductase	Vitamin K epoxide reductase	Thrombin	Factor Xa	Factor Xa
Pro-drug	No	No	No	Yes, active metabolite is dabigatran	No	No
Half-life (hours)	20–60	8–11	120–144	12–17	5–9	9–14
Onset time peak effect (hours)	72–96	36–48	48–72	2	2–3	3
Duration of action	2–5 days	<48 h	7–14 days	24–36 h	24 h	24 h
Metabolism	Via cytochrome P 450	Via cytochrome P 450	Via cytochrome P 450	Via P-Glucoprotein transporter	Via cytochrome P450 (30%), and P-Glucoprotein transporter	Via cytochrome P450 (15%), and P-Glucoprotein transporter
Elimination	Hepatical metabolized	60% Renal 29% Fecal	63% Renal 33% Fecal	85% Renal 6% Fecal	66% Renal 28% Fecal	25% Renal
Bioavailability	79%–100%	60%	>99%	6.5%	80%	66%

2.3. Factor Xa Inhibitors

The idea of using FXa inhibitors as clinical anticoagulants also originates from naturally occurring inhibitors. The first FXa inhibitor to be studied was a compound called antistasin, originally isolated from the Mexican leech *haementeria officinalis* [33]. However, the concept of FXa inhibitors as anticoagulant drugs was not supported until a second FXa inhibitor called the tick anticoagulant peptide (TAP) had been isolated from the soft tick *ornithodors moubata* [34]. *In vitro* and *in vivo* studies demonstrated that FXa inhibitors block the activity of FXa generated via both intrinsic and extrinsic pathways and thus subsequently block the formation of thrombin [35,36].

In 2012 the FXa inhibitor called rivaroxaban was approved for clinical use (Table 2). Rivaroxaban acts via inhibition of the active site of FXa (Figure 1c) [35], and has predictable pharmacokinetic and dynamics [30]. Peak activity of rivaroxaban occurs 2–3 h after intake, with a half-life of 5–9 h [30]. The short half-life suggests that rivaroxaban needs to be taken twice daily, however guidelines for rivaroxaban usage recommend once daily. This recommendation comes from both clinical phase II and III trials, which provided evidence that once daily administration is most beneficial with respect to the balance between safety and efficacy [37]. In addition, the duration of rivaroxaban inhibiting FXa lasts 24 h thereby supporting the once daily policy. Rivaroxaban is mainly excreted by the kidneys (66% with 36% as unchanged drug) with a smaller fraction excreted in the faeces (28% with 7% unchanged) [31].

To date, the most recently approved DOAC is another FXa inhibitor called apixaban (Table 2). Like rivaroxaban, apixaban inhibits both bound and free FXa (Figure 1c). Apixaban activity peaks 3 h after intake and has a half life of 9–14 h [32]. Bioavailability of apixaban is 66%, and apixaban is partly (25%) excreted by the kidneys.

3. Clinical Trials with Oral Anticoagulation Drugs

3.1. Vitamin K Antagonists (VKA)

The promise and later importance of VKA as oral anticoagulant drugs for clinical use became apparent in a randomized trial performed in the 1960s [38]. In this trial, patients with pulmonary embolism were divided in two groups receiving either the anticoagulant drug or placebo control. Of the group receiving anticoagulation therapy none of the patients died, whereas 5 patients in the placebo group died of pulmonary embolism [38].

Ever since the clinical introduction of VKA, their clinical efficacy and safety have been monitored through measuring the coagulation activity of the blood, mainly using the prothrombin time (PT) test or a close variant of this test [39]. A central ingredient of the PT test is a biological tissue reagent called thromboplastin. It quickly became apparent that innate variations in the source and batch of thromboplastin led to significant variabilities in PT results which were usually reported as a prothrombin time ratio (PTR) representing the patient's PT divided by normal PT [39]. In principle, when a high or low laboratory PTR is reported, the anticoagulant dosage is adjusted accordingly to reach the target coagulation ratio [39]. In the early 1960s it became apparent that some commercial thromboplastins were insufficiently responsive to the anticoagulant-induced effect leading to an underestimation of the dose of VKA required to achieve the target PTR. The subsequent overdosing with VKA led to an increase in bleeding complications and indicated the importance of using sensitive thromboplastin-based assays to prevent over or under dosing with VKA. Comparison of thromboplastin assays between North America and the UK revealed that increased sensitivity of assays reduced the incidence of hemorrhage [39,40]. These results also addressed the need for increased standardization of PT assays and international guidelines for monitoring anticoagulation therapy. In 1983, the World Health Organization (WHO) adopted a universally standardized system of reporting patient PT data during VKA therapy called the international normalized ratio (INR) which is still used today [41].

3.2. DOACs

With the approval of DOACs for clinical use, an alternative to VKA or heparin treatment became available. Recent clinical trials have investigated efficacy and safety profiles of DOACs in comparison to VKA treatment. The outcomes of these comparative trials are briefly described below.

3.2.1. Dabigatran Etexilate

The RE-LY and RE-COVER clinical trials demonstrated non-inferiority of dabigatran etexilate compared to warfarin in atrial fibrillation (AF) patients and patients with acute venous thromboembolism, respectively [25,42]. Additionally, the RE-MODEL clinical trial demonstrated non-inferiority of dabigatran compared to enoxaparin treatment with respect to preventing venous thromboembolism after total knee replacement surgery [43]. Taken together these clinical trials demonstrated the non-inferiority of dabigatran compared to VKA treatment. Thus, dabigatran etexilate seems a suitable alternative for VKA for the treatment of patients with increased thrombosis risk.

3.2.2. Rivaroxaban

The clinical trials ROCKET AF, RECORD, EINSTEIN-DVT and EINSTEIN-Extension demonstrated the non-inferiority of rivaroxaban as compared to VKA and heparin treatment in patients with non-valvular atrial fibrillation, symptomatic venous thromboembolism, deep-vein thrombosis, and recurrent thrombosis in deep-vein thrombosis patients [44–46]. Moreover, rivaroxaban demonstrated no difference in risk for major bleedings in patients undergoing elective hip/knee replacement, though rivaroxaban was more effective in preventing symptomatic venous thromboembolism [47].

3.2.3. Apixaban

The ARISTOTLE and ADVANCE clinical trials showed non-inferiority of apixaban as compared to VKA and heparin in AF patients and for thromboprophylaxis in patients after hip replacement, respectively [48,49]. Similar to dabigatran and rivaroxaban, apixaban showed no difference as compared to VKA treatment with respect to risk for major bleedings.

These clinical trials did not demonstrate superiority of DOACs over VKA, questioning whether DOACs should replace VKA as standard treatment. A meta-analysis comparing DOACs with VKA provided additional insight and showed the superiority over DOACs compared to VKA treatment with respect to major bleedings [50]. However, care is required interpreting these results and more research is needed.

4. Advantages and Disadvantages of VKA and DOACs

The use of VKA treatment over 60 years is one of the major advantages, since this revealed both short and long-term effects in humans. Disadvantages of VKA include the narrow therapeutic window and thus indirectly safety and efficacy. Therefore, VKA therapy requires regular monitoring by measuring the INR [21,51]. Additionally, the pharmacokinetic and pharmacodynamics are unpredictable through drug interactions, cytochrome P450-dependent mechanisms, and the influence of dietary vitamin K intake [10,52]. All the coumarin VKA listed in Table 2 (*i.e.*, warfarin, acenocoumarol, and phenprocoumon) have a slow onset, taking *ca.* two to seven days to be effective in inducing anticoagulation [10,21]. Therefore, VKA therapy requires initial co-administration with other anticoagulants, such as heparin. Moreover, it has been shown recently that patients taking VKA treatment display hitherto unreported non-hemostasis side effects [53]. One of these side effects is VKA-induced vascular calcification. Vascular calcification is associated with an increased risk for cardiovascular disease [53–55]. In addition, VKA treatment is associated with arterial stiffness, which in turn is related to vascular calcification [56,57].

DOACs were developed to circumvent the disadvantages of VKA therapy without negatively influencing safety profiles. Initially, the manufacturers of DOACs promoted the view that a major advantage of DOACs was that they did not require routine coagulation testing (as needed for VKA) or the measurement of circulating drug concentrations. However, data from the dabigatran RE-LY trial suggested that adjusting the dosage of dabigatran based on measurements of plasma dabigatran concentrations may reduce major bleeding events by as much as 30%–40% as compared to well-controlled warfarin [58]. Moreover, monitoring dabigatran plasma concentrations has the potential to improve safety and efficacy profiles as compared to fixed dosage [58,59]. Therapeutic drug monitoring of DOACs is supported by population studies which demonstrated a wide range of plasma dabigatran concentrations in different patient groups and at different time points although drug concentrations remained within the putative therapeutic range [60]. Variations in plasma concentration are ascribed to drug interactions, differences in absorption in the gastrointestinal tract, and clearance by the liver and kidneys [61]. These issues raise the question whether DOAC treatment should be regularly monitored.

A major issue of oral anticoagulation using VKA and DOACs is the need for reversal agents and coagulation assays to monitor the precise degree of anticoagulation. This is of importance in the event of bleeding and to allow surgical procedures or to counteract overdosing. The importance of reversal agents is illustrated by warfarin-related bleeding events, in which 50% of patients die within 90 days, mainly due to intracranial hemorrhage [62]. In the case of VKA, guidelines for the reversal of over-anticoagulation are well established with effective reversal agents (phylloquinone, and prothrombin complex concentrates) and sensitive coagulation assays (e.g., INR) to monitor haemostasis [62]. Vitamin K can counteract the effect of VKA via a

NAD(P)H-dependent quinone reductase, the precise identity of which is uncertain. The enzyme that counteracts VKA is predominantly active in the liver and unlike VKOR is not inhibited by VKA thereby enabling the reduction of vitamin K into KH_2 cofactors needed for γ-glutamyl carboxylation (Figure 1b) [63]. Reversal agents for DOACs were initially lacking, but are currently under development (idarucizumab for dabigatran, and andexanet and PER977 for FXa) [64]. Idarucizumab was developed to inactivate dabigatran, and works by binding to dabigatran with an affinity 350 times higher than thrombin. Recently, the clinical trial RE-VERSE AD investigated the capability and safety of idarucizumab as a reversal agent, and demonstrated a complete reversal of the anticoagulation effect of dabigatran within minutes. Of note, a major limitation in the RE-VERSE AD trial is the lack of a control group [65].

It should be noted that all DOACs are partially excreted by the kidneys (80%, 65%, and 25% for dabigatran, rivaroxaban and apixaban, respectively) [66,67] and are therefore unsuitable for patients with severe renal deficiency. In contrast, VKA are predominantly metabolized through the liver and are thus the best option for anticoagulation with this patient population.

5. Vitamin K Dependent Proteins and Atherosclerosis

5.1. Coagulation and Atherosclerosis

Coagulation factors are effective activators of the vascular system independent of their effects on coagulation and exhibit pleiotropic effects on the vasculature that contribute to cardiovascular disease. More specifically, coagulation factors can affect the vessel wall through regulation of the proliferation, migration and differentiation of vascular smooth muscle cells (VSMCs) as well as by inducing oxidative stress, inflammation and apoptosis [66,67], all processes that contribute to the development of atherosclerosis. In addition, micro plaque ruptures and subclinical thrombosis are pivotal to the progression and increased vulnerability of plaques, thereby increasing the risk for atherothrombosis [67].

5.2. Thrombin and Atherosclerosis

Thrombin is the central player in the coagulation cascade and influences non-hemostasis signaling via the protease-activated receptors (PAR-1, PAR-2, PAR-3, PAR-4) [66]. Thrombin activates these receptors via proteolytic cleavage of the N-terminal domain of PAR-1, PAR-3 and PAR-4 resulting in a tethered ligand activating the receptor [68,69]. In the vasculature, endothelial cells express PAR-1, PAR-2 and PAR-4, whereas VSMCs express PAR-1 and PAR-2 [70]. The effects of thrombin on the different PARs are likely to induce different effects, of which PAR-1 related effects have been most studied [66,71].

Human atherosclerotic plaques express elevated levels of PAR-1 [72], suggesting that PAR-1 plays a role in atherosclerosis development. In line with this hypothesis, thrombin induced PAR-1 activation can lead to VSMC migration and proliferation (Figure 2b). Moreover, thrombin elevates collagen production by VSMCs in a PAR-1 dependent manner [73], indicating a possible role for thrombin in plaque stability. Another feature of atherosclerotic plaque development is apoptosis. VSMCs that undergo apoptosis can generate thrombin via a process that accelerates the assembly of the prothrombinase complex [74]. In addition, thrombin generation is associated with vascular calcification [75].

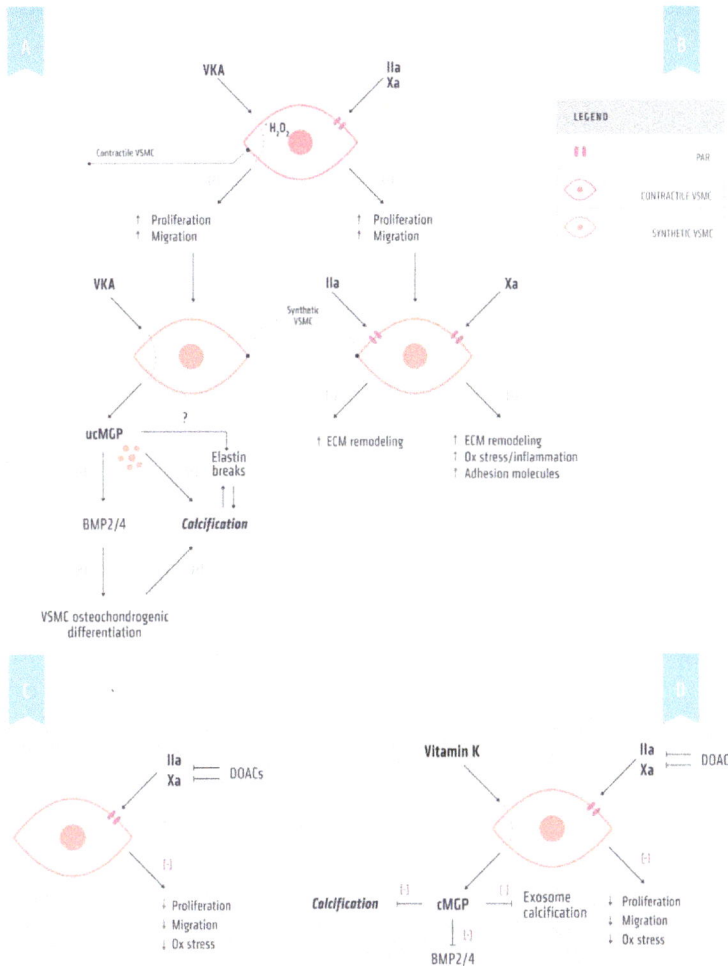

Figure 2. Effects of anticoagulants and vitamin K on vascular calcification. (**A**) Mechanism by which vitamin K antagonist (VKA) induces calcification. VKA induces phenotypic switching of contractile to synthetic vascular smooth muscle cells (VSMCs) by increasing oxidative stress resulting in increased proliferation and migration. Synthetic VSMCs secrete uncarboxylated matrix Gla protein (ucMGP) as a result of vitamin K depletion induced by VKA. ucMGP is unable to inhibit bone morphogenetic protein (BMP) 2 and 4, a marker for osteochondrogenic differentiation. Osteochondrogenic VSMCs are prone to calcification. Additionally, ucMGP is directly associated with increased calcification; (**B**) Thrombin and factor Xa induce non-hemostasis signaling via protease-activated receptors (PARs). Activation of PARs on contractile VSMCs can induce phenotypic switching resulting in increased proliferation and migration. PAR signaling in these synthetic VSMCs increases oxidative stress and adhesion molecules and induces extracellular (ECM) remodeling thereby facilitating calcification; (**C**) DOAC treatment in combination with (**D**) supplemental vitamin K administration has the potential to prevent both hypercoagulability and inhibit vascular calcification.

Of note, rodents lack PAR-1 expression on platelets [71]. Therefore, experiments targeting PAR-1 in rodents can be directly ascribed to PAR-1 expressed by the vessel wall. Indeed, vascular injury is altered in PAR-1 deficient mice possibly via extracellular matrix formation and remodeling [72]. In line with these results, *in vitro* stimulation of VSMCs by thrombin stimulates extracellular matrix production [70].

Dabigatran inhibits thrombin mediated PAR1 function by inhibiting N-terminal cleavage and internalization [76]. The inhibition of thrombin activity by dabigatran may thus inhibit the development of cardiovascular disease by reducing pro-inflammatory signaling [67]. Indeed, dabigatran was shown to attenuate atherosclerosis development [77] and promote plaque stability [78].

5.3. Factor Xa and Atherosclerosis

Like thrombin, FXa induces non-hemostatic signaling via PARs. However, in contrast to thrombin FXa interacts only with PAR-1 and PAR-2 [70,79]. As with PAR-1, the expression of PAR-2 is upregulated in human vascular lesions [70,80]. FXa has been linked to pathophysiological conditions, including inflammation, tissue fibrosis and vascular remodeling [81]. In line with this link, FXa has been shown to induce inflammatory signaling and increase expression of cell adhesion molecules [67]. Moreover, FXa induces proliferation and migration of VSMCs via activation of PAR-2 thereby altering the composition and accumulation of extracellular matrix [82,83]. The *in vivo* importance of PAR-2 in the inflammation process is suggested by findings that PAR-2 deficient mice display lower inflammation in a model of arthritis [84] and from rat studies in which lipopolysaccharide and oxidative stress increased the expression of PAR-2 [85,86].

Taken together, the available data suggests that FXa has a role in atherosclerosis via its interaction with PAR-1 and PAR-2. Recently, treatment of atherosclerosis prone apoE$^{-/-}$ mice with rivaroxaban resulted in increased plaque stability [87]. Since FXa activates prothrombin it is tempting to speculate that inhibition of FXa also prevents thrombin-mediated effects in atherothrombosis.

6. Vitamin K Dependent Proteins and Calcification

Originally, vascular calcification was thought to be a passive process. The discovery of calcification inhibitors that actively prevent vascular calcification showed that it is a highly regulated process involving proteins and cellular components. The VKDP matrix Gla protein (MGP) is a local calcification inhibitor associated with calcifications in human lesions [88,89]. Other VKDP associated with vascular calcification are osteocalcin (OC) and the more recently discovered Gla Rich Protein (GRP) [90]. Moreover, MGP, OC and the downstream regulator bone morphogenetic proteins (BMP) 2 and 4 are associated with microcalcifications in early human atherosclerotic lesions [88]. Microcalcifications in atherosclerosis are associated with increased plaque vulnerability [91–94].

6.1. Osteocalcin

Like all VKDP proteins, OC requires vitamin K for the γ-glutamylcarboxylation of three glutamate-residues, which in turn confers functional protein activity. In tissues and the circulation OC is present in both the carboxylated (cOC) and uncarboxylated (ucOC) conformations. OC is mostly associated with bone metabolism [95] where it promotes bone growth [96–98]. The processes of bone metabolism and soft tissue calcification are closely related, suggesting a possible role of osteocalcin in vascular calcification (Figure 3). As in bone metabolism, OC is thought to both promote [99] and inhibit [100–103] soft tissue calcification in order to regulate remodeling and mineralization [104]. It has been suggested that the inhibitory effect of OC on calcification is via mechanisms that prevent calcium and phosphate precipitation [17].

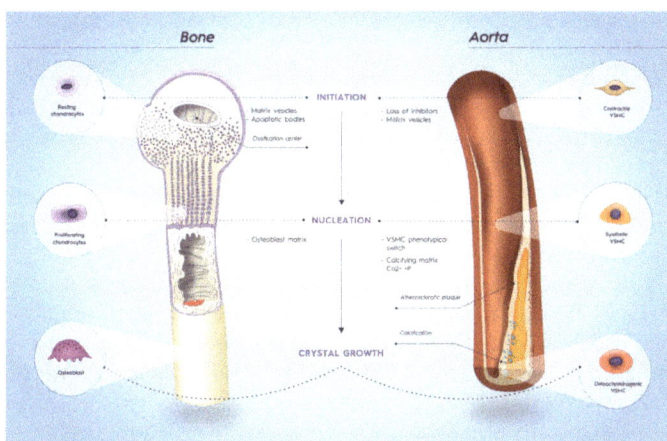

Figure 3. Similarities in bone metabolism and vascular calcification. The calcification process can be divided into three stages: initiation, nucleation and crystal growth. In order to initiate mineralization resting chondrocytes and contractile vascular smooth muscle cells (VSMCs) lose calcification inhibitors. Moreover, vesicles derived from chondrocytes and VSMCs form a nidus for calcification. In both bone metabolism and vascular calcification the matrix plays an important role in the nucleation stage. In bone metabolism, an osteoblast matrix results in proliferation of chondrocytes. Likewise, a calcifying matrix consisting of elastin, collagen and Ca^{2+} and P accompany vascular calcification. Additionally, contractile VSMCs undergo phenotypic switching resulting in synthetic VSMCs, which have increased proliferation and migration in comparison to contractile VSMCs. Finally, osteoblasts and osteochondrogenic VSMCs induce crystal growth in bone metabolism and vascular calcification, respectively.

The role of OC in vascular calcification suggests the possibility that OC measurements can be used as a biomarker of calcification. OC-positive endothelial progenitor cells are elevated in patients with a history of cardiovascular events and were associated with calcification of coronary arteries [105, 106]. During atherosclerosis, VSMCs undergo phenotypic switching resulting in osteoblast-like VSMCs, which are prone to calcification. Calcifying VSMCs express OC [107] and thus increased circulating concentrations of OC may reflect vascular calcification. Indeed, calcification of osteoblast-like VSMCs is associated with OC synthesis [108]. Furthermore, circulating levels of ucOC could provide insights into the relationship between vitamin K status and calcification. Indeed, it has been shown that ucOC concentrations are an independent predictor of carotid artery calcification [109].

6.2. Matrix Gla Protein

MGP is found in a wide range of tissues including heart, lungs, skin and the vasculature. In the vessel wall MGP is secreted by VSMCs [110]. Besides posttranslational carboxylation, MGP can also undergo serine phosphorylation. The precise role of the latter modification is not fully understood, but is thought to play a role in the secretion of MGP [111].

The pivotal role of MGP became clear from MGP-deficient mice, which all died within eight weeks after birth due to rupture of severely calcified arteries [112]. Analyses of the arteries revealed fragmented and calcified elastic fibers and the presence of osteochondrogenic-like cells. Surprisingly, the calcification phenotype of $MGP^{-/-}$ mice was not rescued by restoring circulating levels of MGP via hepatic MGP expression [113]. In contrast, restoring MGP expression in VSMCs rescued the vascular phenotype completely [113]. These data demonstrated that only VSMCs synthesis of carboxylated MGP (cMGP) is able to inhibit vascular calcification. MGP deficiency is also present in humans resulting in

Keutel syndrome. Patients with Keutel syndrome suffer from abnormal soft tissue calcification [104] and have low levels of circulating cMGP [114].

Administration of warfarin results in similar calcification of arteries as observed in MGP$^{-/-}$ mice suggesting that warfarin-induced calcification is via impairment of MGP function [115]. Additionally, since warfarin chemically knocks down γ-carboxylated MGP it can be used as a model to investigate the role of MGP in vascular calcification [115].

There are several routes by which cMGP may inhibit calcification [110]. MGP is present in matrix vesicles and apoptopic bodies released from VSMCs [116]. In the presence of increased extracellular calcium MGP levels initially increase. However, when calcium levels are chronically elevated, MGP levels decrease [110]. Furthermore, MGP blocks VSMC phenotypic switching. Under physiological conditions, VSMCs display a contractile phenotype supporting vascular tone, and are not prone to calcify. In contrast, VSMCs undergoing synthetic or osteochondrogenic differentiation are susceptible to vascular calcification [17]. MGP$^{-/-}$ mice had decreased VSMC contractile markers and increased osteochondrogenic markers [112,117]. The phenotypic switching of VSMCs is under the regulation of BMP 2 and 4, which in turn are inhibited by cMGP [118,119]. MGP also directly inhibits calcium crystal growth by its ability to block nucleation sites through the binding of the negatively charged Gla domain and phosphorylated serine residues of MGP with growing hydroxyapatite crystals [120,121]. Finally, MGP prevents mineralization of elastin fibers by shedding nucleation sites, this process being facilitated by the low molecular weight and small size of MGP allowing it to prevent mineralization within the elastin fibers [122,123].

6.3. Gla Rich Protein

GRP, also termed Upper zone of growth plate and Cartilage Matrix Associated protein (UCMA), is a recently discovered VKDP highly conserved in animals and humans and involved in the inhibition of vascular calcification. Human gene expression and protein accumulation of GRP was shown in the fetal growth plate, vascular system and skin [124]. In human pathological conditions, GRP expression is associated with calcification of skin and arteries [90]. GRP has, like MGP, calcium-binding properties and acts as a calcification inhibitor [125]. The calcification-inhibitory effect of GRP is dose-dependent, requires γ-glutamylcarboxylation, and is thought to act via inhibition of osteochondrogenic switching of VSMCs [125]. GRP knockout mice, however lack phenotypic alterations [126].

7. Role for Vitamin K in Cardiovascular Disease

The first evidence that vitamin K is associated with vascular health came from data from the Rotterdam study [127]. In this observational study the risk for cardiovascular disease was some 50% lower in people in the highest tertile for menaquinone dietary intake (MK4 through MK10) [127]. In epidemiological studies, dietary intakes of menaquinones (MK-4 through MK-10) have been reported to be associated with a reduced risk for cardiovascular mortality [127,128]. Additionally, higher menaquinone intakes (MK-4 through MK-10) or supplementation with MK-7 were associated with reduced calcification, which is presumed to be due to the improved γ-carboxylation and greater functional activity of VKDP [129,130]. Finally, the long chain menaquinone isoprenologue MK-7 has been shown to have a greater impact on restoring coagulation compared to phylloquinone in VKA treated healthy volunteers indicating the overall better efficacy of MK-7 for the γ-carboxylation of the coagulation VKDP synthesized in the liver [14,131]. Explanations for the putative beneficial effect of MK-7 on the vascular system for the γ-carboxylation of MGP and GRP is that long chain menaquinones such as MK7 are mainly transported via low-density lipoproteins and have a slower clearance rate from the circulation [13] as well as a higher co-factor activity for the γ glutamyl-carboxylase [132].

In order to investigate the effect of vitamin K on the vascular system in humans a biomarker that reflects vitamin K status is required. Since vitamin K is essential for carboxylation of VKDP, the carboxylation status of VKDP can be used as a biomarker for vitamin K status. Dialysis patients have significantly increased levels of circulating uncarboxylated MGP (ucMGP) and reduced levels of cMGP indicative of a subclinical vascular vitamin K deficiency [133]. Moreover, circulating levels of ucMGP are positively associated with vascular calcification. Taken together, ucMGP seems a promising biomarker for vascular vitamin K status in relation to vascular calcification [89,133–135]. Therefore, clinical studies investigating the effect of vitamin K on the vascular system and calcification use the carboxylation status of MGP as a biomarker [130]. Currently, clinical trials are ongoing to assess the effect of high intake of vitamin K on vascular calcification progression [136]. In these clinical studies both phylloquinone and menaquinones are under investigation and can therefore provide novel insights into the differential effect of vitamin K forms on vascular calcification.

8. Vitamin K and Direct oral Anticoagulation

Treating patients with hypercoagulability and vascular disease requires personalized medicine. Whereas both VKA and DOACs are equally suitable for treating hypercoagulability, VKA induces vascular calcification thereby affecting the vessel wall in a negative way (Figure 2a). Effects of DOACs on vascular calcification are not known yet, but are unlikely to affect VKDP activity (Figure 2b) [137]. Moreover, high intake of vitamin K has shown to inhibit and even reverse warfarin-induced vascular calcification in experimental animals [56,138] and in adenine treated rats [52]. It is tempting to speculate that co-administration of vitamin K with anticoagulation therapy can target both coagulation and calcification. Since this co-administration is unsuitable with VKA [131], it should be investigated whether combining DOACs and vitamin K can be beneficial for both coagulation and calcification (Figure 2c). Presently, clinical trials assessing these aspects of co-administration are being conducted and the results of these studies should provide novel insights into personalized anticoagulation therapy [136].

9. Conclusions

Currently, VKA are still the most widely prescribed drugs used for anticoagulation therapy. However, owing to the unfavorable pharmacokinetics and actions of VKA, direct thrombin and FXa inhibitors have been introduced as alternatives to VKA. Clinical studies have demonstrated that DOACs are non-inferior to VKA but are likely to lack the calcification-inducing side effect of VKA. Additionally, DOACs exert beneficial effects on atherogenesis via PAR signaling. Presently, ongoing clinical trials are addressing whether vitamin K supplementation can halt or regress vascular calcification. The outcome of these trials will pave the way to test whether co-supplementation of vitamin K with DOACs can benefit both coagulation and calcification.

Acknowledgments: This work was supported in part by research funding from the Trombose Stichting Nederland (grant 2014.02) and by the Norwegian Research Council and NattoPharma ASA.

Author Contributions: Rick van Gorp and Leon Schurgers wrote the manuscript. Leon Schurgers had primary responsibility for the final content.

Conflicts of Interest: Nattopharma ASA received an industrial PhD grant from the Norwegian Research Council to conduct research on vitamin K in collaboration with the Maastricht University. Rick van Gorp has been employed as PhD student to work on this project. Nattopharma ASA is a pharmaceutical company with interest in vitamin K_2.

References

1. Mann, K.G. Biochemistry and physiology of blood coagulation. *Thromb. Haemost.* **1999**, *82*, 165–174. [PubMed]
2. Macfarlane, R.G. An enzyme cascade in the blood clotting mechanism, and its function as a biochemical amplifier. *Nature* **1964**, *202*, 498–499. [CrossRef] [PubMed]
3. Colman, R.W. Are hemostasis and thrombosis two sides of the same coin? *J. Exp. Med.* **2006**, *203*, 493–495. [CrossRef] [PubMed]
4. Badimon, L. Atherosclerosis and thrombosis: Lessons from animal models. *Thromb. Haemost.* **2001**, *86*, 356–365. [PubMed]

5. Fuster, V.; Stein, B.; Ambrose, J.A.; Badimon, L.; Badimon, J.J.; Chesebro, J.H. Atherosclerotic plaque rupture and thrombosis. Evolving concepts. *Circulation* **1990**, *82*, II47–II59. [PubMed]
6. Rosendaal, F.R. Venous thrombosis: A multicausal disease. *Lancet* **1999**, *353*, 1167–1173. [CrossRef]
7. Schofield, F.W. A brief account of a disease in cattle simulating hemorrhagic septicaemia due to feeding sweet clover. *Can. Vet. J. Rev. Vétérinaire Can.* **1984**, *25*, 453–455.
8. Link, K. The discovery of dicumarol and its sequels. *Circulation* **1959**, *19*, 97–107. [CrossRef] [PubMed]
9. Shapiro, S.; Ciferri, F.E. Intramuscular administration of the anticoagulant warfarin (coumadin) sodium. *J. Am. Med. Assoc.* **1957**, *165*, 1377–1380. [CrossRef] [PubMed]
10. Beinema, M.; Brouwers, J.R.B.J.; Schalekamp, T.; Wilffert, B. Pharmacogenetic differences between warfarin, acenocoumarol and phenprocoumon. *Thromb. Haemost.* **2008**, *100*, 1052–1057. [CrossRef] [PubMed]
11. Beulens, J.W.J.; Booth, S.L.; van den Heuvel, E.G.H.M.; Stoecklin, E.; Baka, A.; Vermeer, C. The role of menaquinones (vitamin K2) in human health. *Br. J. Nutr.* **2013**, *110*, 1357–1368. [CrossRef] [PubMed]
12. Schurgers, L.J.; Vermeer, C. Determination of phylloquinone and menaquinones in food. *Eff. Food Matrix Circ. Vitam. K Conc.* **2000**, *30*, 298–307. [CrossRef]
13. Schurgers, L.J.; Vermeer, C. Differential lipoprotein transport pathways of K-vitamins in healthy subjects. *Biochim. Biophys. Acta* **2002**, *1570*, 27–32. [CrossRef]
14. Schurgers, L.J.; Teunissen, K.J.F.; Hamulyak, K.; Knapen, M.H.J.; Vik, H.; Vermeer, C. Vitamin K-containing dietary supplements: Comparison of synthetic vitamin K1 and natto-derived menaquinone-7. *Blood* **2007**, *109*, 3279–3283. [CrossRef] [PubMed]
15. Thijssen, H.H.W.; Vervoort, L.M.T.; Schurgers, L.J.; Shearer, M.J. Menadione is a metabolite of oral vitamin K. *Br. J. Nutr.* **2006**, *95*, 260–266. [CrossRef] [PubMed]
16. Esmon, C.; Sadowski, J.; Suttie, J. A new carboxylation reaction. The vitamin K-dependent incorporation of H-14-CO3- into prothrombin. *J. Biol. Chem.* **1975**, *250*, 4744–4748. [PubMed]
17. Willems, B.A.G.; Vermeer, C.; Reutelingsperger, C.P.M.; Schurgers, L.J. The realm of vitamin K dependent proteins: Shifting from coagulation toward calcification. *Mol. Nutr. Food Res.* **2014**, *58*, 1620–1635. [CrossRef] [PubMed]
18. Van Horn, W.D. Structural and functional insights into human vitamin K epoxide reductase and vitamin K epoxide reductase-like1. *Crit. Rev. Biochem. Mol. Biol.* **2013**, *48*, 357–372. [CrossRef] [PubMed]
19. Stafford, D. The vitamin K cycle. *J. Thromb. Haemost.* **2005**, *3*, 1873–1878. [CrossRef] [PubMed]
20. Weitz, J.I.; Hirsh, J. New antithrombotic agents. *Chest* **1998**, *114*, 715S–727S. [CrossRef] [PubMed]
21. Van Aken, H.; Bode, C.; Darius, H.; Diehm, C.; Encke, A.; Gulba, D.C.; Haas, S.; Hacke, W.; Puhl, W.; Quante, M.; *et al.* State-of-the-art review: Anticoagulation: The present and future. *Clin. Appl. Thromb. Hemost.* **2001**, *7*, 195–204. [CrossRef] [PubMed]
22. Greinacher, A.; Warkentin, T.E. The direct thrombin inhibitor hirudin. *Thromb. Haemost.* **2008**, *99*, 819–829. [CrossRef] [PubMed]
23. Eriksson, B.I.; Wille-Jørgensen, P.; Kälebo, P.; Mouret, P.; Rosencher, N.; Bösch, P.; Baur, M.; Ekman, S.; Bach, D.; Lindbratt, S.; *et al.* A comparison of recombinant hirudin with a low-molecular-weight heparin to prevent thromboembolic complications after total hip replacement. *N. Engl. J. Med.* **1997**, *337*, 1329–1335. [CrossRef] [PubMed]
24. Investigators, G.L. Randomized trial of intravenous heparin *versus* recombinant hirudin for acute coronary syndromes. The Global Use of Strategies to Open Occluded Coronary Arteries (GUSTO) IIa Investigators. *Circulation* **1994**, *90*, 1631–1637.
25. Schulman, S.; Kearon, C.; Kakkar, A.K.; Mismetti, P.; Schellong, S.; Eriksson, H.; Baanstra, D.; Schnee, J.; Goldhaber, S.Z. RE-COVER Study Group Dabigatran *versus* warfarin in the treatment of acute venous thromboembolism. *N. Engl. J. Med.* **2009**, *361*, 2342–2352. [CrossRef] [PubMed]
26. Schulman, S.; Wåhlander, K.; Lundström, T.; Clason, S.B.; Eriksson, H. THRIVE III Investigators Secondary prevention of venous thromboembolism with the oral direct thrombin inhibitor ximelagatran. *N. Engl. J. Med.* **2003**, *349*, 1713–1721. [CrossRef] [PubMed]
27. Laizure, S.C.; Parker, R.B.; Herring, V.L.; Hu, Z.-Y. Identification of carboxylesterase-dependent dabigatran etexilate hydrolysis. *Drug Metab. Dispos. Biol. Fate Chem.* **2014**, *42*, 201–206. [CrossRef] [PubMed]
28. Akwaa, F.; Spyropoulos, A.C. The potential of target-specific oral anticoagulants for the acute and long-term treatment of venous thromboembolism. *Curr. Med. Res. Opin.* **2014**, *30*, 2179–2190. [CrossRef] [PubMed]

29. Yeh, C.H.; Hogg, K.; Weitz, J.I. Overview of the New Oral Anticoagulants: Opportunities and Challenges. *Arterioscler. Thromb. Vasc. Biol.* **2015**, *35*, 1056–1065. [CrossRef] [PubMed]

30. Kubitza, D.; Becka, M.; Wensing, G.; Voith, B.; Zuehlsdorf, M. Safety, pharmacodynamics, and pharmacokinetics of BAY 59–7939—An oral, direct Factor Xa inhibitor—After multiple dosing in healthy male subjects. *Eur. J. Clin. Pharmacol.* **2005**, *61*, 873–880. [CrossRef] [PubMed]

31. Kubitza, D.; Haas, S. Novel factor Xa inhibitors for prevention and treatment of thromboembolic diseases. *Expert Opin. Investig. Drugs* **2006**, *15*, 843–855. [CrossRef] [PubMed]

32. Weitz, J.I. Emerging anticoagulants for the treatment of venous thromboembolism. *Thromb. Haemost.* **2006**, *96*, 274–284. [CrossRef] [PubMed]

33. Nutt, E.M.; Jain, D.; Lenny, A.B.; Schaffer, L.; Siegl, P.K.; Dunwiddie, C.T. Purification and characterization of recombinant antistasin: A leech-derived inhibitor of coagulation factor Xa. *Arch. Biochem. Biophys.* **1991**, *285*, 37–44. [CrossRef]

34. Yeh, C.H.; Fredenburgh, J.C.; Weitz, J.I. Oral direct factor Xa inhibitors. *Circ. Res.* **2012**, *111*, 1069–1078. [CrossRef] [PubMed]

35. Perzborn, E.; Strassburger, J.; Wilmen, A.; Pohlmann, J.; Roehrig, S.; Schlemmer, K.-H.; Straub, A. *In vitro* and *in vivo* studies of the novel antithrombotic agent BAY 59-7939—An oral, direct Factor Xa inhibitor. *J. Thromb. Haemost.* **2005**, *3*, 514–521. [CrossRef] [PubMed]

36. Schurgers, L.J.; Spronk, H.M.H. Differential cellular effects of old and new oral anticoagulants: Consequences to the genesis and progression of atherosclerosis. *Thromb. Haemost.* **2014**, *112*, 909–917. [CrossRef] [PubMed]

37. Kreutz, R. A clinical and pharmacologic assessment of once-daily *versus* twice-daily dosing for rivaroxaban. *J. Thromb. Thrombolysis* **2014**, *38*, 137–149. [CrossRef] [PubMed]

38. Barritt, D.W.; Jordan, S.C. Anticoagulant drugs in the treatment of pulmonary embolism. A controlled trial. *Lancet* **1960**, *1*, 1309–1312. [CrossRef]

39. Duxbury, B.M.; Poller, L. The oral anticoagulant saga: Past, present, and future. *Clin. Appl. Thromb. Hemost.* **2001**, *7*, 269–275. [CrossRef] [PubMed]

40. Hull, R.; Hirsh, J.; Jay, R.; Carter, C.; England, C.; Gent, M.; Turpie, A.G.; McLoughlin, D.; Dodd, P.; Thomas, M.; *et al.* Different intensities of oral anticoagulant therapy in the treatment of proximal-vein thrombosis. *N. Engl. J. Med.* **1982**, *307*, 1676–1681. [CrossRef] [PubMed]

41. Guyatt, G.H.; Akl, E.A.; Crowther, M.; Gutterman, D.D.; Schuünemann, H.J. Executive summary: Antithrombotic therapy and prevention of thrombosis, 9th ed.: American college of chest physicians evidence-based clinical practice guidelines. *Chest* **2012**, *141*, 7S–47S. [CrossRef] [PubMed]

42. Connolly, S.J.; Ezekowitz, M.D.; Yusuf, S.; Eikelboom, J.; Oldgren, J.; Parekh, A.; Pogue, J.; Reilly, P.A.; Themeles, E.; Varrone, J.; *et al.* RE-LY Steering Committee and Investigators Dabigatran *versus* warfarin in patients with atrial fibrillation. *N. Engl. J. Med.* **2009**, *361*, 1139–1151. [CrossRef] [PubMed]

43. Eriksson, B.I.; Dahl, O.E.; Rosencher, N.; Kurth, A.A.; van Dijk, C.N.; Frostick, S.P.; Kälebo, P.; Christiansen, A.V.; Hantel, S.; Hettiarachchi, R.; *et al.* RE-MODEL Study Group Oral dabigatran etexilate *vs.* subcutaneous enoxaparin for the prevention of venous thromboembolism after total knee replacement: The RE-MODEL randomized trial. *J. Thromb. Haemost.* **2007**, *5*, 2178–2185. [CrossRef] [PubMed]

44. Patel, M.R.; Mahaffey, K.W.; Garg, J.; Pan, G.; Singer, D.E.; Hacke, W.; Breithardt, G.; Halperin, J.L.; Hankey, G.J.; Piccini, J.P.; *et al.* ROCKET AF Investigators Rivaroxaban *versus* warfarin in nonvalvular atrial fibrillation. *N. Engl. J. Med.* **2011**, *365*, 883–891. [CrossRef] [PubMed]

45. Eriksson, B.I.; Borris, L.C.; Friedman, R.J.; Haas, S.; Huisman, M.V.; Kakkar, A.K.; Bandel, T.J.; Beckmann, H.; Muehlhofer, E.; Misselwitz, F.; *et al.* RECORD1 Study Group Rivaroxaban *versus* enoxaparin for thromboprophylaxis after hip arthroplasty. *N. Engl. J. Med.* **2008**, *358*, 2765–2775. [CrossRef] [PubMed]

46. EINSTEIN Investigators; Bauersachs, R.; Berkowitz, S.D.; Brenner, B.; Büller, H.R.; Decousus, H.; Gallus, A.S.; Lensing, A.W.; Misselwitz, F.; Prins, M.H.; *et al.* Oral rivaroxaban for symptomatic venous thromboembolism. *N. Engl. J. Med.* **2010**, *363*, 2499–2510.

47. Eriksson, B.I.; Kakkar, A.K.; Turpie, A.G.G.; Gent, M.; Bandel, T.-J.; Homering, M.; Misselwitz, F.; Lassen, M.R. Oral rivaroxaban for the prevention of symptomatic venous thromboembolism after elective hip and knee replacement. *J. Bone Joint Surg. Br.* **2009**, *91*, 636–644. [CrossRef] [PubMed]

48. Granger, C.B.; Alexander, J.H.; McMurray, J.J.V.; Lopes, R.D.; Hylek, E.M.; Hanna, M.; Al-Khalidi, H.R.; Ansell, J.; Atar, D.; Avezum, A.; *et al.* ARISTOTLE Committees and Investigators Apixaban *versus* warfarin in patients with atrial fibrillation. *N. Engl. J. Med.* **2011**, *365*, 981–992. [CrossRef] [PubMed]

49. Lassen, M.R.; Gallus, A.; Raskob, G.E.; Pineo, G.; Chen, D.; Ramirez, L.M. ADVANCE-3 Investigators Apixaban *versus* enoxaparin for thromboprophylaxis after hip replacement. *N. Engl. J. Med.* **2010**, *363*, 2487–2498. [CrossRef] [PubMed]

50. Van Es, N.; Coppens, M.; Schulman, S.; Middeldorp, S.; Büller, H.R. Direct oral anticoagulants compared with vitamin K antagonists for acute venous thromboembolism: Evidence from phase 3 trials. *Blood* **2014**, *124*, 1968–1975. [CrossRef] [PubMed]

51. Haas, S. Medical indications and considerations for future clinical decision making. *Thromb. Res.* **2003**, *109* (Suppl. 1), S31–S37. [CrossRef]

52. McCabe, K.M.; Booth, S.L.; Fu, X.; Shobeiri, N.; Pang, J.J.; Adams, M.A.; Holden, R.M. Dietary vitamin K and therapeutic warfarin alter the susceptibility to vascular calcification in experimental chronic kidney disease. *Kidney Int.* **2013**, *83*, 835–844. [CrossRef] [PubMed]

53. Chatrou, M.L.L.; Winckers, K.; Hackeng, T.M.; Reutelingsperger, C.P.; Schurgers, L.J. Vascular calcification: The price to pay for anticoagulation therapy with vitamin K-antagonists. *Blood Rev.* **2012**, *26*, 155–166. [CrossRef] [PubMed]

54. Rosenhek, R.; Binder, T.; Porenta, G.; Lang, I.; Christ, G.; Schemper, M.; Maurer, G.; Baumgartner, H. Predictors of outcome in severe, asymptomatic aortic stenosis. *N. Engl. J. Med.* **2000**, *343*, 611–617. [CrossRef] [PubMed]

55. Rennenberg, R.J.M.W.; Kessels, A.G.H.; Schurgers, L.J.; van Engelshoven, J.M.A.; de Leeuw, P.W.; Kroon, A.A. Vascular calcifications as a marker of increased cardiovascular risk: A meta-analysis. *Vasc. Health Risk Manag.* **2009**, *5*, 185–197. [CrossRef] [PubMed]

56. Schurgers, L.J.; Spronk, H.M.; Soute, B.A.; Schiffers, P.; DeMey, J.G.R.; Vermeer, C. Regression of warfarin-induced medial elastocalcinosis by high intake of vitamin K in rats. *Blood* **2007**, *109*, 2823–2831. [CrossRef] [PubMed]

57. Mac-Way, F.; Poulin, A.; Utescu, M.S.; De Serres, S.A.; Marquis, K.; Douville, P.; Desmeules, S.; Larivière, R.; Lebel, M.; Agharazii, M. The impact of warfarin on the rate of progression of aortic stiffness in hemodialysis patients: A longitudinal study. *Nephrol. Dial. Transplant.* **2014**, *29*, 2113–2120. [CrossRef] [PubMed]

58. Cohen, D. Dabigatran: How the drug company withheld important analyses. *BMJ (Clin. Res. ed.)* **2014**, *349*. [CrossRef] [PubMed]

59. Moore, T.J.; Cohen, M.R.; Mattison, D.R. Dabigatran, bleeding, and the regulators. *BMJ (Clin. Res. ed.)* **2014**, *349*. [CrossRef] [PubMed]

60. Favaloro, E.J.; Lippi, G. Laboratory testing in the era of direct or non-vitamin K antagonist oral anticoagulants: A practical guide to measuring their activity and avoiding diagnostic errors. *Semin. Thromb. Hemost.* **2015**, *41*, 208–227. [PubMed]

61. Lippi, G.; Favaloro, E.J.; Mattiuzzi, C. Combined administration of antibiotics and direct oral anticoagulants: A renewed indication for laboratory monitoring? *Semin. Thromb. Hemost.* **2014**, *40*, 756–765. [PubMed]

62. Bauer, K.A. Targeted Anti-Anticoagulants. *N. Engl. J. Med.* **2015**, *373*, 569–571. [CrossRef] [PubMed]

63. Shearer, M.J.; Newman, P. Metabolism and cell biology of vitamin K. *Thromb. Haemost.* **2008**, *100*, 530–547. [CrossRef] [PubMed]

64. Crowther, M.; Crowther, M.A. Antidotes for Novel Oral Anticoagulants: Current Status and Future Potential. *Arterioscler. Thromb. Vasc. Biol.* **2015**, *35*, 1736–1745. [CrossRef] [PubMed]

65. Pollack, C.V.; Reilly, P.A.; Eikelboom, J.; Glund, S.; Verhamme, P.; Bernstein, R.A.; Dubiel, R.; Huisman, M.V.; Hylek, E.M.; Kamphuisen, P.W.; *et al.* Idarucizumab for Dabigatran Reversal. *N. Engl. J. Med.* **2015**, *373*, 511–520. [CrossRef] [PubMed]

66. Patterson, C.; Stouffer, G.A.; Madamanchi, N.; Runge, M.S. New tricks for old dogs: Nonthrombotic effects of thrombin in vessel wall biology. *Circ. Res.* **2001**, *88*, 987–997. [CrossRef] [PubMed]

67. Borissoff, J.I.; Spronk, H.M.H.; Ten Cate, H. The hemostatic system as a modulator of atherosclerosis. *N. Engl. J. Med.* **2011**, *364*, 1746–1760. [PubMed]

68. Ma, L.; Dorling, A. The roles of thrombin and protease-activated receptors in inflammation. *Semin. Immunopathol.* **2012**, *34*, 63–72. [CrossRef] [PubMed]

69. Kalz, J.; Ten Cate, H.; Spronk, H.M.H. Thrombin generation and atherosclerosis. *J. Thromb. Thrombolysis* **2014**, *37*, 45–55. [CrossRef] [PubMed]

70. Alberelli, M.A.; De Candia, E. Functional role of protease activated receptors in vascular biology. *Vasc. Pharmacol.* **2014**, *62*, 72–81. [CrossRef] [PubMed]

71. Martorell, L.; Martínez-González, J.; Rodríguez, C.; Gentile, M.; Calvayrac, O.; Badimon, L. Thrombin and protease-activated receptors (PARs) in atherothrombosis. *Thromb. Haemost.* **2008**, *99*, 305–315. [CrossRef] [PubMed]

72. Cheung, W.M.; D'Andrea, M.R.; Andrade-Gordon, P.; Damiano, B.P. Altered vascular injury responses in mice deficient in protease-activated receptor-1. *Arterioscler. Thromb. Vasc. Biol.* **1999**, *19*, 3014–3024. [CrossRef] [PubMed]

73. Dabbagh, K.; Laurent, G.J.; McAnulty, R.J.; Chambers, R.C. Thrombin stimulates smooth muscle cell procollagen synthesis and mRNA levels via a PAR-1 mediated mechanism. *Thromb. Haemost.* **1998**, *79*, 405–409. [PubMed]

74. Flynn, P.; Byrne, C.; Baglin, T.; Weissberg, P.; Bennett, M. Thrombin generation by apoptotic vascular smooth muscle cells. *Blood* **1997**, *89*, 4378–4384. [PubMed]

75. Borissoff, J.I.; Joosen, I.A.; Versteylen, M.O.; Spronk, H.M.; ten Cate, H.; Hofstra, L. Accelerated *In Vivo* Thrombin Formation Independently Predicts the Presence and Severity of CT Angiographic Coronary Atherosclerosis. *JACC Cardiovasc. Imaging* **2012**, *5*, 1201–1210. [CrossRef] [PubMed]

76. Chen, B.; Soto, A.G.; Coronel, L.J.; Goss, A.; van Ryn, J.; Trejo, J. Characterization of Thrombin-Bound Dabigatran Effects on Protease-Activated Receptor-1 Expression and Signaling *In Vitro. Mol. Pharmacol.* **2015**, *88*, 95–105. [CrossRef] [PubMed]

77. Pingel, S.; Tiyerili, V.; Mueller, J.; Werner, N.; Nickenig, G.; Mueller, C. Thrombin inhibition by dabigatran attenuates atherosclerosis in ApoE deficient mice. *Arch. Med. Sci.* **2014**, *10*, 154–160. [CrossRef] [PubMed]

78. Kadoglou, N.P.E.; Moustardas, P.; Katsimpoulas, M.; Kapelouzou, A.; Kostomitsopoulos, N.; Schafer, K.; Kostakis, A.; Liapis, C.D. The beneficial effects of a direct thrombin inhibitor, dabigatran etexilate, on the development and stability of atherosclerotic lesions in apolipoprotein E-deficient mice: Dabigatran etexilate and atherosclerosis. *Cardiovasc. Drugs Ther. Spons. Int. Soc. Cardiovasc. Pharmacother.* **2012**, *26*, 367–374. [CrossRef] [PubMed]

79. Borensztajn, K.; Peppelenbosch, M.P.; Spek, C.A. Factor Xa: At the crossroads between coagulation and signaling in physiology and disease. *Trends Mol. Med.* **2008**, *14*, 429–440. [CrossRef] [PubMed]

80. Lee, H.; Hamilton, J.R. Physiology, pharmacology, and therapeutic potential of protease-activated receptors in vascular disease. *Pharmacol. Ther.* **2012**, *134*, 246–259. [CrossRef] [PubMed]

81. Esmon, C.T. Targeting factor Xa and thrombin: Impact on coagulation and beyond. *Thromb. Haemost.* **2014**, *111*, 625–633. [CrossRef] [PubMed]

82. Böhm, A.; Flößer, A.; Ermler, S.; Fender, A.C.; Lüth, A.; Kleuser, B.; Schrör, K.; Rauch, B.H. Factor-Xa-induced mitogenesis and migration require sphingosine kinase activity and S1P formation in human vascular smooth muscle cells. *Cardiovasc. Res.* **2013**, *99*, 505–513. [CrossRef] [PubMed]

83. Borensztajn, K.; Spek, C.A. Blood coagulation factor Xa as an emerging drug target. *Expert Opin. Ther. Targets* **2011**, *15*, 341–349. [CrossRef] [PubMed]

84. Ferrell, W.R.; Lockhart, J.C.; Kelso, E.B.; Dunning, L.; Plevin, R.; Meek, S.E.; Smith, A.J.H.; Hunter, G.D.; McLean, J.S.; McGarry, F.; *et al.* Essential role for proteinase-activated receptor-2 in arthritis. *J. Clin. Investig.* **2003**, *111*, 35–41. [CrossRef] [PubMed]

85. Aman, M.; Hirano, M.; Kanaide, H.; Hirano, K. Upregulation of proteinase-activated receptor-2 and increased response to trypsin in endothelial cells after exposure to oxidative stress in rat aortas. *J. Vasc. Res.* **2010**, *47*, 494–506. [CrossRef] [PubMed]

86. Cicala, C.; Pinto, A.; Bucci, M.; Sorrentino, R.; Walker, B.; Harriot, P.; Cruchley, A.; Kapas, S.; Howells, G.L.; Cirino, G. Protease-activated receptor-2 involvement in hypotension in normal and endotoxemic rats *in vivo*. *Circulation* **1999**, *99*, 2590–2597. [CrossRef] [PubMed]

87. Zhou, Q.; Bea, F.; Preusch, M.; Wang, H.; Isermann, B.; Shahzad, K.; Katus, H.A.; Blessing, E. Evaluation of plaque stability of advanced atherosclerotic lesions in apo E-deficient mice after treatment with the oral factor Xa inhibitor rivaroxaban. *Mediat. Inflamm.* **2011**, *2011*, 1–9. [CrossRef] [PubMed]

88. Roijers, R.B.; Debernardi, N.; Cleutjens, J.P.M.; Schurgers, L.J.; Mutsaers, P.H.A.; van der Vusse, G.J. Microcalcifications in early intimal lesions of atherosclerotic human coronary arteries. *Am. J. Pathol.* **2011**, *178*, 2879–2887. [CrossRef] [PubMed]

89. Schurgers, L.J.; Teunissen, K.J.F.; Knapen, M.H.J.; Kwaijtaal, M.; van Diest, R.; Appels, A.; Reutelingsperger, C.P.; Cleutjens, J.P.M.; Vermeer, C. Novel conformation-specific antibodies against matrix γ-carboxyglutamic acid (Gla) protein: Undercarboxylated matrix Gla protein as marker for vascular calcification. *Arterioscler. Thromb. Vasc. Biol.* **2005**, *25*, 1629–1633. [CrossRef] [PubMed]

90. Viegas, C.S.B.; Cavaco, S.; Williamson, M.K.; Price, P.A.; Cancela, M.L.; Simes, D.C. Gla-rich protein is a novel vitamin K-dependent protein present in serum that accumulates at sites of pathological calcifications. *Am. J. Pathol.* **2009**, *175*, 2288–2298. [CrossRef] [PubMed]

91. Joshi, N.V.; Vesey, A.T.; Williams, M.C.; Shah, A.S.V.; Calvert, P.A.; Craighead, F.H.M.; Yeoh, S.E.; Wallace, W.; Salter, D.; Fletcher, A.M.; *et al.* 18F-fluoride positron emission tomography for identification of ruptured and high-risk coronary atherosclerotic plaques: A prospective clinical trial. *Lancet* **2014**, *383*, 705–713. [CrossRef]

92. Ehara, S.; Kobayashi, Y.; Yoshiyama, M.; Shimada, K.; Shimada, Y.; Fukuda, D.; Nakamura, Y.; Yamashita, H.; Yamagishi, H.; Takeuchi, K.; *et al.* Spotty calcification typifies the culprit plaque in patients with acute myocardial infarction: An intravascular ultrasound study. *Circulation* **2004**, *110*, 3424–3429. [CrossRef] [PubMed]

93. Bluestein, D.; Alemu, Y.; Avrahami, I.; Gharib, M.; Dumont, K.; Ricotta, J.J.; Einav, S. Influence of microcalcifications on vulnerable plaque mechanics using FSI modeling. *J. Biomech.* **2008**, *41*, 1111–1118. [CrossRef] [PubMed]

94. Vengrenyuk, Y.; Carlier, S.; Xanthos, S.; Cardoso, L.; Ganatos, P.; Virmani, R.; Einav, S.; Gilchrist, L.; Weinbaum, S. A hypothesis for vulnerable plaque rupture due to stress-induced debonding around cellular microcalcifications in thin fibrous caps. *Proc. Natl. Acad. Sci. USA* **2006**, *103*, 14678–14683. [CrossRef] [PubMed]

95. Lombardi, G.; Perego, S.; Luzi, L.; Banfi, G. A four-season molecule: Osteocalcin. Updates in its physiological roles. *Endocrine* **2014**, *48*, 394–404. [CrossRef] [PubMed]

96. Schlieper, G.; Schurgers, L.; Brandenburg, V.; Reutlingsperger, C.; Floege, J. Vascular calcification in chronic kidney disease: An update. *Nephrol. Dial. Transplant.* **2015**. [CrossRef] [PubMed]

97. Yamada, S.; Taniguchi, M.; Tokumoto, M.; Toyonaga, J.; Fujisaki, K.; Suehiro, T.; Noguchi, H.; Iida, M.; Tsuruya, K.; Kitazono, T. The antioxidant tempol ameliorates arterial medial calcification in uremic rats: Important role of oxidative stress in the pathogenesis of vascular calcification in chronic kidney disease. *J. Bone Miner. Res.* **2012**, *27*, 474–485. [CrossRef] [PubMed]

98. Ndip, A.; Wilkinson, F.L.; Jude, E.B.; Boulton, A.J.; Alexander, M.Y. RANKL-OPG and RAGE modulation in vascular calcification and diabetes: Novel targets for therapy. *Diabetologia* **2014**, *57*, 2251–2260. [CrossRef] [PubMed]

99. Lei, Y.; Sinha, A.; Nosoudi, N.; Grover, A.; Vyavahare, N. Hydroxyapatite and calcified elastin induce osteoblast-like differentiation in rat aortic smooth muscle cells. *Exp. Cell Res.* **2014**, *323*, 198–208. [CrossRef] [PubMed]

100. Hunter, G.K.; Hauschka, P.V.; Poole, A.R.; Rosenberg, L.C.; Goldberg, H.A. Nucleation and inhibition of hydroxyapatite formation by mineralized tissue proteins. *Biochem. J.* **1996**, *317*, 59–64. [CrossRef] [PubMed]

101. Ducy, P.; Desbois, C.; Boyce, B.; Pinero, G.; Story, B.; Dunstan, C.; Smith, E.; Bonadio, J.; Goldstein, S.; Gundberg, C.; *et al.* Increased bone formation in osteocalcin-deficient mice. *Nature* **1996**, *382*, 448–452. [CrossRef] [PubMed]

102. Kavukcuoglu, N.B.; Patterson-Buckendahl, P.; Mann, A.B. Effect of osteocalcin deficiency on the nanomechanics and chemistry of mouse bones. *J. Mech. Behav. Biomed. Mater.* **2009**, *2*, 348–354. [CrossRef] [PubMed]

103. Roy, M.E.; Nishimoto, S.K.; Rho, J.Y.; Bhattacharya, S.K.; Lin, J.S.; Pharr, G.M. Correlations between osteocalcin content, degree of mineralization, and mechanical properties of *C. carpio* rib bone. *J. Biomed. Mater. Res.* **2001**, *54*, 547–553. [CrossRef]

104. Evrard, S.; Delanaye, P.; Kamel, S.; Cristol, J.-P.; Cavalier, E. SFBC/SN joined working group on vascular calcifications vascular calcification: From pathophysiology to biomarkers. *Clin. Chim. Acta* **2015**, *438*, 401–414. [CrossRef] [PubMed]

105. Price, P.A.; Otsuka, A.A.; Poser, J.W.; Kristaponis, J.; Raman, N. Characterization of a γ-carboxyglutamic acid-containing protein from bone. *Proc. Natl. Acad. Sci. USA* **1976**, *73*, 1447–1451. [CrossRef] [PubMed]

106. Van de Loo, P.G.F.; Soute, B.; van Haarlem, L.; Vermeer, C. The effect of Gla-containing proteins on the precipitation of insoluble salts. *Biochem. Biophys. Res. Commun.* **1987**, *142*, 113–119. [CrossRef]

107. Kapustin, A.N.; Shanahan, C.M. Osteocalcin: A novel vascular metabolic and osteoinductive factor? *Arterioscler. Thromb. Vasc. Biol.* **2011**, *31*, 2169–2171. [CrossRef] [PubMed]

108. Aikawa, E.; Nahrendorf, M.; Sosnovik, D.; Lok, V.M.; Jaffer, F.A.; Aikawa, M.; Weissleder, R. Multimodality molecular imaging identifies proteolytic and osteogenic activities in early aortic valve disease. *Circulation* **2007**, *115*, 377–386. [CrossRef] [PubMed]

109. Okura, T.; Kurata, M.; Enomoto, D.; Jotoku, M.; Nagao, T.; Desilva, V.R.; Higaki, J. Undercarboxylated osteocalcin is a biomarker of carotid calcification in patients with essential hypertension. *Kidney Blood Press. Res.* **2010**, *33*, 66–71. [CrossRef] [PubMed]

110. Schurgers, L.J.; Uitto, J.; Reutelingsperger, C.P. Vitamin K-dependent carboxylation of matrix Gla-protein: A crucial switch to control ectopic mineralization. *Trends Mol. Med.* **2013**, *19*, 217–226. [CrossRef] [PubMed]

111. Wajih, N.; Borras, T.; Xue, W.; Hutson, S.M.; Wallin, R. Processing and transport of matrix γ-carboxyglutamic acid protein and bone morphogenetic protein-2 in cultured human vascular smooth muscle cells: Evidence for an uptake mechanism for serum fetuin. *J. Biochem.* **2004**, *279*, 43052–43060. [CrossRef] [PubMed]

112. Luo, G.; Ducy, P.; McKee, M.; Pinero, G.; Loyer, E.; Behringer, R.; Karsenty, G. Spontaneous calcification of arteries and cartilage in mice lacking matrix GLA protein. *Nature* **1997**, *385*, 78–81. [CrossRef] [PubMed]

113. Murshed, M.; Schinke, T.; McKee, M.D.; Karsenty, G. Extracellular matrix mineralization is regulated locally; different roles of two gla-containing proteins. *J. Cell Biol.* **2004**, *165*, 625–630. [CrossRef] [PubMed]

114. Cranenburg, E.C.M.; van Spaendonck-Zwarts, K.Y.; Bonafe, L.; Mittaz Crettol, L.; Rödiger, L.A.; Dikkers, F.G.; van Essen, A.J.; Superti-Furga, A.; Alexandrakis, E.; Vermeer, C.; *et al.* Circulating matrix γ-carboxyglutamate protein (MGP) species are refractory to vitamin K treatment in a new case of Keutel syndrome. *J. Thromb. Haemost.* **2011**, *9*, 1225–1235. [CrossRef] [PubMed]

115. Price, P.; Faus, S.; Williamson, M. Warfarin causes rapid calcification of the elastic lamellae in rat arteries and heart valves. *Arterioscler. Thromb. Vasc. Biol.* **1998**, *18*, 1400–1407. [CrossRef] [PubMed]

116. Reynolds, J.L.; Joannides, A.J.; Skepper, J.N.; McNair, R.; Schurgers, L.J.; Proudfoot, D.; Jahnen-Dechent, W.; Weissberg, P.L.; Shanahan, C.M. Human vascular smooth muscle cells undergo vesicle-mediated calcification in response to changes in extracellular calcium and phosphate concentrations: A potential mechanism for accelerated vascular calcification in ESRD. *J. Am. Soc. Nephrol.* **2004**, *15*, 2857–2867. [CrossRef] [PubMed]

117. Steitz, S.A.; Speer, M.Y.; Curinga, G.; Yang, H.Y.; Haynes, P.; Aebersold, R.; Schinke, T.; Karsenty, G.; Giachelli, C.M. Smooth muscle cell phenotypic transition associated with calcification: Upregulation of Cbfa1 and downregulation of smooth muscle lineage markers. *Circ. Res.* **2001**, *89*, 1147–1154. [CrossRef] [PubMed]

118. Yao, Y.; Bennett, B.J.; Wang, X.; Rosenfeld, M.E.; Giachelli, C.; Lusis, A.J.; Boström, K.I. Inhibition of bone morphogenetic proteins protects against atherosclerosis and vascular calcification. *Circ. Res.* **2010**, *107*, 485–494. [CrossRef] [PubMed]

119. Boström, K.I.; Rajamannan, N.M.; Towler, D.A. The regulation of valvular and vascular sclerosis by osteogenic morphogens. *Circ. Res.* **2011**, *109*, 564–577. [CrossRef] [PubMed]

120. O'Young, J.; Liao, Y.; Xiao, Y.; Jalkanen, J.; Lajoie, G.; Karttunen, M.; Goldberg, H.A.; Hunter, G.K. Matrix Gla protein inhibits ectopic calcification by a direct interaction with hydroxyapatite crystals. *J. Am. Chem. Soc.* **2011**, *133*, 18406–18412. [CrossRef] [PubMed]

121. Schurgers, L.J.; Spronk, H.M.H.; Skepper, J.N.; Hackeng, T.M.; Shanahan, C.M.; Vermeer, C.; Weissberg, P.L.; Proudfoot, D. Post-translational modifications regulate matrix Gla protein function: Importance for inhibition of vascular smooth muscle cell calcification. *J. Thromb. Haemost.* **2007**, *5*, 2503–2511. [CrossRef] [PubMed]

122. Khavandgar, Z.; Roman, H.; Li, J.; Lee, S.; Vali, H.; Brinckmann, J.; Davis, E.C.; Murshed, M. Elastin haploinsufficiency impedes the progression of arterial calcification in MGP-deficient mice. *J. Bone Miner. Res.* **2014**, *29*, 327–337. [CrossRef] [PubMed]

123. Price, P.A.; Toroian, D.; Lim, J.E. Mineralization by inhibitor exclusion: The calcification of collagen with fetuin. *J. Biol. Chem.* **2009**, *284*, 17092–17101. [CrossRef] [PubMed]

124. Cancela, M.L.; Conceição, N.; Laizé, V. Gla-rich protein, a new player in tissue calcification? *Adv. Nutr.* **2012**, *3*, 174–181. [CrossRef] [PubMed]

125. Viegas, C.S.B.; Rafael, M.S.; Enriquez, J.L.; Teixeira, A.; Vitorino, R.; Luís, I.M.; Costa, R.M.; Santos, S.; Cavaco, S.; Neves, J.; *et al.* Gla-rich protein acts as a calcification inhibitor in the human cardiovascular system. *Arterioscler. Thromb. Vasc. Biol.* **2015**, *35*, 399–408. [CrossRef] [PubMed]

126. Eitzinger, N.; Surmann-Schmitt, C.; Bösl, M.; Schett, G.; Engelke, K.; Hess, A.; von der Mark, K.; Stock, M. Ucma is not necessary for normal development of the mouse skeleton. *Bone* **2012**, *50*, 670–680. [CrossRef] [PubMed]

127. Geleijnse, J.M.; Vermeer, C.; Grobbee, D.E.; Schurgers, L.J.; Knapen, M.H.J.; van der Meer, I.M.; Hofman, A.; Witteman, J.C.M. Dietary intake of menaquinone is associated with a reduced risk of coronary heart disease: The Rotterdam Study. *J. Nutr.* **2004**, *134*, 3100–3105. [PubMed]

128. Juanola-Falgarona, M.; Salas-Salvadó, J.; Martínez-González, M.Á.; Corella, D.; Estruch, R.; Ros, E.; Fitó, M.; Arós, F.; Gómez-Gracia, E.; Fiol, M.; *et al.* Dietary intake of vitamin k is inversely associated with mortality risk. *J. Nutr.* **2014**, *144*, 743–750. [CrossRef] [PubMed]

129. Beulens, J.W.; Bots, M.L.; Atsma, F.; Bartelink, M.L.E.; Prokop, M.; Geleijnse, J.M.; Van Der Schouw, Y.T. High dietary menaquinone intake is associated with reduced coronary calcification. *Atherosclerosis* **2009**, *203*, 489–493. [CrossRef] [PubMed]

130. Westenfeld, R.; Krueger, T.; Schlieper, G.; Cranenburg, E.C.M.; Magdeleyns, E.J.; Heidenreich, S.; Holzmann, S.; Vermeer, C.; Jahnen-Dechent, W.; Ketteler, M.; *et al.* Effect of vitamin K_2 supplementation on functional vitamin K deficiency in hemodialysis patients: A randomized trial. *Am. J. Kidney Dis.* **2012**, *59*, 186–195. [CrossRef] [PubMed]

131. Theuwissen, E.; Teunissen, K.J.; Spronk, H.M.H.; Hamulyak, K.; ten Cate, H.; Shearer, M.J.; Vermeer, C.; Schurgers, L.J. Effect of low-dose supplements of menaquinone-7 (vitamin K_2) on the stability of oral anticoagulant treatment: Dose-response relationship in healthy volunteers. *J. Thromb. Haemost.* **2013**, *11*, 1085–1092. [CrossRef] [PubMed]

132. Buitenhuis, H.C.; Soute, B.A.; Vermeer, C. Comparison of the vitamins K1, K2 and K3 as cofactors for the hepatic vitamin K-dependent carboxylase. *Biochim. Biophys. Acta* **1990**, *1034*, 170–175. [CrossRef]

133. Schlieper, G.; Westenfeld, R.; Krüger, T.; Cranenburg, E.C.; Magdeleyns, E.J.; Brandenburg, V.M.; Djuric, Z.; Damjanovic, T.; Ketteler, M.; Vermeer, C.; *et al.* Circulating nonphosphorylated carboxylated matrix Gla protein predicts survival in ESRD. *J. Am. Soc. Nephrol.* **2011**, *22*, 387–395. [CrossRef] [PubMed]

134. Ueland, T.; Dahl, C.P.; Gullestad, L.; Aakhus, S.; Broch, K.; Skårdal, R.; Vermeer, C.; Aukrust, P.; Schurgers, L.J. Circulating levels of non-phosphorylated undercarboxylated matrix Gla protein are associated with disease severity in patients with chronic heart failure. *Clin. Sci.* **2011**, *121*, 119–127. [CrossRef] [PubMed]

135. Cranenburg, E.C.M.; Vermeer, C.; Koos, R.; Boumans, M.-L.; Hackeng, T.M.; Bouwman, F.G.; Kwaijtaal, M.; Brandenburg, V.M.; Ketteler, M.; Schurgers, L.J. The circulating inactive form of matrix Gla Protein (ucMGP) as a biomarker for cardiovascular calcification. *J. Vasc. Res.* **2008**, *45*, 427–436. [CrossRef] [PubMed]

136. Brandenburg, V.M.; Schurgers, L.J.; Kaesler, N.; Püsche, K.; van Gorp, R.H.; Leftheriotis, G.; Reinartz, S.; Koos, R.; Krüger, T. Prevention of vasculopathy by vitamin K supplementation: Can we turn fiction into fact? *Atherosclerosis* **2015**, *240*, 10–16. [CrossRef] [PubMed]

137. Morishima, Y.; Kamisato, C.; Honda, Y.; Furugohri, T.; Shibano, T. The effects of warfarin and edoxaban, an oral direct factor Xa inhibitor, on γcarboxylated (Gla-osteocalcin) and undercarboxylated osteocalcin (uc-osteocalcin) in rats. *Thromb. Res.* **2013**, *131*, 59–63. [CrossRef] [PubMed]

138. Krüger, T.; Oelenberg, S.; Kaesler, N.; Schurgers, L.J.; van de Sandt, A.M.; Boor, P.; Schlieper, G.; Brandenburg, V.M.; Fekete, B.C.; Veulemans, V.; *et al.* Warfarin induces cardiovascular damage in mice. *Arterioscler. Thromb. Vasc. Biol.* **2013**, *33*, 2618–2624. [CrossRef] [PubMed]

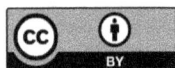

nutrients

MDPI

Review

Concepts and Controversies in Evaluating Vitamin K Status in Population-Based Studies

M. Kyla Shea and Sarah L. Booth *

USDA Human Nutrition Research Center on Aging, Tufts University, Boston, MA 02111, USA
* Correspondence: sarah.booth@tufts.edu; Tel.: +617-556-3231

Received: 25 September 2015; Accepted: 9 December 2015; Published: 2 January 2016

Abstract: A better understanding of vitamin K's role in health and disease requires the assessment of vitamin K nutritional status in population and clinical studies. This is primarily accomplished using dietary questionnaires and/or biomarkers. Because food composition databases in the US are most complete for phylloquinone (vitamin K1, the primary form in Western diets), emphasis has been on phylloquinone intakes and associations with chronic diseases. There is growing interest in menaquinone (vitamin K2) intakes for which the food composition databases need to be expanded. Phylloquinone is commonly measured in circulation, has robust quality control schemes and changes in response to phylloquinone intake. Conversely, menaquinones are generally not detected in circulation unless large quantities are consumed. The undercarboxylated fractions of three vitamin K-dependent proteins are measurable in circulation, change in response to vitamin K supplementation and are modestly correlated. Since different vitamin K dependent proteins are implicated in different diseases the appropriate vitamin K-dependent protein biomarker depends on the outcome under study. In contrast to other nutrients, there is no single biomarker that is considered a gold-standard measure of vitamin K status. Most studies have limited volume of specimens. Strategic decisions, guided by the research question, need to be made when deciding on choice of biomarkers.

Keywords: vitamin K; epidemiology; vitamin K intake; biomarkers; review

1. Introduction

Vitamin K is a class of structurally-similar compounds, all of which function as an enzymatic co-factor in the γ-carboxylation of vitamin K-dependent proteins [1]. While the best known vitamin K-dependent proteins are clotting proteins, vitamin K-dependent proteins are also present in many extra-hepatic tissues that have been implicated in many chronic diseases [2]. As new roles for vitamin K in health and disease emerge, so has interest in measuring vitamin K status in population-based studies. The purpose of this review is to evaluate the methods currently available to assess vitamin K status in human studies.

2. Vitamin K Intakes

A seemingly straightforward approach to estimate nutrient status is to estimate how much of the nutrient is being consumed [3]. Dietary forms of vitamin K fall into two general categories: Phylloquinone (vitamin K1) and menaquinones (collectively referred to as vitamin K2), which are comprised of at least 10 compounds (menaquinone-4 to menaquinone-13) that differ from phylloquinone in the length and saturation of their side-chain (Figure 1).

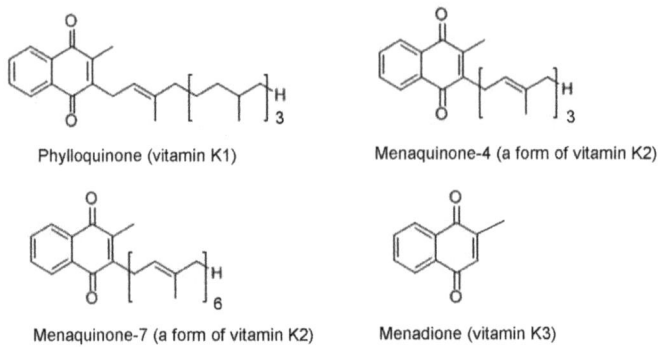

Figure 1. Forms of vitamin K.

Phylloquinone is plant-based, and concentrated in green leafy vegetables and certain plant oils (1). Longer chain menaquinones (menaquinone-7–menaquinone-13) have a bacterial origin, and are primarily concentrated in animal meats and fermented foods. Menaquinone-4, which is the most similar structurally to phylloquinone, is unique among the menaquinones in that it is not produced by bacteria, but instead is either formed from phylloquinone or a pro-vitamin menadione form used in animal feed. In the human diet, menaquinone-4 is concentrated in animal meats and dairy products.

The United States Institute of Medicine's Adequate Intake of vitamin K is set at 90 and 120 μg/day for adult women and men respectively [4]. These are based on median intakes reported in NHANES III [4]. Globally, dietary recommendations for vitamin K vary from 50 to 120 μg/day [5]. These recommendations do not differentiate phylloquinone intake from menaquinone intake. However, at the time the recommendations were set, the food composition databases from which they are based only contained the phylloquinone content of foods. Hence, the current vitamin K recommendations are based on phylloquinone, which is the primary form in Western diets [6–10]. As reviewed elsewhere, there is insufficient scientific knowledge at this time to determine an independent dietary recommendation for menaquinones [11].

Assessment of dietary intakes of vitamin K in population studies has relied on the use of the food frequency questionnaire (FFQ). There are many types of dietary questionnaires, which have been reviewed extensively [12,13]. In epidemiological studies, the FFQ is most commonly used because it is efficient in terms of cost and time, and imposes minimal burden on the study participant [3]. The FFQ appears to be suitable to rank individuals in terms of micronutrient intakes, but its ability to estimate absolute intakes of single nutrients is limited. The FFQ (similar to most diet questionnaires) is subjective and relies on individuals' recall ability and perceptions, which can bias the estimates of nutrient intake [14]. Nonetheless, the FFQ has been used to estimate phylloquinone and/or menaquinone intakes as measures of vitamin K status in several studies [9,14–18].

The findings of population-based studies that have related phylloquinone intake to chronic disease are inconsistent (Table 1).

Table 1. Population-based studies of vitamin K intake and disease.

Population	Region/Cohort	Vitamin K Form and Reported Intakes	Outcome	Results	References
1836 men and 2971 women, >55 years	Rotterdam, The Netherlands (Rotterdam Study)	PK: 257 ± 116 µg/day (men); 244 µg/day (women); MK (total): 31 ± 19 µg/day (men); 33 ± 16 µg/day (women)	CHD	Highest MK tertile had lower CHD risk; PK intake not associated with CHD	[9]
807 army personnel, 39–45 years, 82% male	United States	PK: 115 ± 79 µg/day	CAC	No association	[19]
564 post-menopausal women	Utrecht, The Netherlands (PROSPECT-EPIC)	PK: 217 ± 92 µg/day; MK: 32 ± 12 µg/day	CAC	Highest MK quartile (34 ± 3 µg/day) had lower prevalence CAC; PK intake not associated with CAC prevalence	[15]
16,057 post-menopausal women	Utrecht, The Netherlands (PROSPECT-EPIC)	PK: 212 ± 100 µg/day; MK: 29 ± 13 µg/day	CHD	Higher MK intake associated with lower CHD risk; PK intake not associated with CHD	[17]
72,874 women, 38–65 years	United States (Nurse's Health Study)	PK: 184 ± 106 µg/day	CHD	PK intake not associated with CHD once adjusted for healthy lifestyle characteristics	[20]
40,087 men, 40–75 years	United States (Physicians Health Study)	PK: 165 (67–383) µg/day (median, 5%–95%ile)	CHD	PK intake not associated with CHD once adjusted for healthy lifestyle characteristics	[8]
1112 men and 1479 women, 58 ± 9 years	Framingham, MA, United States (Framingham Offspring)	PK: 153 ± 115 µg/day (men); 171 ± 103 µg/day (women)	BMD	Higher PK intake associated with higher BMD in women, but not in men	[21]
898 women, 45–54 years	Scotland	PK: 109 ± 54 µg/day	BMD	Higher PK intake associated with higher BMD and less bone resorption	[22]
335 men and 553 women, 75 ± 5 years	Framingham, MA, United States (Framingham Heart Study)	PK: 143 ± 97 µg/day (men); 163 ± 115 µg/day (women)	BMD and hip fracture	Higher PK intake associated with lower fracture risk; not associated with BMD	[16]
72,327 women aged 38–63 years	United States (Nurse's Health Study)	PK: 169 (41–604) µg/day (median, 1%–99%ile)	Hip fracture	Higher quintiles PK intake (≥109 µg/day) associated with lower hip fracture risk (RR: 0.70; 95% CI: 0.53, 0.93)	[23]
1605 men, 1339 women	Hong Kong	PK: 254 (157–362) µg/day (median (range), men); 239 (162–408) µg/day (median (range), women)	Hip and non-vertebral fracture	PK intake not associated with any fracture outcome	[24]
1800 women, peri-menopausal, 43–58 years	Denmark (Danish Osteoporosis Prevention Study)	PK: baseline: 67 (45–105) µg/day (median, 25%–75%iles); 5 year followup: 60 (37–99) µg/day (median, 25%–75%iles)	BMD and fracture	PK intake not associated with BMD or fracture	[25]
1238 men, 1569 women, 71–75 years	Norway (Hordaland)	PK: 69 (67) µg/day (median (IQR), women); 75(62) µg/day (men); MK: 10 (7) µg/day (women); 12 (8) µg/day (men)	Hip fracture	Higher PK intake associated with lower fracture risk; no association between MK intake and fracture	[26]

Table 1. *Cont.*

Population	Region/Cohort	Vitamin K Form and Reported Intakes	Outcome	Results	References
625 men and women, 40–80 years	The Netherlands (PROSPECT-EPIC)	PK: 210 ± 127 μg/day; MK: 31 ± 13 μg/day	Metabolic Syndrome	Higher MK intake associated with lower prevalence MetSyn; PK intake not associated with MetSyn	[27]
510 men and women, diabetic and/or at risk for CHD, 67 ± 6 years	Spain (PREDIMED)	PK: 398 ± 201 μg/day	Insulin resistance and inflammation	Higher PK intake associated with improvements in IR and inflammation	[28]
662 men and women, 62 ± 10 years	United States (MESA)	PK: 93 ± 107 μg/day	Inflammation	No association between PK intake and inflammation	[29]
1247 men and 1472 women, 26–81 years	Framingham, MA, United States (Framingham Offspring)	PK: 139 (10 to 1975) μg/day (median (range))	Insulin resistance, sensitivity, glycemic status	Higher PK intake associated with better insulin sensitivity and glucose tolerance	[30]
11,319 men 40–64 years	Europe (EPIC-Heidelberg)	PK: 94 (71–124) μg/day (median (25%–75%ile); MK4-14: 35 (25–76) μg/day (median (25%–75%ile))	Prostate cancer	MK intake inversely associated with prostate cancer (*p*-trend = 0.06) and advanced prostate cancer (*p*-trend = 0.02)	[18]
24,340 men and women, 40–64 years	Europe (EPIC-Heidelberg)	PK 35 μg/day (median, men); MK 35 μg/day (median, men); PK 32 μg/day (median, women); MK 32 μg/day (median, women)	Cancer—lung, colorectal, breast, prostate	MK intake inversely associated with cancer incidence in men and mortality in men and women	[31]
7216 men and women, diabetic and/or at risk for CHD, 67 ± 6 years	Spain (PREDIMED)	PK: mean 356 μg/day; MK: mean 36 μg/day	Cardiovascular, cancer, all-cause mortality	Higher PK intake associated with lower cancer and all-cause mortality; MK intake not associated with mortality	[32]

Some found higher phylloquinone intake to be associated with higher BMD and lower fracture risk [16,26], lower cardiovascular disease (CVD) risk [8,20], improved insulin sensitivity [28,30], and lower mortality risk [32,33]. Others found phylloquinone intake was not associated with BMD [21,25], fracture [24], metabolic syndrome [27], or CVD [15,17,19,34]. The use of phylloquinone intake as the sole indicator of vitamin K status needs to be interpreted cautiously because phylloquinone intake also reflects healthy diets and lifestyles, given its concentration in green leafy vegetables and plant oils [8,20,35]. This residual confounding may not be completely eliminated when adjustments for healthy diet and/or lifestyle characteristics are made. When phylloquinone intake was estimated using the FFQ and a 5-day diet record, FFQ estimates were consistently higher, which may be due to over-reporting of vegetables [36,37]. In addition, the ability of the FFQ to accurately capture phylloquinone intakes greater than 200 µg/day is of concern. In the Framingham Offspring Study, which used the Harvard FFQ to estimate phylloquinone intake, plasma phylloquinone positively correlated with intakes up to 200 µg/d, above which the association between plasma phylloquinone and phylloquinone intake plateaued [38]. A similar pattern was observed in a separate cohort of older community-dwelling men and women in the U.S. participating in a phylloquinone supplementation trial when analyzed at baseline [39] (Figure 2).

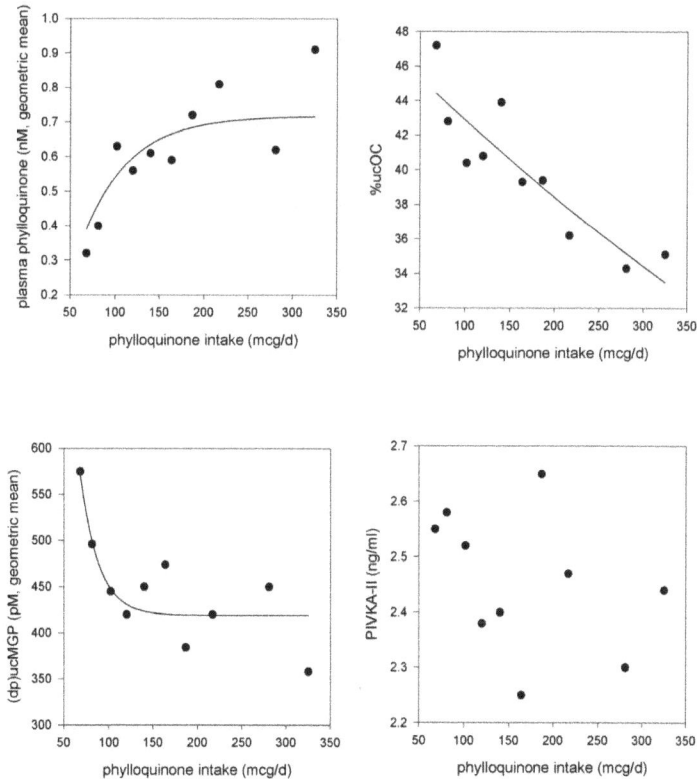

Figure 2. Association between food frequency questionnaire (FFQ)-estimated phylloquinone intake and circulating biomarkers of vitamin K status (at baseline) in community-dwelling older men and women participating in a phylloquinone supplementation trial [39,40]. The geometric mean of each biomarker is plotted at the median intake within each decile category. Adjustment was made for age, sex, BMI, energy intake (kcals/day), season, and triglycerides (for plasma phylloquinone).

While this plateau could reflect a saturation at the intakes >200 μg/day, circulating phylloquinone concentrations have been shown to increase to >2.0 nM in response to 500 μg/day and to >20 nM in response to 5000 μg/day of phylloquinone supplementation [39,41]. Therefore, it appears the FFQ may not be an appropriate method to estimate intakes in populations where phylloquinone intakes typically exceed 200 μg/day and results of studies doing so need to be interpreted accordingly.

Higher intakes of menaquinones were reported to be associated with less subclinical and clinical CVD, metabolic syndrome and some forms of cancer [9,15,17,18,27,31]. These associations may not be prone to confounding by a healthy diet because menaquinones are not found in foods that are typically characteristic of a healthy diet. However, the difference in total menaquinone intake between the highest and lowest categories of intake has been reported to be as narrow as ~20 μg/day [9,15,17,27]. The potential protective influence of a difference of 20 μg/day of total menaquinone is uncertain, and merits further research. It is also important to consider the food sources of menaquinones. Some cheeses rich in long-chain menaquinones are consumed in European countries more than in the US [42,43], and cheese intake itself has been associated with lower risk for type 2 diabetes, CVD, and mortality [44–47]. It is plausible menaquinone intake tracks intake of other nutrients and/or fatty acids found in cheese that have also been associated with cardiovascular disease [44,48].

The contribution of menaquinones, both in terms of forms and amounts to overall vitamin K intake varies regionally. In Western diets the relative contribution of menaquinones is thought to be much less than that of phylloquinone. However, food composition databases used in most countries do not quantify menaquinones specifically [11,49]. The most recent release of the USDA National Nutrient Database contains menaquinone-4 contents of a limited number of dairy and meat products [49]. Databases used in the Netherlands quantify individual menaquinones (menaquinone 4–10) in a limited number of foods, but are being updated [11,50]. Reported intakes of long-chain menaquinones are high in eastern Japan because *natto*, a bacterially-fermented soy food rich in menaquinone-7, is commonly eaten in that region [51]. Some have also suggested consumption of bacterially-fermented cheese, which is rich in long-chain menaquinones, is higher in the Netherlands, which may account for the long-chain menaquinone content of their diets [11]. However, a comparison of dairy intakes across EPIC study locations does not confirm this assertion [52].

Some have proposed dietary menaquinones to be more beneficial to cardiovascular and metabolic health than dietary phylloquinone [9,15,17,27]. However, the relative validity of the FFQ used in these studies was better for menaquinone than for phylloquinone [9,15,17,27]. Validity was assessed in reference to twelve 24-h recalls, but menaquinone intake validity has not yet been assessed in reference to any biomarkers. In contrast, the validity of the FFQ used to assess phylloquinone intake in these studies was poor, as acknowledged by the investigators, and the reported phylloquinone intakes were double what the current US recommendations are (means ranged from 212 to 257 μg/day) [9,17,27]. This may have blunted any ability to detect associations with dietary phylloquinone given the observed plateau effect. Furthermore, adjustment for intakes of cheese and/or other nutritional components of cheese associated with reduced CVD risk could be important but has not yet been done. Given the limitations inherent to using self-reported methods to estimate dietary intakes [3,53,54], population-based studies relating vitamin K status to chronic disease could be strengthened by the addition of vitamin K status biomarkers to dietary intake estimates.

3. Vitamin K Status Biomarkers

Nutritional biomarkers are biochemical measures measured in blood, urine, feces, adipose tissue or other tissues that reflect nutrient status [55]. Nutritional biomarkers are not limited by incomplete food composition databases, and are independent of recall, interviewer and social acceptance biases [55]. In contrast to dietary questionnaires which only estimate intake and generally do not account for relative bioavailability, biomarkers reflect intake, absorption and metabolism [55]. However, a thorough understanding of the biomarker's underlying biology is required in order to consider all the physiological factors that may influence its relationship to the intake of a specific nutrient. For a comprehensive review of vitamin K bioavailability, refer to Shearer *et al.* [5]. Biomarkers can be affected by health status, including the disease outcome of interest, which can lead to misclassification and erroneous conclusions in studies that aim to identify nutritional risk factors for disease. Temporal variability needs to be considered, since many biomarkers can vary post-prandially and/or diurnally [3]. Biomarkers represent nutrient status at one point in time, which may limit extrapolation to long-term status unless repeated measures are made. In addition, biomarker analyses require rigorous laboratory standardization and quality control procedures to reduce measurement error and misclassification [56]. Nonetheless biomarkers can provide valuable estimates of nutrient status in population studies when the studies' results are interpreted in the context of the strengths and limitations of the biomarker measured.

3.1. Circulating Vitamin K

Phylloquinone is the primary circulating form of vitamin K, and has been successfully measured to rank individuals' vitamin K status in population-based and clinic-based studies worldwide (Table 2). These studies also demonstrate the large variability in circulating vitamin K in most populations.

Table 2. Reported circulating concentrations of vitamin K in population- or clinic-based individuals not taking vitamin K supplements (Data are mean ± SD, unless otherwise indicated.).

Participants	Region	Phylloquinone	Menaquinone	Fasted	References
Post-menopausal women: generally healthy, 52–93 years (n = 23)	Japan	0.22 ± 0.32 nM[d]	MK4: 0.02 ± 0.001 nM[d]; MK7: 0.54 ± 1.00 nM[d]	not specified	[57]
with hip or vertebral fracture history, 66–93 years (n = 51)	Japan	0.21 ± 0.18 nM[d]	MK4: non-detectable[d]; MK7: 0.66 ± 1.00 nM[d]	not specified	
Pre-menopausal women generally healthy, 30–49 years (n = 52)	Nagano, Japan	0.68 ± 0.45 nM[d]	MK4: 0.03 ± 0.06 nM[d]; MK7: 2.23 ± 3.12 nM[d]	yes	[58]
Post-menopausal women generally healthy, 50–80 years (n = 344)		0.70 ± 0.53 nM[d]	MK4: 0.05 ± 0.08 nM[d]; MK7: 3.04 ± 4.32 nM[d]	yes	
Post-menopausal women: normal BMD, 54 ± 0.8 years (n = 52)	Osaka, Japan	0.29 ± 0.03 nM[d]	MK7: 2.44 ± 0.15 nM[d]	yes	[59]
low BMD, 55 ± 1.3 years, (n = 19)		0.18 ± 0.02 nM[d]	MK7: 1.67 ± 0.07 nM[d]	yes	
	Tokyo, Japan (n = 49; 50–84 years)	0.33 ± 0.21 nM[d]	MK7: 2.37 ± 2.75 nM[d]	yes	[51]
Post-menopausal women	Hiroshima, Japan (n = 25; 51–66 years)	0.33 ± 0.26 nM[d]	MK7: 0.55 ± 0.83 nM[d]	yes	
	London & Nottingham, United Kingdom (n = 31; 48–84 years)	0.23 ± 0.24 nM[d]	MK7: 0.17 ± 0.09 nM[d]	yes	
Older men, nursing home residents: normal BMD, 74 ± 10 years (n = 15)	Japan	0.85 ± 0.73 nM	MK7: 1.44 ± 0.85 nM		[60]
low BMD, 74 ± 11 years (n = 12)		0.60 ± 0.73 nM	MK7: 0.71 ± 0.35 nM		
Free living older adults: men, ≥65 years (n = 385)	Great Britain	0.34 (0.06–1.84) nM[a]	NR	yes	[61]
women, ≥65 years (n = 493)		0.37(0.06–2.06) nM[a]	NR		
Institution-living older adults: men, ≥65 years (n = 60)		0.26 (0.06–1.73) nM[a]	NR		
women, ≥65 years (n = 165)		0.23 (0.06–0.89) nM[a]	NR		
Free living older adults: men, 19–64 years (n = 530)	Great Britain	1.13 (0.20–8.80) nM[a]	NR	yes	[62]
women, 19–64 years (n = 624)		0.81 (0.02–8.71) nM[a]	NR		
Free living older adults: men, 65–75 years (n = 86)	Shenyang, China	1.88 ± 2.19 nM	NR	yes	[63]
women, 65–75 years (n = 92)		2.48 ± 2.88 nM	NR		
men, 60–83 years (n = 67)	Cambridge, United Kingdom	0.66 ± 0.75 nM	NR		
women, 60–83 years (n = 67)		0.73 ± 0.84 nM	NR		

Table 2. Cont.

Participants	Region	Phylloquinone	Menaquinone	Fasted	References
Free-living women: Pre-menopausal, 31 ± 11 years (n = 11)	Shenyang, China	0.28 ± 0.04 nM [b,d]	NR	yes	[64]
Post-menopausal, 68 ± 3 years (n = 23)		0.45 ± 0.06 nM [b,d]	NR		
Pre-menopausal, 36 ± 11 years (n = 11)	Cambridge, United Kingdom	0.14 ± 0.02 nM [b,d]	NR		
Post-menopausal, 67 ± 7 years (n = 31)		0.14 ± 0.01 nM [b,d]	NR		
Pre-menopausal, 37 ± 4 years (n = 11)	Keneba, Gambia	0.27 ± 0.05 nM [b,d]	NR		
Post-menopausal, 68 ± 8 years (n = 50)		0.16 ± 0.02 nM [b,d]	NR		
Post-menopausal women, 57 ± 5 years (n = 508)	Utrecht, The Netherlands	18% non-detectable; among detectable: 1.08 ± 1.03 nM	NR	no	[65]
Hemodialysis patients, 64 ± 14 years, 63% male (n = 387)	Italy	0.44 ± 0.44 nM [d]	MK4: 0.30 ± 0.33 nM [d]; MK5: 0.45 ± 0.35 nM [d]; MK6: 0.28 ± 0.45 nM [d]; MK7: 0.52 ± 0.45 nM [d]	yes	[66]
Healthy Controls, 57 ± 4 years, 70% male (n = 62)		0.61 ± 0.45 nM [d]	MK4: 0.41 ± 0.38 nM [d]; MK5: 0.58 ± 0.50 nM [d]; MK6: 0.50 ± 0.51 nM [d]; MK7: 0.88 ± 0.62 nM [d]		
Patients with stage 3–5 CKD, 61 ± 14 years, 61% male (n = 162)	Kingston Ontario, Canada	2.1 ± 2.4 nM	NR		[67]
Patients with ESKD, 64 ± 15 years, 66% male (n = 44)	Kingston Ontario, Canada	1.25 ± 1.17 nM	NR		[68]
Free-living men and women: Men, 59 ± 9 years (n = 741)	Framingham, MA, United States	1.54 ± 2.00 nM	NR	yes	[69]
Premenopausal women, 47 ± 7 years, (n = 170)		1.05 ± 1.04 nM			
Postmenopausal women: Current estrogen use, 58 ± 7 years (n = 269)		1.46 ± 1.25 nM			
No current estrogen use, 63 ± 8 years (n = 424)		1.41 ± 1.54 nM			
Free-living adults: White, 62 ± 10 years, 45% male (n = 262)	6 communities across United States	1.3 ± 0.1 nM	NR	yes	[70]
African American, 63 ± 10 years, 47% male (n = 180)		1.5 ± 0.1 nM			
Hispanic, 60 ± 10 years, 51% male (n = 169)		1.2 ± 0.1 nM			
Chinese-American, 62 ± 10 years, 45% male (n = 93)		2.4 ± 0.2 nM			
Older free-living adults, 70–79 years, 38% male, 46% black (n = 791)	Memphis TN and Pittsburgh PA, United States	0.8 ± 0.9 nM [c]	NR		[71]

[a] geometric mean (inner 95% range); [b] geometric mean ± SEM; [c] median ± interquartile range; [d] reported as ng/mL, converted to nmol/L by multiplying ng/mL by 2.22; NR: Not reported.

However, the number of studies that have evaluated circulating phylloquinone in relation to chronic disease is relatively few compared to the studies that assessed dietary vitamin K intake. Higher circulating phylloquinone has been associated with less bone loss and fracture [66,69,72], less osteoarthritis [71,73,74], and less coronary calcium progression is some [75] but not all [65] cohorts. Circulating concentrations of phylloquinone are 50 to 25,000 times lower than other fat-soluble nutrients, which has historically presented technological challenges in its measurement [76]. Sensitive HPLC and mass spectrometry assays have been developed to measure phylloquinone in blood but there is considerable variability in the separation techniques and assay standards used, some of which leads to erroneous reporting. However external quality assurance programs are now available to standardize assays used from one laboratory to the next and monitor inter-laboratory variation, and any study measuring circulating phylloquinone should be an active member of these programs to verify accuracy of the measures reported [76].

Phylloquinone is transported on triglyceride-rich lipoproteins in circulation, with smaller fractions carried on HDL and LDL cholesterol [77] (Figure 3).

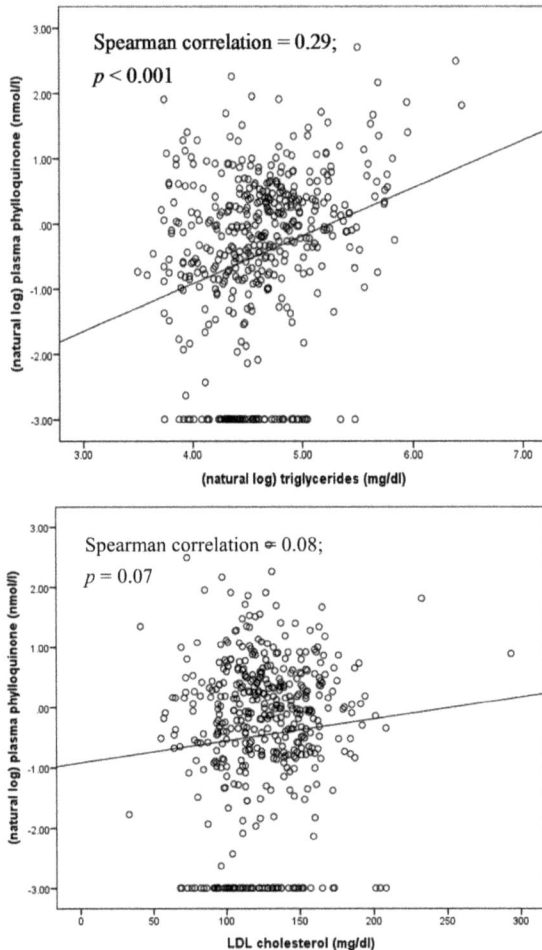

Figure 3. *Cont.*

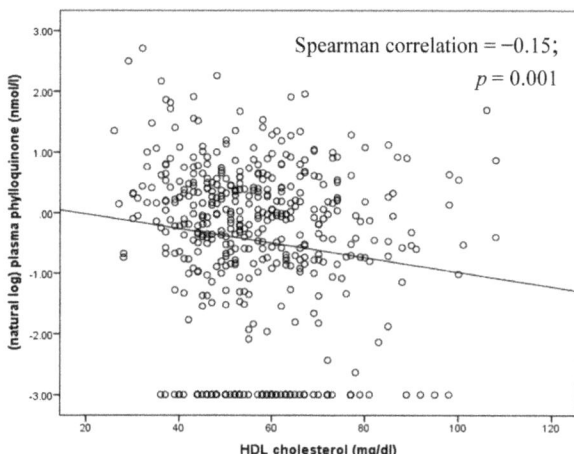

Figure 3. Correlation between circulating phylloquinone and lipids at baseline in community-dwelling older men and women participating in a phylloquinone supplementation trial [39,40].

Circulating phylloquinone responds to changes in dietary phylloquinone intake [78,79], and concentrations peak 6–10 h post-prandially [80]. There is also some indication that the response of circulating concentrations of phylloquinone vary with the type of meal pattern [81]. Given the physiology underlying phylloquinone absorption and transport, circulating phylloquinone should be measured in fasting samples and corrected for triglycerides to better reflect overall nutritional status. In population-based studies, adjustment for triglycerides strengthened associations between circulating phylloquinone and bone mineral density [69] and coronary calcium progression [75]. In studies that have not adjusted plasma phylloquinone for triglycerides, the data are more difficult to interpret. For example, in a sub-study of the Dutch Prospect cohort, post-menopausal women with the higher plasma phylloquinone had a higher prevalence of coronary calcium (CAC, an indicator of subclinical CVD) [65]. However, the plasma samples from which phylloquinone was measured were not obtained in a fasted state and triglyceride measures were unavailable. The investigators adjusted for cholesterol instead, but cholesterol is weakly correlated with circulating phylloquinone (Figure 3), and does not reflect its absorption. Since hypertriglyceridemia is a risk factor for CVD [82], it is plausible the phylloquinone tracked elevated triglycerides.

There is currently no established threshold of plasma/serum phylloquinone that indicates insufficiency or deficiency. When the Adequate Intake is met in controlled feeding studies, circulating phylloquinone concentrations approximate 1.0 nM [83]. However, it is not currently known if the Adequate Intake is sufficient to meet all physiological needs, especially health outcomes not related to coagulation [2]. As a corollary, it is not known if 1.0 nM of circulating phylloquinone is similarly sufficient. As such, low circulating phylloquinone has not been consistently defined in the scientific literature [71–75], making it difficult to clarify a threshold for insufficiency. Additional research in this area is needed.

Circulating phylloquinone appears to be influenced by more than dietary vitamin K intake and triglycerides [38,70,84], and much of the variability remains to be explained. In a multi-ethnic US cohort, race-ethnicity was identified as a significant predictor of serum phylloquinone with Chinese-Americans and African-Americans having higher concentrations than Caucasians and Hispanics [70]. In a primarily Caucasian cohort, plasma phylloquinone was not found to be significantly heritable [84]. However, a subsequent GWAS analysis of Caucasian participants in three US cohorts identified multiple candidate genes as potential determinants of circulating phylloquinone [85]. Since none of the variants achieved significance at the GWA level of $<1 \times 10^8$ larger studies are needed to confirm these findings, and more diverse cohorts are needed to expand these findings to include other race/ethnic groups. This requires more studies that measure plasma/serum phylloquinone, which to date has not been a common biomarker in large-scale population studies.

Studies reporting circulating menaquinones as a biomarker of vitamin K status are more limited (Table 2) because menaquinones are generally not detected in circulation unless supplements are taken or large quantities of menaquinone-rich foods are consumed. In women from Nagano Japan, circulating menaquinone-7 is reported to exceed 10 nM, which likely reflects natto consumption in that region. In these same women, the average concentration of menaquinone-4 was 0.2 nM, although >50% had non-detectable concentrations despite use of highly sensitive instrumentation [58]. In two studies using less sensitive HPLC methods with post-column reduction and fluorescence detection (lower limit of detection ~0.1 ng/mL), menaquinone-4 was detected in only 10% of 105 postmenopausal women from Japan or the United Kingdom [51] and in none of 440 postmenopausal Canadian women with osteopenia, half of whom were consuming daily doses of 5 mg of phylloquinone [41] (Booth *et al.*, unpublished data). These observational data are also consistent with a recent intervention study that showed single or consecutive oral administration of menaquinone-4 failed to increase serum menaquinone-4 concentrations [86]. At odds to the collective observations of others, in a study conducted in Italy, Fusaro *et al.* reported relatively high plasma concentrations of menaquinones 4–7 in chronic kidney disease patients and healthy controls not taking supplements, with chronic kidney disease patients having lower average menaquinone and phylloquinone concentrations [66]. In this same study, low concentrations of menaquinone-4 and menaquinone-7 were associated with significantly higher odds of aortic artery and iliac artery calcification respectively, and low menaquinone-5 concentrations were found to be associated with lower odds for abdominal aorta calcification. The concentration of menaquinone-5 was reported to be relatively equal to that of circulating phylloquinone, even though menaquinone-5 is not found in many foods and is rarely synthesized by bacteria [49]. No other study has reported such high concentrations of circulating menaquinone concentrations among individuals not taking menaquinone supplements and there are no other studies that have reported detectable menaquinone-5 concentrations in circulation despite concerted efforts to find circulating menaquinones using very sensitive mass spectrometry instrumentation [87]. Given the contradictory associations of menaquinone-5 with aortic calcification does not fit our current understanding of the role of vitamin K-dependent proteins in calcification, there are sufficient doubts regarding the validity of these findings. Until the findings of the study by Fusaro *et al.* [66] are independently replicated, use of circulating menaquinones as a measure of vitamin K status in population studies is uncertain.

3.2. Undercarboxylated Vitamin K-Dependent Proteins

When there is insufficient vitamin K due to low vitamin K intake or vitamin K antagonism with oral anticoagulants such as warfarin, the post-translational carboxylation of vitamin K dependent proteins is reduced, which means the undercarboxylated (inactive) fractions of these proteins increases. Of the known vitamin K-dependent proteins, clotting proteins are the most recognized [1]. As reviewed elsewhere [88] prothrombin time, also expressed as international normalized ratio, is a routine clinical assay that can reflect clinical deficiency of vitamin K. However, these tests are non-specific, have low sensitivity for detecting low vitamin K status [89] and do not reflect intakes in generally healthy adults (Figure 2), so are not used in population studies as a measure of vitamin K status. Undercarboxylated prothrombin, known as PIVKA-II (proteins induced in vitamin K absence or antagonism-factor II), is measurable in circulation, and PIVKA-II concentrations change in response to dietary vitamin K depletion [83] and warfarin use [90]. Commercially-available PIVKA-II assays have low sensitivity for detecting variation in normal vitamin K intakes, which limits its utility in ranking individuals in population studies. One exception is in patients with chronic kidney disease, given the high prevalence of vitamin K deficiency in this patient population. PIVKA-II is not affected by reduced kidney function so circulating concentrations should not be influenced by the disease itself [68].

Osteocalcin (OC) is a vitamin K-dependent protein synthesized exclusively in bone during bone formation. OC is also detectable in serum and is used as a bone formation biomarker [91–93]. During dietary vitamin K depletion, the undercarboxylated fraction of OC (ucOC) increases whereas it decreases in response to vitamin K supplementation [83,94]. UcOC is detectable in circulation even when vitamin K intakes are sufficient to maintain coagulation, suggesting the storage of vitamin K in extra-hepatic organs is secondary to hepatic storage, as demonstrated in animal models [95,96]. For this reason, ucOC reflects vitamin K intake more so than PIVKA-II and is thought to be a more sensitive indicator of vitamin K status in community-based individuals (Figure 2). There are two immunoassay methods available to measure undercarboxylated OC: the hydroxyapatite binding assay or a commercially available immunoassay, which measures fully undercarboxylated OC directly (Takara Inc., Kyoto, Japan) [91,97]. More recently, a mass spectrometric immunoassay was developed that can provide qualitative and relative percent abundance information on the molecular variants of OC present in serum [94]. The absolute concentration of ucOC is positively correlated with total OC ($r = 0.78$) (Table 3). Because of this, when serum ucOC is used as a measure of vitamin K status it should be expressed as a% of total OC (%ucOC; when measured using a hydroxyapatite binding assay) or as a ratio to the carboxylated OC when measured directly (using immunoassay) [91], but not all studies have done so [98].

Table 3. Correlations among phylloquinone intake and biomarkers of vitamin K status in community-dwelling primarily Caucasian older adults ($n = 443$). Data are presented as Pearson correlation coefficients (*p*-value).

	Phylloquinone Intake (µg/Day) [a,b]	Plasma Phylloquinone (nM) [a,c]	PIVKA (ng/mL) [d]	%ucOC [e]	ucOC (ng/mL) [e]	Total OC (ng/mL) [e]	(dp)ucMGP (pM) [a,f]
plasma phylloquinone (nM) [a,c]	0.17 (<0.001) [h,i]						
PIVKA (ng/mL) [d]	−0.05 (0.30) [h]	−0.17 (<0.001) [i]					
%ucOC [e]	−0.14 (0.003) [h]	−0.23 (<0.001) [i]	0.08 (0.11)				
ucOC (ng/mL) [e]	−0.06 (0.19) [h]	−0.18 (<0.001) [i]	0.04 (0.42)	0.78 (<0.001)			
Total OC (ng/mL) [e]	0.02 (0.64) [h]	−0.08 (0.09) [i]	−0.02 (0.74)	0.41 (<0.001)	0.84 (<0.001)		
(dp)ucMGP (pM) [af]	−0.14 (<0.001) [h]	−0.32 (<0.001)	−0.06 (0.24)	0.26 (<0.001)	0.22 (<0.001)	0.08 (0.08)	
Total MGP (ng/mL) [g]	0.08 (0.10) [h]	0.04 (0.46) [i]	−0.06 (0.24)	−0.10 (0.03)	−0.03 (0.52)	0.05 (0.29)	0.29 (<0.001)

[a] natural log transformed to reduce skewness; [b] estimated using the Harvard Food Frequency Questionnaire [39]; [c] measured using reverse-phase HPLC [39]; [d] measured using enzyme-linked immunoassay (ELISA) (Diagnostica Stago) [99]; [e] measured using radioimmunoassay [39,91]; [f] measured using sandwich ELISA [100,101]; [g] measured using radioimmunoassay [40,102]; [h] $n = 438$; [i] adjusted for triglycerides.

Because osteocalcin is synthesized in bone, the early studies of %ucOC as a functional indicator of vitamin K status focused on bone. Observational evidence suggested lower %ucOC to be associated with higher bone mineral density and reduced hip fracture risk [69,103–106], leading to the hypothesis that reducing %ucOC with vitamin K supplementation would decrease age-related bone loss. While some randomized trials reported a beneficial effect of vitamin K on bone health [41,107,108], others did not, even though vitamin K supplementation effectively reduced %ucOC [39,109–112]. Hence, the relevance of %ucOC to bone health is equivocal, as previously reviewed [97].

There has been recent interest in ucOC and its putative role in regulating glucose homeostasis. This theory was developed based on animal models which found injection of ucOC reduced blood glucose and improved insulin sensitivity in mice [113,114]. Several [115–120], but not all [117,121], studies that sought to extrapolate this finding to humans, found circulating ucOC to be inversely correlated to measures of insulin resistance. This could suggest a protective role for ucOC and therefore infer a detrimental role for vitamin K in metabolic disease because vitamin K promotes OC carboxylation. Since the primary dietary sources of vitamin K are green leafy vegetables and vegetable oils, this would represent a paradigm shift with respect to health benefits of vitamin K-rich foods. However, these studies did not correct for total osteocalcin, hence did not differentiate between an overall bone effect, as indicated by changes in the osteocalcin molecule, and a vitamin K effect, which would have been isolated if expressed as %ucOC. The limitations of these earlier population studies have been reinforced by the results of a recent meta-analysis, which found total OC and ucOC to be similarly inversely associated with fasting plasma glucose and glycosylated hemoglobin. Collectively, these suggest that the OC, but not its carboxylation status, hence vitamin K status, may be relevant to insulin resistance [122].

Matrix gla protein (MGP) is a vitamin K-dependent protein that functions as a calcification inhibitor in vascular tissue and cartilage [123]. In addition to being post-translationally carboxylated, MGP is also phosphorylated [124]. Assays that measure different forms of MGP in plasma are available [100], and the different circulating species appear to be differentially associated with health outcomes related to calcification (Supplementary Table S1). Only the dephosphorylated undercarboxylated form ((dp)ucMGP) responds to vitamin K supplementation [100,101,125,126]. When plotted against FFQ-estimated vitamin K intake, (dp)ucMGP decreased up an intake of 100–150 µg/day at which point the association plateaued (Figure 2), which may reflect the limitations of estimating vitamin K intake using FFQs previously discussed. (Dp)ucMGP has been suggested to be a functional indicator of vitamin K status in tissues that utilize MGP [100,127], such that higher amounts of (dp)ucMGP reflect lower vitamin K status. Several [128–134], but not all [135,136] population-based studies found higher plasma (dp)ucMGP was associated with more arterial calcification, arterial stiffness (which is positively associated with calcification) and CVD. In a post hoc analysis of a randomized controlled trial that found phylloquinone supplementation reduced CAC progression over 3 years in older men and women, dp-ucMGP was reduced by phylloquinone supplementation, but the change in (dp)ucMGP did not correlate with change in CAC [101]. Recently menaquinone-7 was reported to reduce plasma (dp)ucMGP and have a beneficial effect on arterial stiffness in post-menopausal women. At baseline (dp)ucMGP was positively correlated with stiffness, but the investigators did not report if changes in (dp)ucMGP correlated with changes in stiffness [137]. Because the majority of studies that measured (dp)ucMGP were done in primarily Caucasian groups (Supplementary Table S1), the relevance of (dp)ucMGP to vitamin K status and health outcomes in non-Caucasian groups merits investigation.

Similar to the situation with osteocalcin, the amount of (dp)ucMGP in circulation also depends on the total amount of MGP available [91,101]. It may be inappropriate, therefore, to extrapolate the association of higher (dp)ucMGP with more adverse health outcomes as being related to vitamin K insufficiency because the associations may be related to overall MGP status. For example, total MGP increases with age, independent of vitamin K intake [102], and given that age is an independent predictor of CVD and other chronic diseases, MGP may simply be a strong biomarker for age. It is also plausible that diseases characterized by calcification and/or cardiac dysfunction affect the synthesis of MGP because calcium as well as cardiac overload can promote MGP expression [138–140]. This could suggest elevated MGP is a consequence of CVD rather than causal. Much remains to be understood about the physiology underlying MGPs role in health and disease, which cannot be ascertained using observational studies. It is premature to conclude increasing MGP carboxylation with vitamin K will reduce risk for CVD and other outcomes related to calcification until this is tested using well-designed clinical trials.

3.3. Urinary Biomarkers

In addition to the blood measures, methods have been developed to measure urinary biomarkers of vitamin K metabolism. Y-Carboxyglutamic acid (gla) is an indicator of the turnover of all vitamin K-dependent proteins. Some [83,141], but not all [79,142] studies found urinary gla decreased when vitamin K intake is decreased. As vitamin K is catabolized, 5 carbon and 7 carbon aglycone metabolites are produced, which are water soluble and excreted in urine. These metabolites increase in response to vitamin K supplementation [143] and repletion, with a concomitant decrease in response to vitamin K depletion [143]. Menadione (vitamin K3; Figure 1) is the naphthoquinone ring metabolite of vitamin K that is thought to be an intermediary in the tissue-specific conversion of phylloquinone to menaquinone-4. Menadione is detectable in urine [144] and was found to change in response to vitamin K depletion and repletion more than urinary gla [141]. Because these urinary measures ideally require 24 h urine collection, their utility in clinic-based or in large-scale population-based studies is very limited. To the best of our knowledge, there are no studies that have examined the association of any of these measures with health outcomes for which a role for vitamin K has been suggested.

3.4. Interrelatedness of Vitamin K Status Biomarkers

Although there are multiple biomarkers available to estimate vitamin K status, it is apparent that no single biomarker is valid for use across all population-based studies. Since most population-based studies have limited volume of specimens, strategic decisions need to be made when deciding on choice of biomarkers.

After three years of supplementation with 500 µg/day of phylloquinone, plasma phylloquinone increased by >100% and %ucOC (and ucOC ng/mL) and (dp)ucMGP decreased by 50%–80% (Figure 4) [39,40]. The total MGP decreased 3.5% in the placebo group and increased 3.5% in the phylloquinone supplemented group, and the between group difference in this change reached statistical significance. However, the biological relevance of this difference is uncertain.

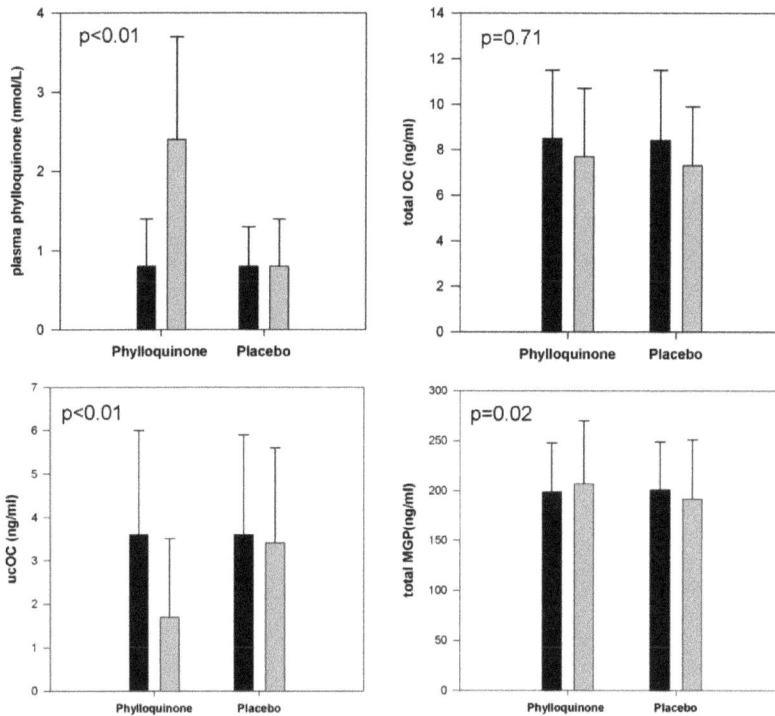

Figure 4. *Cont.*

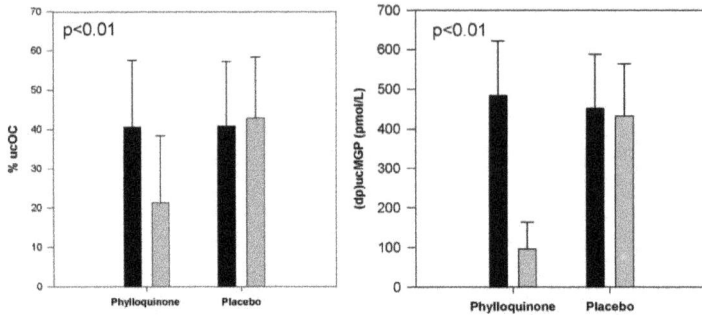

Figure 4. Circulating biomarkers at baseline (■) and after 3 years (□) of supplementation with 500 μg/day phylloquinone (*n* = 229) or placebo (*n* = 223) in primarily Caucasian community-dwelling men and women 65–80 years old. (Because of skewed distributions, plasma phylloquinone and (dp)ucMgp are presented as median values with error bars representing inter-quartile ranges. Otherwise data are presented as means with error bars representing standard deviations. *p*-values reflect the between-group difference for change in the biomarker in response to phylloquinone supplementation *versus* placebo).

PIVKA-II amounts were overall within the normal range at baseline [99], hence were not examined in response to supplementation given the low sensitivity of PIVKA-II to vitamin K supplementation in healthy individuals. Relative changes of urinary gla were more subtle compared to changes in circulating phylloquinone or undercarboxylated vitamin K-dependent proteins [83,141]. In this same cohort [39,40] observed at baseline, with the exception of PIVKA-II, circulating biomarkers of vitamin K significantly correlated with phylloquinone intake and with one another, but the correlations were overall not strong (Table 3). Unfortunately there are no urinary measures of vitamin K status available for comparison in population studies. Interestingly, in a racially diverse cohort, (dp)ucMGP was significantly correlated with plasma phylloquinone in whites but not in blacks (Figure 5) [145].

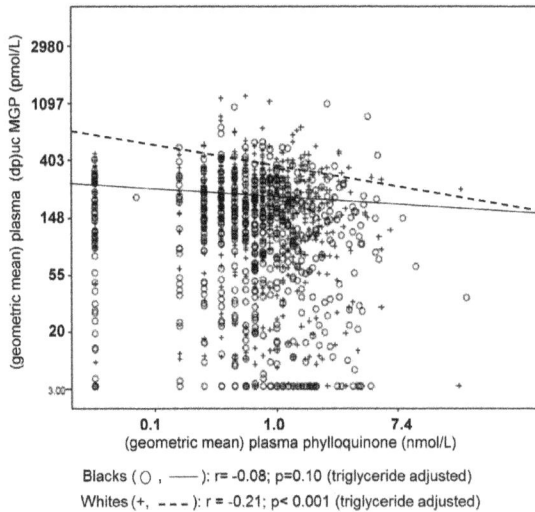

Blacks (○, —): r= -0.08; p=0.10 (triglyceride adjusted)
Whites (+, - - -): r = -0.21; p< 0.001 (triglyceride adjusted)

Figure 5. Correlation between circulating phylloquinone and (dp)ucMGP in black (*n* = 507) and white (*n* = 570) men and women 70–79 years old.

This may suggest the different measures of vitamin K status are influenced by physiological factors in addition to vitamin K. At this time, a combination of circulating concentrations of phylloquinone (and menaquinones when detectable), preferably corrected for circulating triglycerides, with an undercarboxylated non-coagulation protein, such as %ucOC (which can be corrected for the non-dietary influences on total protein concentrations), or (dp)ucMGP, would provide the most comprehensive approach to measure vitamin K status in population-based studies at this time, and allow for suitable ranking.

4. Conclusions

In summary, despite the multiple measures available, population- and clinic-based studies of vitamin K status are challenged by the lack of a single gold-standard measure. Dietary intake assessment by FFQ is convenient and easily implemented. Food composition databases are being expanded to include multiple menaquinone forms, so dietary questionnaires will no longer be limited to phylloquinone intake. Because menaquinones are generally not detected in circulation unless very large amounts are consumed, correlating menaquinone intake to circulating levels is problematic. While the use of biomarkers to estimate vitamin K status is not subject to the same limitations as the use dietary intake measures [3,53,54], there are limitations to each of the available biomarkers that need to be considered when studies are designed and interpreted. Circulating phylloquinone is carried on triglyceride-rich lipoproteins, which necessitates the use of fasting samples and concomitant measurement of triglycerides to reduce confounding. The amount of undercarboxylated vitamin K-dependent proteins in circulation depends on the total amount of protein, in addition to vitamin K availability. If these measures are not corrected for the total amount of the protein under study, they may reflect total protein status as well as vitamin K status which can confound the interpretation of the results. At this time, none of the urinary measures have been applied large cohorts so their utility epidemiologically is uncertain. Given the strengths and limitations of the available measures, and their modest inter-relatedness, vitamin K status may be estimated more accurately if multiple biomarkers, or biomarkers in combination with dietary intake are used.

Supplementary Materials: Supplementary materials can be accessed at: http://www.mdpi.com/2072-6643/7/12/5554/s1.

Acknowledgments: This study was supported in part by the U.S. Department of Agriculture, Agricultural Research Service under Cooperative Agreement No. 58-1950-7-707, the National Institute of Aging (R01AG14759), the National Heart Lung and Blood Institute (R01HL69272), the National Institute of Arthritis Musculoskeletal and Skin Diseases (R21AR062284 and K01AR063167), and a New Investigator Grant from the Arthritis Foundation.

Author Contributions: M.K.S. and S.L.B. generated the concept of the review. M.K.S. drafted the manuscript and S.L.B. reviewed and edited the manuscript.

Conflicts of Interest: The authors declare no conflicts of interest.

Abbreviations

BMD: bone mineral density, **CAC**: coronary artery calcium, **CHD**: coronary heart disease, **(dp)ucMGP**: dephosphorylated undercarboxylated matrix gla protein, **ELISA**: enzyme-linked immunoassay, **EPIC**: European Prospective Investigation into Cancer and Nutrition Study, **FFQ**: food frequency questionnaire, **HPLC**: high performance liquid chromatography, **IR**: insulin resistance, **MESA**: Multi-ethnic Study of Atherosclerosis, **MGP**: matrix gla protein, **MK**: menaquinone, **PIVKA-II**: proteins induced in vitamin K absence or antagonism-factor II, **PK**: phylloquinone, **ucOC**: undercarboxylated osteocalcin, **%ucOC**: percent undercarboxylated osteocalcin.

References

1. Suttie, J.W. *Vitamin K in Health and Disease*; CRC Press: Boca Raton, FL, USA, 2009.
2. McCann, J.C.; Ames, B.N. Vitamin K, an example of triage theory: Is micronutrient inadequacy linked to diseases of aging? *Am. J. Clin. Nutr.* **2009**, *90*, 889–907. [CrossRef] [PubMed]

3.   Willett, W.C. *Nutritional Epidemiology*, 3rd ed.; Oxford University Press: Oxford, UK, 2013.
4.   Food and Nutrition Board, Insititue of Medicne. *Dietary Reference Intakes for Vitamin A, Vitamin K, Arsenic, Boron, Chromium, Copper, Iodine, Iron, Manganese, Molybdenum, Nickel, Silicon, Vanadium, and Zinc;* National Academy Press: Washington, DC, USA, 2002.
5.   Shearer, M.J.; Fu, X.; Booth, S.L. Vitamin K nutrition, metabolism, and requirements: Current concepts and future research. *Adv. Nutr.* **2012**, *3*, 182–195. [CrossRef] [PubMed]
6.   Booth, S.L.; Pennington, J.A.; Sadowski, J.A. Food sources and dietary intakes of vitamin K-1 (phylloquinone) in the American diet: Data from the FDA Total Diet Study. *J. Am. Diet. Assoc.* **1996**, *96*, 149–154. [CrossRef]
7.   Duggan, P.; Cashman, K.D.; Flynn, A.; Bolton-Smith, C.; Kiely, M. Phylloquinone (vitamin K1) intakes and food sources in 18–64-year-old Irish adults. *Br. J. Nutr.* **2004**, *92*, 151–158. [CrossRef] [PubMed]
8.   Erkkila, A.T.; Booth, S.L.; Hu, F.B.; Jacques, P.F.; Lichtenstein, A.H. Phylloquinone intake and risk of cardiovascular diseases in men. *Nutr. Metab. Cardiovasc. Dis.* **2007**, *17*, 58–62. [CrossRef] [PubMed]
9.   Geleijnse, J.M.; Vermeer, C.; Grobbee, D.E.; Schurgers, L.J.; Knapen, M.H.; van der Meer, I.M.; Hofman, A.; Witteman, J.C. Dietary intake of menaquinone is associated with a reduced risk of coronary heart disease: The Rotterdam Study. *J. Nutr.* **2004**, *134*, 3100–3105. [PubMed]
10. Thane, C.W.; Bolton-Smith, C.; Coward, W.A. Comparative dietary intake and sources of phylloquinone (vitamin K1) among British adults in 1986–1987 and 2000–2001. *Br. J. Nutr.* **2006**, *96*, 1105–1115. [CrossRef] [PubMed]
11. Beulens, J.W.; Booth, S.L.; van den Heuvel, E.G.; Stoecklin, E.; Baka, A.; Vermeer, C. The role of menaquinones (vitamin K2) in human health. *Br. J. Nutr.* **2013**, *110*, 1357–1368. [CrossRef] [PubMed]
12. Tucker, K.L.; Smith, C.E.; Lai, C.Q.; Ordovas, J.M. Quantifying diet for nutrigenomic studies. *Annu. Rev. Nutr.* **2013**, *33*, 349–371. [CrossRef] [PubMed]
13. Barrett-Connor, E. Nutrition epidemiology: How do we know what they ate? *Am. J. Clin. Nutr.* **1991**, *54* (Suppl. S1), 182S–187S. [CrossRef]
14. Westerterp, K.R.; Goris, A.H. Validity of the assessment of dietary intake: Problems of misreporting. *Curr. Opin. Clin. Nutr. Metab. Care* **2002**, *5*, 489–493. [CrossRef] [PubMed]
15. Beulens, J.W.; Bots, M.L.; Atsma, F.; Bartelink, M.L.; Prokop, M.; Geleijnse, J.M.; Witteman, J.C.; Grobbee, D.E.; van der Schouw, Y.T. High dietary menaquinone intake is associated with reduced coronary calcification. *Atherosclerosis* **2009**, *203*, 489–493. [CrossRef] [PubMed]
16. Booth, S.L.; Tucker, K.L.; Chen, H.; Hannan, M.T.; Gagnon, D.R.; Cupples, L.A.; Wilson, P.W.; Ordovas, J.; Schaefer, E.J.; Dawson-Hughes, B.; *et al.* Dietary vitamin K intakes are associated with hip fracture but not with bone mineral density in elderly men and women. *Am. J. Clin. Nutr.* **2000**, *71*, 1201–1208. [PubMed]
17. Gast, G.C.; de Roos, N.M.; Sluijs, I.; Bots, M.L.; Beulens, J.W.; Geleijnse, J.M.; Witteman, J.C.; Grobbee, D.E.; Peeters, P.H.; van der Schouw, Y.T. A high menaquinone intake reduces the incidence of coronary heart disease. *Nutr. Metab. Cardiovasc. Dis.* **2009**, *19*, 504–510. [CrossRef] [PubMed]
18. Nimptsch, K.; Rohrmann, S.; Linseisen, J. Dietary intake of vitamin K and risk of prostate cancer in the Heidelberg cohort of the European Prospective Investigation into Cancer and Nutrition (EPIC-Heidelberg). *Am. J. Clin. Nutr.* **2008**, *87*, 985–992. [PubMed]
19. Villines, T.C.; Hatzigeorgiou, C.; Feuerstein, I.M.; O'Malley, P.G.; Taylor, A.J. Vitamin K1 intake and coronary calcification. *Coron. Artery Dis.* **2005**, *16*, 199–203. [CrossRef] [PubMed]
20. Erkkila, A.T.; Booth, S.L.; Hu, F.B.; Jacques, P.F.; Manson, J.E.; Rexrode, K.M.; Stampfer, M.J.; Lichtenstein, A.H. Phylloquinone intake as a marker for coronary heart disease risk but not stroke in women. *Eur. J. Clin. Nutr.* **2005**, *59*, 196–204. [CrossRef] [PubMed]
21. Booth, S.L.; Broe, K.E.; Gagnon, D.R.; Tucker, K.L.; Hannan, M.T.; McLean, R.R.; Dawson-Hughes, B.; Wilson, P.W.; Cupples, L.A.; Kiel, D.P. Vitamin K intake and bone mineral density in women and men. *Am. J. Clin. Nutr.* **2003**, *77*, 512–516. [PubMed]
22. Macdonald, H.M.; McGuigan, F.E.; Lanham-New, S.A.; Fraser, W.D.; Ralston, S.H.; Reid, D.M. Vitamin K1 intake is associated with higher bone mineral density and reduced bone resorption in early postmenopausal Scottish women: No evidence of gene-nutrient interaction with apolipoprotein E polymorphisms. *Am. J. Clin. Nutr.* **2008**, *87*, 1513–1520. [PubMed]
23. Feskanich, D.; Weber, P.; Willett, W.C.; Rockett, H.; Booth, S.L.; Colditz, G.A. Vitamin K intake and hip fractures in women: A prospective study. *Am. J. Clin. Nutr.* **1999**, *69*, 74–79. [PubMed]

24. Chan, R.; Leung, J.; Woo, J. No association between dietary vitamin K intake and fracture risk in chinese community-dwelling older men and women: A prospective study. *Calcif. Tissue Int.* **2012**, *90*, 396–403. [CrossRef] [PubMed]

25. Rejnmark, L.; Vestergaard, P.; Charles, P.; Hermann, A.P.; Brot, C.; Eiken, P.; Mosekilde, L. No effect of vitamin K1 intake on bone mineral density and fracture risk in perimenopausal women. *Osteoporos. Int.* **2006**, *17*, 1122–1132. [CrossRef] [PubMed]

26. Apalset, E.M.; Gjesdal, C.G.; Eide, G.E.; Tell, G.S. Intake of vitamin K1 and K2 and risk of hip fractures: The Hordaland Health Study. *Bone* **2011**, *49*, 990–995. [CrossRef] [PubMed]

27. Dam, V.; Dalmeijer, G.W.; Vermeer, C.; Drummen, N.E.; Knapen, M.H.; van der Schouw, Y.T.; Beulens, J.W. The association between vitamin K and the metabolic syndrome: A ten year follow-up study in adults. *J. Clin. Endocrinol. Metab.* **2015**, *100*, 2472–2479. [CrossRef] [PubMed]

28. Juanola-Falgarona, M.; Salas-Salvado, J.; Estruch, R.; Portillo, M.P.; Casas, R.; Miranda, J.; Martinez-Gonzalez, M.A.; Bullo, M. Association between dietary phylloquinone intake and peripheral metabolic risk markers related to insulin resistance and diabetes in elderly subjects at high cardiovascular risk. *Cardiovasc. Diabetol.* **2013**, *12*, 58–61. [CrossRef] [PubMed]

29. Shea, M.K.; Cushman, M.; Booth, S.L.; Burke, G.L.; Chen, H.; Kritchevsky, S.B. Associations between vitamin K status and haemostatic and inflammatory biomarkers in community-dwelling adults. The Multi-Ethnic Study of Atherosclerosis. *Thromb. Haemost.* **2014**, *112*, 438–444. [CrossRef] [PubMed]

30. Yoshida, M.; Booth, S.L.; Meigs, J.B.; Saltzman, E.; Jacques, P.F. Phylloquinone intake, insulin sensitivity, and glycemic status in men and women. *Am. J. Clin. Nutr.* **2008**, *88*, 210–215. [PubMed]

31. Nimptsch, K.; Rohrmann, S.; Kaaks, R.; Linseisen, J. Dietary vitamin K intake in relation to cancer incidence and mortality: Results from the Heidelberg cohort of the European Prospective Investigation into Cancer and Nutrition (EPIC-Heidelberg). *Am. J. Clin. Nutr.* **2010**, *91*, 1348–1358. [CrossRef] [PubMed]

32. Juanola-Falgarona, M.; Salas-Salvado, J.; Martinez-Gonzalez, M.A.; Corella, D.; Estruch, R.; Ros, E.; Fito, M.; Aros, F.; Gomez-Gracia, E.; Fiol, M.; *et al.* Dietary intake of vitamin K is inversely associated with mortality risk. *J. Nutr.* **2014**, *144*, 743–750. [CrossRef] [PubMed]

33. Cheung, C.L.; Sahni, S.; Cheung, B.M.; Sing, C.W.; Wong, I.C. Vitamin K intake and mortality in people with chronic kidney disease from NHANES III. *Clin. Nutr.* **2015**, *34*, 235–240. [CrossRef] [PubMed]

34. Geisen, C.; Watzka, M.; Sittinger, K.; Steffens, M.; Daugela, L.; Seifried, E.; Muller, C.R.; Wienker, T.F.; Oldenburg, J. VKORC1 haplotypes and their impact on the inter-individual and inter-ethnical variability of oral anticoagulation. *Thromb. Haemost.* **2005**, *94*, 773–779. [PubMed]

35. Braam, L.; McKeown, N.; Jacques, P.; Lichtenstein, A.; Vermeer, C.; Wilson, P.; Booth, S. Dietary phylloquinone intake as a potential marker for a heart-healthy dietary pattern in the Framingham Offspring cohort. *J. Am. Diet. Assoc.* **2004**, *104*, 1410–1414. [CrossRef] [PubMed]

36. Feskanich, D.; Rimm, E.B.; Giovannucci, E.L.; Colditz, G.A.; Stampfer, M.J.; Litin, L.B.; Willett, W.C. Reproducibility and validity of food intake measurements from a semiquantitative food frequency questionnaire. *J. Am. Diet. Assoc.* **1993**, *93*, 790–796. [CrossRef]

37. Presse, N.; Shatenstein, B.; Kergoat, M.J.; Ferland, G. Validation of a semi-quantitative food frequency questionnaire measuring dietary vitamin K intake in elderly people. *J. Am. Diet. Assoc.* **2009**, *109*, 1251–1255. [CrossRef] [PubMed]

38. McKeown, N.M.; Jacques, P.F.; Gundberg, C.M.; Peterson, J.W.; Tucker, K.L.; Kiel, D.P.; Wilson, P.W.; Booth, S.L. Dietary and nondietary determinants of vitamin K biochemical measures in men and women. *J. Nutr.* **2002**, *132*, 1329–1334. [PubMed]

39. Booth, S.L.; Dallal, G.; Shea, M.K.; Gundberg, C.; Peterson, J.W.; Dawson-Hughes, B. Effect of vitamin K supplementation on bone loss in elderly men and women. *J. Clin. Endocrinol. Metab.* **2008**, *93*, 1217–1223. [CrossRef] [PubMed]

40. Shea, M.K.; O'Donnell, C.J.; Hoffmann, U.; Dallal, G.E.; Dawson-Hughes, B.; Ordovas, J.M.; Price, P.A.; Williamson, M.K.; Booth, S.L. Vitamin K supplementation and progression of coronary artery calcium in older men and women. *Am. J. Clin. Nutr.* **2009**, *89*, 1799–1807. [CrossRef] [PubMed]

41. Cheung, A.M.; Tile, L.; Lee, Y.; Tomlinson, G.; Hawker, G.; Scher, J.; Hu, H.; Vieth, R.; Thompson, L.; Jamal, S.; *et al.* Vitamin K supplementation in postmenopausal women with osteopenia (ECKO trial): A randomized controlled trial. *PLoS Med.* **2008**, *5*, e196. [CrossRef] [PubMed]

42. Elder, S.J.; Haytowitz, D.B.; Howe, J.; Peterson, J.W.; Booth, S.L. Vitamin K contents of meat, dairy, and fast food in the U.S. Diet. *J. Agric. Food. Chem.* **2006**, *54*, 463–467. [CrossRef]
43. Manoury, E.; Jourdon, K.; Boyaval, P.; Fourcassie, P. Quantitative measurement of vitamin K2 (menaquinones) in various fermented dairy products using a reliable high-performance liquid chromatography method. *J. Dairy Sci.* **2013**, *96*, 1335–1346. [CrossRef] [PubMed]
44. Praagman, J.; Dalmeijer, G.W.; van der Schouw, Y.T.; Soedamah-Muthu, S.S.; Monique Verschuren, W.M.; Bas Bueno-de-Mesquita, H.; Geleijnse, J.M.; Beulens, J.W. The relationship between fermented food intake and mortality risk in the European Prospective Investigation into Cancer and Nutrition-Netherlands cohort. *Br. J. Nutr.* **2015**, *113*, 498–506. [CrossRef] [PubMed]
45. Sluijs, I.; Forouhi, N.G.; Beulens, J.W.; van der Schouw, Y.T.; Agnoli, C.; Arriola, L.; Balkau, B.; Barricarte, A.; Boeing, H.; Bueno-de-Mesquita, H.B.; *et al.* The amount and type of dairy product intake and incident type 2 diabetes: Results from the EPIC-InterAct Study. *Am. J. Clin. Nutr.* **2012**, *96*, 382–390. [CrossRef] [PubMed]
46. Aune, D.; Norat, T.; Romundstad, P.; Vatten, L.J. Dairy products and the risk of type 2 diabetes: A systematic review and dose-response meta-analysis of cohort studies. *Am. J. Clin. Nutr.* **2013**, *98*, 1066–1083. [CrossRef] [PubMed]
47. Sonestedt, E.; Wirfalt, E.; Wallstrom, P.; Gullberg, B.; Orho-Melander, M.; Hedblad, B. Dairy products and its association with incidence of cardiovascular disease: The Malmo diet and cancer cohort. *Eur. J. Epidemiol.* **2011**, *26*, 609–618. [CrossRef] [PubMed]
48. Farvid, M.S.; Ding, M.; Pan, A.; Sun, Q.; Chiuve, S.E.; Steffen, L.M.; Willett, W.C.; Hu, F.B. Dietary linoleic acid and risk of coronary heart disease: A systematic review and meta-analysis of prospective cohort studies. *Circulation* **2014**, *130*, 1568–1578. [CrossRef] [PubMed]
49. Walther, B.; Karl, J.P.; Booth, S.L.; Boyaval, P. Menaquinones, bacteria, and the food supply: The relevance of dairy and fermented food products to vitamin K requirements. *Adv. Nutr.* **2013**, *4*, 463–473. [CrossRef] [PubMed]
50. Schurgers, L.J.; Vermeer, C. Determination of phylloquinone and menaquinones in food. Effect of food matrix on circulating vitamin K concentrations. *Haemostasis* **2000**, *30*, 298–307. [PubMed]
51. Kaneki, M.; Hodges, S.J.; Hosoi, T.; Fujiwara, S.; Lyons, A.; Crean, S.J.; Ishida, N.; Nakagawa, M.; Takechi, M.; Sano, Y.; *et al.* Japanese fermented soybean food as the major determinant of the large geographic difference in circulating levels of vitamin K2: Possible implications for hip-fracture risk. *Nutrition* **2001**, *17*, 315–321. [CrossRef]
52. Hjartaker, A.; Lagiou, A.; Slimani, N.; Lund, E.; Chirlaque, M.D.; Vasilopoulou, E.; Zavitsanos, X.; Berrino, F.; Sacerdote, C.; Ocke, M.C.; *et al.* Consumption of dairy products in the European Prospective Investigation into Cancer and Nutrition (EPIC) cohort: Data from 35,955 24-h dietary recalls in 10 European countries. *Public Health Nutr.* **2002**, *5*, 1259–1271. [CrossRef] [PubMed]
53. Thompson, F.E.; Byers, T. Dietary assessment resource manual. *J. Nutr.* **1994**, *124* (Suppl. S11), 2245S–2317S. [PubMed]
54. Miller, T.M.; Abdel-Maksoud, M.F.; Crane, L.A.; Marcus, A.C.; Byers, T.E. Effects of social approval bias on self-reported fruit and vegetable consumption: A randomized controlled trial. *Nutr. J.* **2008**, *7*, 18588696. [CrossRef] [PubMed]
55. Potischman, N. Biologic and methodologic issues for nutritional biomarkers. *J. Nutr.* **2003**, *133* (Suppl. S3), 875S–880S. [PubMed]
56. Blanck, H.M.; Bowman, B.A.; Cooper, G.R.; Myers, G.L.; Miller, D.T. Laboratory issues: Use of nutritional biomarkers. *J. Nutr.* **2003**, *133* (Suppl. S3), 888S–894S. [PubMed]
57. Kawana, K.; Takahashi, M.; Hoshino, H.; Kushida, K. Circulating levels of vitamin K1, menaquinone-4, and menaquinone-7 in healthy elderly Japanese women and patients with vertebral fractures and patients with hip fractures. *Endocr. Res.* **2001**, *27*, 337–343. [CrossRef] [PubMed]
58. Tsugawa, N.; Shiraki, M.; Suhara, Y.; Kamao, M.; Tanaka, K.; Okano, T. Vitamin K status of healthy Japanese women: Age-related vitamin K requirement for gamma-carboxylation of osteocalcin. *Am. J. Clin. Nutr.* **2006**, *83*, 380–386. [PubMed]
59. Kanai, T.; Takagi, T.; Masuhiro, K.; Nakamura, M.; Iwata, M.; Saji, F. Serum vitamin K level and bone mineral density in post-menopausal women. *Int. J. Gynaecol. Obstet.* **1997**, *56*, 25–30. [CrossRef]

60. Tamatani, M.; Morimoto, S.; Nakajima, M.; Fukuo, K.; Onishi, T.; Kitano, S.; Niinobu, T.; Ogihara, T. Decreased circulating levels of vitamin K and 25-hydroxyvitamin D in osteopenic elderly men. *Metabolism* **1998**, *47*, 195–199. [CrossRef]

61. Thane, C.W.; Bates, C.J.; Shearer, M.J.; Unadkat, N.; Harrington, D.J.; Paul, A.A.; Prentice, A.; Bolton-Smith, C. Plasma phylloquinone (vitamin K1) concentration and its relationship to intake in a national sample of British elderly people. *Br. J. Nutr.* **2002**, *87*, 615–622. [CrossRef] [PubMed]

62. Thane, C.W.; Wang, L.Y.; Coward, W.A. Plasma phylloquinone (vitamin K1) concentration and its relationship to intake in British adults aged 19–64 years. *Br. J. Nutr.* **2006**, *96*, 1116–1124. [CrossRef] [PubMed]

63. Yan, L.; Zhou, B.; Greenberg, D.; Wang, L.; Nigdikar, S.; Prynne, C.; Prentice, A. Vitamin K status of older individuals in northern China is superior to that of older individuals in the UK. *Br. J. Nutr.* **2004**, *92*, 939–945. [CrossRef] [PubMed]

64. Beavan, S.R.; Prentice, A.; Stirling, D.M.; Dibba, B.; Yan, L.; Harrington, D.J.; Shearer, M.J. Ethnic differences in osteocalcin gamma-carboxylation, plasma phylloquinone (vitamin K1) and apolipoprotein E genotype. *Eur. J. Clin. Nutr.* **2005**, *59*, 72–81. [CrossRef] [PubMed]

65. Dalmeijer, G.W.; van der Schouw, Y.T.; Booth, S.L.; de Jong, P.A.; Beulens, J.W. Phylloquinone concentrations and the risk of vascular calcification in healthy women. *Arterioscler. Thromb. Vasc. Biol.* **2014**, *34*, 1587–1590. [CrossRef] [PubMed]

66. Fusaro, M.; Noale, M.; Viola, V.; Galli, F.; Tripepi, G.; Vajente, N.; Plebani, M.; Zaninotto, M.; Guglielmi, G.; Miotto, D.; *et al.* Vitamin K, vertebral fractures, vascular calcifications, and mortality: VItamin K Italian (VIKI) dialysis study. *J. Bone Miner. Res.* **2012**, *27*, 2271–2278. [CrossRef] [PubMed]

67. Holden, R.M.; Morton, A.R.; Garland, J.S.; Pavlov, A.; Day, A.G.; Booth, S.L. Vitamins K and D status in stages 3–5 chronic kidney disease. *Clin. J. Am. Soc. Nephrol.* **2010**, *5*, 590–597. [CrossRef] [PubMed]

68. Elliott, M.J.; Booth, S.L.; Hopman, W.M.; Holden, R.M. Assessment of potential biomarkers of subclinical vitamin K deficiency in patients with end-stage kidney disease. *Can. J. Kidney Health Dis.* **2014**, *1*. [CrossRef] [PubMed]

69. Booth, S.L.; Broe, K.E.; Peterson, J.W.; Cheng, D.M.; Dawson-Hughes, B.; Gundberg, C.M.; Cupples, L.A.; Wilson, P.W.; Kiel, D.P. Associations between vitamin K biochemical measures and bone mineral density in men and women. *J. Clin. Endocrinol. Metab.* **2004**, *89*, 4904–4909. [CrossRef] [PubMed]

70. Shea, M.K.; Booth, S.L.; Nettleton, J.A.; Burke, G.L.; Chen, H.; Kritchevsky, S.B. Circulating phylloquinone concentrations of adults in the United States differ according to race and ethnicity. *J. Nutr.* **2012**, *142*, 1060–1066. [CrossRef] [PubMed]

71. Shea, M.K.; Kritchevsky, S.B.; Hsu, F.C.; Nevitt, M.; Booth, S.L.; Kwoh, C.K.; McAlindon, T.E.; Vermeer, C.; Drummen, N.; Harris, T.B.; *et al.* The association between vitamin K status and knee osteoarthritis features in older adults: The Health, Aging and Body Composition Study. *Osteoarthr. Cartil.* **2015**, *23*, 370–378. [CrossRef] [PubMed]

72. Tsugawa, N.; Shiraki, M.; Suhara, Y.; Kamao, M.; Ozaki, R.; Tanaka, K.; Okano, T. Low plasma phylloquinone concentration is associated with high incidence of vertebral fracture in Japanese women. *J. Bone Miner. Metab.* **2008**, *26*, 79–85. [CrossRef] [PubMed]

73. Neogi, T.; Booth, S.L.; Zhang, Y.Q.; Jacques, P.F.; Terkeltaub, R.; Aliabadi, P.; Felson, D.T. Low vitamin K status is associated with osteoarthritis in the hand and knee. *Arthritis Rheum.* **2006**, *54*, 1255–1261. [CrossRef] [PubMed]

74. Misra, D.; Booth, S.L.; Tolstykh, I.; Felson, D.T.; Nevitt, M.C.; Lewis, C.E.; Torner, J.; Neogi, T. Vitamin K deficiency is associated with incident knee osteoarthritis. *Am. J. Med.* **2013**, *126*, 243–248. [CrossRef] [PubMed]

75. Shea, M.K.; Booth, S.L.; Miller, M.E.; Burke, G.L.; Chen, H.; Cushman, M.; Tracy, R.P.; Kritchevsky, S.B. Association between circulating vitamin K1 and coronary calcium progression in community-dwelling adults: The Multi-Ethnic Study of Atherosclerosis. *Am. J. Clin. Nutr.* **2013**, *98*, 197–208. [CrossRef] [PubMed]

76. Card, D.J.; Shearer, M.J.; Schurgers, L.J.; Harrington, D.J. The external quality assurance of phylloquinone (vitamin K(1)) analysis in human serum. *Biomed. Chromatogr.* **2009**, *23*, 1276–1282. [CrossRef] [PubMed]

77. Lamon-Fava, S.; Sadowski, J.A.; Davidson, K.W.; O'Brien, M.E.; McNamara, J.R.; Schaefer, E.J. Plasma lipoproteins as carriers of phylloquinone (vitamin K1) in humans. *Am. J. Clin. Nutr.* **1998**, *67*, 1226–1231. [PubMed]

78. Booth, S.L.; Tucker, K.L.; McKeown, N.M.; Davidson, K.W.; Dallal, G.E.; Sadowski, J.A. Relationships between dietary intakes and fasting plasma concentrations of fat-soluble vitamins in humans. *J. Nutr.* **1997**, *127*, 587–592. [PubMed]

79. Booth, S.L.; O'Brien-Morse, M.E.; Dallal, G.E.; Davidson, K.W.; Gundberg, C.M. Response of vitamin K status to different intakes and sources of phylloquinone-rich foods: Comparison of younger and older adults. *Am. J. Clin. Nutr.* **1999**, *70*, 368–377. [PubMed]

80. Novotny, J.A.; Kurilich, A.C.; Britz, S.J.; Baer, D.J.; Clevidence, B.A. Vitamin K absorption and kinetics in human subjects after consumption of 13C-labelled phylloquinone from kale. *Br. J. Nutr.* **2010**, *104*, 858–862. [CrossRef] [PubMed]

81. Jones, K.S.; Bluck, L.J.; Wang, L.Y.; Stephen, A.M.; Prynne, C.J.; Coward, W.A. The effect of different meals on the absorption of stable isotope-labelled phylloquinone. *Br. J. Nutr.* **2009**, *102*, 1195–1202. [CrossRef] [PubMed]

82. Nordestgaard, B.G.; Varbo, A. Triglycerides and cardiovascular disease. *Lancet* **2014**, *384*, 626–635. [CrossRef]

83. Booth, S.L.; Martini, L.; Peterson, J.W.; Saltzman, E.; Dallal, G.E.; Wood, R.J. Dietary phylloquinone depletion and repletion in older women. *J. Nutr.* **2003**, *133*, 2565–2569. [PubMed]

84. Shea, M.K.; Benjamin, E.J.; Dupuis, J.; Massaro, J.M.; Jacques, P.F.; D'Agostino, R.B., Sr.; Ordovas, J.M.; O'Donnell, C.J.; Dawson-Hughes, B.; *et al.* Genetic and non-genetic correlates of vitamins K and D. *Eur. J. Clin. Nutr.* **2009**, *63*, 458–464. [CrossRef] [PubMed]

85. Dashti, H.S.; Shea, M.K.; Smith, C.E.; Tanaka, T.; Hruby, A.; Richardson, K.; Wang, T.J.; Nalls, M.A.; Guo, X.; Liu, Y.; *et al.* Meta-analysis of genome-wide association studies for circulating phylloquinone concentrations. *Am. J. Clin. Nutr.* **2014**, *100*, 1462–1469. [CrossRef] [PubMed]

86. Sato, T.; Schurgers, L.J.; Uenishi, K. Comparison of menaquinone-4 and menaquinone-7 bioavailability in healthy women. *Nutr. J.* **2012**, *11*. [CrossRef] [PubMed]

87. Karl, J.P.; Fu, X.; Dolnikowski, G.G.; Saltzman, E.; Booth, S.L. Quantification of phylloquinone and menaquinones in feces, serum, and food by high-performance liquid chromatography-mass spectrometry. *J. Chromatogr. B Anal. Technol. Biomed. Life Sci.* **2014**, *963*, 128–133. [CrossRef] [PubMed]

88. Booth, S.L.; Al, R.A. Determinants of vitamin K status in humans. *Vitam. Horm.* **2008**, *78*, 1–22. [PubMed]

89. Suttie, J.W. Vitamin K and human nutrition. *J. Am. Diet. Assoc.* **1992**, *92*, 585–590. [PubMed]

90. Limdi, N.A.; Nolin, T.D.; Booth, S.L.; Centi, A.; Marques, M.B.; Crowley, M.R.; Allon, M.; Beasley, T.M. Influence of kidney function on risk of supratherapeutic international normalized ratio-related hemorrhage in warfarin users: A prospective cohort study. *Am. J. Kidney Dis.* **2015**, *65*, 701–709. [CrossRef] [PubMed]

91. Gundberg, C.M.; Nieman, S.D.; Abrams, S.; Rosen, H. Vitamin K status and bone health: An analysis of methods for determination of undercarboxylated osteocalcin. *J. Clin. Endocrinol. Metab.* **1998**, *83*, 3258–3266. [CrossRef] [PubMed]

92. Greenspan, S.L.; Resnick, N.M.; Parker, R.A. Early changes in biochemical markers of bone turnover are associated with long-term changes in bone mineral density in elderly women on alendronate, hormone replacement therapy, or combination therapy: A three-year, double-blind, placebo-controlled, randomized clinical trial. *J. Clin. Endocrinol. Metab.* **2005**, *90*, 2762–2767. [PubMed]

93. Rosen, C.J.; Chesnut, C.H., III; Mallinak, N.J. The predictive value of biochemical markers of bone turnover for bone mineral density in early postmenopausal women treated with hormone replacement or calcium supplementation. *J. Clin. Endocrinol. Metab.* **1997**, *82*, 1904–1910. [PubMed]

94. Rehder, D.S.; Gundberg, C.M.; Booth, S.L.; Borges, C.R. Gamma-carboxylation and fragmentation of osteocalcin in human serum defined by mass spectrometry. *Mol. Cell. Proteomics* **2015**, *14*, 1546–1555. [CrossRef] [PubMed]

95. Price, P.A.; Kaneda, Y. Vitamin K counteracts the effect of warfarin in liver but not in bone. *Thromb. Res.* **1987**, *46*, 121–131. [CrossRef]

96. Hara, K.; Kobayashi, M.; Akiyama, Y. Comparison of inhibitory effects of warfarin on gamma-carboxylation between bone and liver in rats. *J. Bone Miner. Metab.* **2005**, *23*, 366–372. [CrossRef] [PubMed]

97. Gundberg, C.M.; Lian, J.B.; Booth, S.L. Vitamin K-dependent carboxylation of osteocalcin: Friend or foe? *Adv. Nutr.* **2012**, *3*, 149–157. [CrossRef] [PubMed]

98. Theuwissen, E.; Magdeleyns, E.J.; Braam, L.A.; Teunissen, K.J.; Knapen, M.H.; Binnekamp, I.A.; van Summeren, M.J.; Vermeer, C. Vitamin K status in healthy volunteers. *Food Funct.* **2014**, *5*, 229–234. [CrossRef] [PubMed]

99. Shea, M.K.; Booth, S.L.; Gundberg, C.M.; Peterson, J.W.; Waddell, C.; Dawson-Hughes, B.; Saltzman, E. Adulthood obesity is positively associated with adipose tissue concentrations of vitamin K and inversely associated with circulating indicators of vitamin K status in men and women. *J. Nutr.* **2010**, *140*, 1029–1034. [CrossRef] [PubMed]

100. Cranenburg, E.C.; Koos, R.; Schurgers, L.J.; Magdeleyns, E.J.; Schoonbrood, T.H.; Landewe, R.B.; Brandenburg, V.M.; Bekers, O.; Vermeer, C. Characterisation and potential diagnostic value of circulating matrix Gla protein (MGP) species. *Thromb. Haemost.* **2010**, *104*, 811–822. [PubMed]

101. Shea, M.K.; O'Donnell, C.J.; Vermeer, C.; Magdeleyns, E.J.; Crosier, M.D.; Gundberg, C.M.; Ordovas, J.M.; Kritchevsky, S.B.; Booth, S.L. Circulating uncarboxylated matrix gla protein is associated with vitamin K nutritional status, but not coronary artery calcium, in older adults. *J. Nutr.* **2011**, *141*, 1529–1534. [CrossRef] [PubMed]

102. O'Donnell, C.J.; Shea, M.K.; Price, P.A.; Gagnon, D.R.; Wilson, P.W.; Larson, M.G.; Kiel, D.P.; Hoffmann, U.; Ferencik, M.; Clouse, M.E.; *et al.* Matrix Gla protein is associated with risk factors for atherosclerosis but not with coronary artery calcification. *Arterioscler. Thromb. Vasc. Biol.* **2006**, *26*, 2769–2774. [CrossRef] [PubMed]

103. Liu, G.; Peacock, M. Age-related changes in serum undercarboxylated osteocalcin and its relationships with bone density, bone quality, and hip fracture. *Calcif. Tissue Int.* **1998**, *62*, 286–289. [CrossRef] [PubMed]

104. Szulc, P.; Chapuy, M.C.; Meunier, P.J.; Delmas, P.D. Serum undercarboxylated osteocalcin is a marker of the risk of hip fracture in elderly women. *J. Clin. Invest.* **1993**, *91*, 1769–1774. [CrossRef] [PubMed]

105. Szulc, P.; Arlot, M.; Chapuy, M.C.; Duboeuf, F.; Meunier, P.J.; Delmas, P.D. Serum undercarboxylated osteocalcin correlates with hip bone mineral density in elderly women. *J. Bone Miner. Res.* **1994**, *9*, 1591–1595. [CrossRef] [PubMed]

106. Vergnaud, P.; Garnero, P.; Meunier, P.J.; Breart, G.; Kamihagi, K.; Delmas, P.D. Undercarboxylated osteocalcin measured with a specific immunoassay predicts hip fracture in elderly women: The EPIDOS Study. *J. Clin. Endocrinol. Metab.* **1997**, *82*, 719–724. [CrossRef] [PubMed]

107. Braam, L.A.; Knapen, M.H.; Geusens, P.; Brouns, F.; Hamulyak, K.; Gerichhausen, M.J.; Vermeer, C. Vitamin K1 supplementation retards bone loss in postmenopausal women between 50 and 60 years of age. *Calcif. Tissue Int.* **2003**, *73*, 21–26. [CrossRef] [PubMed]

108. Knapen, M.H.; Drummen, N.E.; Smit, E.; Vermeer, C.; Theuwissen, E. Three-year low-dose menaquinone-7 supplementation helps decrease bone loss in healthy postmenopausal women. *Osteoporos. Int.* **2013**, *24*, 2499–2507. [CrossRef] [PubMed]

109. Binkley, N.; Harke, J.; Krueger, D.; Engelke, J.; Vallarta-Ast, N.; Gemar, D.; Checovich, M.; Chappell, R.; Suttie, J. Vitamin K treatment reduces undercarboxylated osteocalcin but does not alter bone turnover, density, or geometry in healthy postmenopausal North American women. *J. Bone Miner. Res.* **2009**, *24*, 983–991. [CrossRef] [PubMed]

110. Bolton-Smith, C.; McMurdo, M.E.; Paterson, C.R.; Mole, P.A.; Harvey, J.M.; Fenton, S.T.; Prynne, C.J.; Mishra, G.D.; Shearer, M.J. Two-year randomized controlled trial of vitamin K1 (phylloquinone) and vitamin D3 plus calcium on the bone health of older women. *J. Bone Miner. Res.* **2007**, *22*, 509–519. [CrossRef] [PubMed]

111. O'Connor, E.M.; Grealy, G.; McCarthy, J.; Desmond, A.; Craig, O.; Shanahan, F.; Cashman, K.D. Effect of phylloquinone (vitamin K1) supplementation for 12 months on the indices of vitamin K status and bone health in adult patients with Crohn's disease. *Br. J. Nutr.* **2014**, *112*, 1163–1174. [CrossRef] [PubMed]

112. Emaus, N.; Gjesdal, C.G.; Almas, B.; Christensen, M.; Grimsgaard, A.S.; Berntsen, G.K.; Salomonsen, L.; Fonnebo, V. Vitamin K2 supplementation does not influence bone loss in early menopausal women: A randomised double-blind placebo-controlled trial. *Osteoporos. Int.* **2010**, *21*, 1731–1740. [CrossRef] [PubMed]

113. Ferron, M.; Hinoi, E.; Karsenty, G.; Ducy, P. Osteocalcin differentially regulates beta cell and adipocyte gene expression and affects the development of metabolic diseases in wild-type mice. *Proc. Natl. Acad. Sci. USA* **2008**, *105*, 5266–5270. [CrossRef] [PubMed]

114. Ferron, M.; McKee, M.D.; Levine, R.L.; Ducy, P.; Karsenty, G. Intermittent injections of osteocalcin improve glucose metabolism and prevent type 2 diabetes in mice. *Bone* **2012**, *50*, 568–575. [CrossRef] [PubMed]

115. Pollock, N.K.; Bernard, P.J.; Gower, B.A.; Gundberg, C.M.; Wenger, K.; Misra, S.; Bassali, R.W.; Davis, C.L. Lower uncarboxylated osteocalcin concentrations in children with prediabetes is associated with beta-cell function. *J. Clin. Endocrinol. Metab.* **2011**, *96*, E1092–E1099. [CrossRef] [PubMed]

116. Prats-Puig, A.; Mas-Parareda, M.; Riera-Perez, E.; Gonzalez-Forcadell, D.; Mier, C.; Mallol-Guisset, M.; Diaz, M.; Bassols, J.; de Zegher, F.; Ibanez, L.; *et al.* Carboxylation of osteocalcin affects its association with metabolic parameters in healthy children. *Diabetes Care* **2010**, *33*, 661–663. [CrossRef] [PubMed]

117. Lu, C.; Ivaska, K.K.; Alen, M.; Wang, Q.; Tormakangas, T.; Xu, L.; Wiklund, P.; Mikkola, T.M.; Pekkala, S.; Tian, H.; Vaananen, H.K.; *et al.* Serum osteocalcin is not associated with glucose but is inversely associated with leptin across generations of nondiabetic women. *J. Clin. Endocrinol. Metab.* **2012**, *97*, 4106–4114. [CrossRef] [PubMed]

118. Iki, M.; Tamaki, J.; Fujita, Y.; Kouda, K.; Yura, A.; Kadowaki, E.; Sato, Y.; Moon, J.S.; Tomioka, K.; Okamoto, N.; *et al.* Serum undercarboxylated osteocalcin levels are inversely associated with glycemic status and insulin resistance in an elderly Japanese male population: Fujiwara-kyo Osteoporosis Risk in Men (FORMEN) Study. *Osteoporos. Int.* **2012**, *23*, 761–770. [CrossRef] [PubMed]

119. Okuno, S.; Ishimura, E.; Tsuboniwa, N.; Norimine, K.; Yamakawa, K.; Yamakawa, T.; Shoji, S.; Mori, K.; Nishizawa, Y.; Inaba, M. Significant inverse relationship between serum undercarboxylated osteocalcin and glycemic control in maintenance hemodialysis patients. *Osteoporos. Int.* **2013**, *24*, 605–612. [CrossRef] [PubMed]

120. Yeap, B.B.; Alfonso, H.; Chubb, S.A.; Gauci, R.; Byrnes, E.; Beilby, J.P.; Ebeling, P.R.; Handelsman, D.J.; Allan, C.A.; Grossmann, M.; *et al.* Higher serum undercarboxylated osteocalcin and other bone turnover markers are associated with reduced diabetes risk and lower estradiol concentrations in older men. *J. Clin. Endocrinol. Metab.* **2015**, *100*, 63–71. [CrossRef] [PubMed]

121. Shea, M.K.; Gundberg, C.M.; Meigs, J.B.; Dallal, G.E.; Saltzman, E.; Yoshida, M.; Jacques, P.F.; Booth, S.L. Gamma-carboxylation of osteocalcin and insulin resistance in older men and women. *Am. J. Clin. Nutr.* **2009**, *90*, 1230–1235. [CrossRef] [PubMed]

122. Liu, D.M.; Guo, X.Z.; Tong, H.J.; Tao, B.; Sun, L.H.; Zhao, H.Y.; Ning, G.; Liu, J.M. Association between osteocalcin and glucose metabolism: A meta-analysis. *Osteoporos. Int.* **2015**, *26*, 2823–2833. [CrossRef] [PubMed]

123. Luo, G.; Ducy, P.; McKee, M.D.; Pinero, G.J.; Loyer, E.; Behringer, R.R.; Karsenty, G. Spontaneous calcification of arteries and cartilage in mice lacking matrix GLA protein. *Nature* **1997**, *386*, 78–81. [CrossRef] [PubMed]

124. Schurgers, L.J.; Spronk, H.M.; Skepper, J.N.; Hackeng, T.M.; Shanahan, C.M.; Vermeer, C.; Weissberg, P.L.; Proudfoot, D. Post-translational modifications regulate matrix Gla protein function: Importance for inhibition of vascular smooth muscle cell calcification. *J. Thromb. Haemost.* **2007**, *5*, 2503–2511. [CrossRef] [PubMed]

125. Dalmeijer, G.W.; van der Schouw, Y.T.; Magdeleyns, E.; Ahmed, N.; Vermeer, C.; Beulens, J.W. The effect of menaquinone-7 supplementation on circulating species of matrix Gla protein. *Atherosclerosis* **2012**, *225*, 397–402. [CrossRef] [PubMed]

126. Schlieper, G.; Westenfeld, R.; Kruger, T.; Cranenburg, E.C.; Magdeleyns, E.J.; Brandenburg, V.M.; Djuric, Z.; Damjanovic, T.; Ketteler, M.; Vermeer, C.; *et al.* Circulating nonphosphorylated carboxylated matrix gla protein predicts survival in ESRD. *J. Am. Soc. Nephrol.* **2011**, *22*, 387–395. [CrossRef] [PubMed]

127. Westenfeld, R.; Krueger, T.; Schlieper, G.; Cranenburg, E.C.; Magdeleyns, E.J.; Heidenreich, S.; Holzmann, S.; Vermeer, C.; Jahnen-Dechent, W.; Ketteler, M.; *et al.* Effect of vitamin K2 supplementation on functional vitamin K deficiency in hemodialysis patients: A randomized trial. *Am. J. Kidney Dis.* **2012**, *59*, 186–195. [CrossRef] [PubMed]

128. Dalmeijer, G.W.; van der Schouw, Y.T.; Magdeleyns, E.J.; Vermeer, C.; Verschuren, W.M.; Boer, J.M.; Beulens, J.W. Matrix Gla protein species and risk of cardiovascular events in type 2 diabetic patients. *Diabetes Care* **2013**, *36*, 3766–3771. [CrossRef] [PubMed]

129. Liu, Y.P.; Gu, Y.M.; Thijs, L.; Knapen, M.H.; Salvi, E.; Citterio, L.; Petit, T.; Carpini, S.D.; Zhang, Z.; Jacobs, L.; *et al.* Inactive matrix Gla protein is causally related to adverse health outcomes: A Mendelian randomization study in a Flemish population. *Hypertension* **2015**, *65*, 463–470. [CrossRef] [PubMed]

130. Mayer, O., Jr.; Seidlerova, J.; Bruthans, J.; Filipovsky, J.; Timoracka, K.; Vanek, J.; Cerna, L.; Wohlfahrt, P.; Cifkova, R.; Theuwissen, E.; *et al.* Desphospho-uncarboxylated matrix Gla-protein is associated with mortality risk in patients with chronic stable vascular disease. *Atherosclerosis* **2014**, *235*, 162–168. [CrossRef] [PubMed]

131. Mayer, O., Jr.; Seidlerova, J.; Wohlfahrt, P.; Filipovsky, J.; Vanek, J.; Cifkova, R.; Windrichova, J.; Topolcan, O.; Knapen, M.H.; Drummen, N.E.; *et al.* Desphospho-uncarboxylated matrix Gla protein is associated with increased aortic stiffness in a general population. *J. Hum. Hypertens.* **2015**. [CrossRef] [PubMed]

132. Pivin, E.; Ponte, B.; Pruijm, M.; Ackermann, D.; Guessous, I.; Ehret, G.; Liu, Y.P.; Drummen, N.E.; Knapen, M.H.; Pechere-Bertschi, A.; *et al.* Inactive matrix Gla-protein is associated with arterial stiffness in an adult population-based study. *Hypertension* **2015**, *66*, 85–92. [CrossRef] [PubMed]

133. Pivin, E.; Pruijm, M.; Ackermann, D.; Guessous, I.; Ehret, G.; Pechere-Bertschi, A.; Paccaud, F.; Mohaupt, M.; Vermeer, C.; Staessen, J.A.; *et al.* 1D.03: Inactive matrix gla protein is associated with renal resistive index in a population-based study. *J. Hypertens.* **2015**, *33* (Suppl. S1). [CrossRef] [PubMed]

134. van den Heuvel, E.G.; van Schoor, N.M.; Lips, P.; Magdeleyns, E.J.; Deeg, D.J.; Vermeer, C.; den, H.M. Circulating uncarboxylated matrix Gla protein, a marker of vitamin K status, as a risk factor of cardiovascular disease. *Maturitas* **2014**, *77*, 137–141. [CrossRef] [PubMed]

135. Dalmeijer, G.W.; van der Schouw, Y.T.; Vermeer, C.; Magdeleyns, E.J.; Schurgers, L.J.; Beulens, J.W. Circulating matrix Gla protein is associated with coronary artery calcification and vitamin K status in healthy women. *J. Nutr. Biochem.* **2013**, *24*, 624–628. [CrossRef] [PubMed]

136. Dalmeijer, G.W.; van der Schouw, Y.T.; Magdeleyns, E.J.; Vermeer, C.; Verschuren, W.M.; Boer, J.M.; Beulens, J.W. Circulating desphospho-uncarboxylated matrix gamma-carboxyglutamate protein and the risk of coronary heart disease and stroke. *J. Thromb. Haemost.* **2014**, *12*, 1028–1034. [CrossRef] [PubMed]

137. Knapen, M.H.; Braam, L.A.; Drummen, N.E.; Bekers, O.; Hoeks, A.P.; Vermeer, C. Menaquinone-7 supplementation improves arterial stiffness in healthy postmenopausal women: Double-blind randomised clinical trial. *Thromb. Haemost.* **2015**, *113*, 1135–1144. [CrossRef] [PubMed]

138. Farzaneh-Far, A.; Weissberg, P.L.; Proudfoot, D.; Shanahan, C.M. Transcriptional regulation of matrix gla protein. *Z. Kardiol.* **2001**, *90* (Suppl. S3), 38–42. [CrossRef] [PubMed]

139. Mustonen, E.; Pohjolainen, V.; Aro, J.; Pikkarainen, S.; Leskinen, H.; Ruskoaho, H.; Rysa, J. Upregulation of cardiac matrix Gla protein expression in response to hypertrophic stimuli. *Blood Press* **2009**, *18*, 286–293. [CrossRef] [PubMed]

140. Price, P.A.; Thomas, G.R.; Pardini, A.W.; Figueira, W.F.; Caputo, J.M.; Williamson, M.K. Discovery of a high molecular weight complex of calcium, phosphate, fetuin, and matrix gamma-carboxyglutamic acid protein in the serum of etidronate-treated rats. *J. Biol. Chem.* **2002**, *277*, 3926–3934. [CrossRef] [PubMed]

141. Truong, J.T.; Fu, X.; Saltzman, E.; Al, R.A.; Dallal, G.E.; Gundberg, C.M.; Booth, S.L. Age group and sex do not influence responses of vitamin K biomarkers to changes in dietary vitamin K. *J. Nutr.* **2012**, *142*, 936–941. [CrossRef] [PubMed]

142. Bugel, S.; Sorensen, A.D.; Hels, O.; Kristensen, M.; Vermeer, C.; Jakobsen, J.; Flynn, A.; Molgaard, C.; Cashman, K.D. Effect of phylloquinone supplementation on biochemical markers of vitamin K status and bone turnover in postmenopausal women. *Br. J. Nutr.* **2007**, *97*, 373–380. [CrossRef] [PubMed]

143. Harrington, D.J.; Soper, R.; Edwards, C.; Savidge, G.F.; Hodges, S.J.; Shearer, M.J. Determination of the urinary aglycone metabolites of vitamin K by HPLC with redox-mode electrochemical detection. *J. Lipid Res.* **2005**, *46*, 1053–1060. [CrossRef] [PubMed]

144. Al, R.A.; Peterson, J.; Choi, S.W.; Suttie, J.; Barakat, S.; Booth, S.L. Measurement of menadione in urine by HPLC. *J. Chromatogr. B Anal. Technol. Biomed. Life Sci.* **2010**, *878*, 2457–2460.

145. Shea, M.K.; Booth, S.L.; Brinkley, T.E.; Kritchevsky, S.B. Vitamin K status in black and white older adults and its relationship with cardiovascular disease risk. *FASEB J.* **2015**, *29* (Suppl. S1), 906.4.

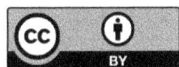

nutrients

MDPI

Article

Phylloquinone and Menaquinone-4 Tissue Distribution at Different Life Stages in Male and Female Sprague–Dawley Rats Fed Different VK Levels Since Weaning or Subjected to a 40% Calorie Restriction since Adulthood

Guylaine Ferland [1,*], **Isabelle Doucet** [1,2] **and Dominique Mainville** [1,3]

1   Département de nutrition, Université de Montréal, Montréal, QC H3C 3J7, Canada;
    isadoucet@me.com (I.D.); dominique.mainville@hotmail.com (D.M.)
2   Hôpital de la Cité-de-la-Santé, Laval, QC H7M 3L9, Canada
3   CIUSSS du Centre-Sud-de-l'Île-de-Montréal, Centre de réadaptation Lucie-Bruneau, Montréal,
    QC H2H 2N8, Canada
*   Correspondence: guylaine.ferland@umontreal.ca; Tel.: +1-514-340-2800 (ext. 3236)

Received: 22 December 2015; Accepted: 19 February 2016; Published: 4 March 2016

Abstract: Whether through the vitamin K-dependent proteins or the individual K vitamers, vitamin K (VK) is associated with a number of age-related conditions (e.g., osteoporosis, atherosclerosis, insulin resistance, cognitive decline). In light of this, we investigated the influence of lifetime dietary VK exposure on the tissue distribution of phylloquinone (K_1) and menaquinone-4 (MK-4) vitamers in 3-, 12- and 22-month-old male and female rats fed different K_1 diets since weaning or subjected to a 40% calorie restricted diet (CR) since adulthood. Dietary K_1 intakes around the minimal amount required for normal blood coagulation had no significant influence on body weights of both male and female rats at different life stages. Tissue contents of the K vitamers differed according to organs, were generally higher in females than in males, and increased with K_1 intake. The MK-4/total VK ratios tended to be increased in old age possibly reflecting an increased physiological demand for MK-4 during aging. Our study also confirmed the greater susceptibility of male rats to low VK containing diet, notably at a younger age. Despite lifelong higher K_1 intakes per unit body weight, tissue K_1 and MK-4 contents at 20 months were generally lower in CR rats compared to their *ad libitum* (*AL*) counterparts. Whether the lower tissue MK-4 content is the result of lower synthesis from K_1 or greater tissue utilization remains to be determined. However, the more youthful coagulation profile observed in old CR rats (*vs. AL* rats) tends to support the notion that CR is associated with greater utilization of the K vitamers to sustain physiological functions.

Keywords: phylloquinone; menaquinone-4; tissue distribution; sex; age; diet; caloric restriction

1. Introduction

As a unique cofactor to the gamma-glutamyl carboxylase (GGCX), an enzyme that converts specific glutamic acid residues to gamma-carboxyglutamic acid in precursor proteins, vitamin K (VK) *i.e.*, all K vitamers, participates in the biological activation of several proteins. The vitamin K-dependent proteins (VKDPs) are notably involved in hemostasis, the calcification process (*i.e.*, bone matrix and vasculature), brain function, and glucose metabolism [1–4]. Compounds with VK activity all have a common 2-methyl-1,4-naphtoquinone ring but differ in structure at the 3-position. Phylloquinone (K_1), derived from plants, is the main dietary form, while the menaquinones, which are of bacterial origin, form a family of compounds with unsaturated isoprenyl side chains of various lengths [5].

One of the menaquinones, menaquinone-4 (MK-4), is not a common product of bacterial synthesis but is synthesized from phylloquinone with menadione as an intermediate [6–8]. In recent years, the human UbiA prenyltransferase containing 1 (UBIAD1) enzyme was shown to be responsible for the MK-4 biosynthesis [9,10].

In addition to its role as enzymatic cofactor in the carboxylation reaction, there is evidence to support other specific actions for VK notably, the K_1 and MK-4 vitamers. Specifically, both vitamers have been involved in the synthesis of sphingolipids, a group of complex lipids present in brain cell membranes and which possess important cell signaling properties [11]. Recent studies also point to protective roles for K_1 and MK-4 against oxidative stress and inflammatory processes. *In vitro*, both vitamers were shown to limit the production of interleukin-6 (IL-6) and other proinflammatory cytokines through the inhibtion of nuclear factor kappaB [12–14] whereas, *in vivo*, MK-4 limited inflammation in encephalomyelitis [15]. Both K_1 and MK-4 have also been shown to prevent glutathione depletion-mediated oxidative injury and cell death in primary culture of oligodendrocyte precursors and immature fetal cortical neurons [16,17]. Menaquinone-4 specifically has also been shown to possess potent anticancer properties, inducing apoptosis in several types of tumor cells [18] and inhibiting growth of hepatocarcinoma cells [19]. At the molecular level, MK-4 is a ligand for the steroid xenobiotic receptor [20,21] and promotes protein kinase A (PKA) activation [22–24], a signaling pathway that has also been associated with enhanced testosterone production in rats [25].

Tissue concentrations of the K vitamers have been investigated in various rat strains and shown to vary according to organs [6–8], dietary intake [7,26–28], and sex [29,30]. The role of age on diet-induced changes in tissue VK distribution was also investigated in animals of various ages (*i.e.*, 3, 12, 24 months) fed different VK diets for short periods of time (about one month) [28,29]. Collectively, these studies have provided essential information on the factors that influence the tissue contents of the K vitamers in rats, and the mechanisms underlying the biotransformation of K_1 to MK-4. However, to our knowledge, no studies have reported on lifetime VK dietary exposure on tissue distribution at distinct life stages.

Aging is a complex process that negatively impacts the development of the different systems and their ability to function. Age-related diseases include cancer, cardiovascular disease, diabetes, osteoporosis, and neurodegenerative diseases such as dementia and Alzheimer's disease [31]. Caloric restriction (CR) is a well-established experimental model, which has been shown to increase longevity and delay the onset of age-related diseases in various experimental models (*i.e.*, invertebrate model organisms, rodents, primates). In rodents, this dietary regimen has been shown to extend lifespan by up to 50% [32,33].

Whether through the VKDPs or the specific actions of K_1 and MK-4, VK is associated with numerous age-associated conditions including osteoporosis, diabetes, cardiovascular disease and cognitive decline [1,2]. In light of this, we endeavoured to investigate the influence of lifetime dietary VK exposure on the tissue distribution of the K_1 and MK-4 vitamers in two models of aging. In the first study (Study 1), we report the tissue VK distribution in 3-, 12- and 22-month-old male and female rats fed different K_1 diets since weaning. In the second study (Study 2), we report the VK tissue distribution in 20-month-old male and females rats, which were fed *ad libitum* (*AL*) throughout their lives or were subjected to a 40% calorie restricted diet (CR) since adulthood.

2. Methods and Materials

2.1. Animals and Diets

Protocols for both studies were approved by the Animal Care Committee of the Université de Montréal in compliance with the guidelines of the Canadian Council on Animal Care.

Study 1. A total of 120 rats were used for this study. 4-week-old male and female Sprague–Dawley rats were obtained from Charles Rivers Canada Inc. (St Constant, QC, Canada) and housed 3 per cage in suspended stainless steel wire-bottom cages (to prevent coprophagy) in a room kept at 22 °C with a 12 h light-dark cycle. Rats were kept in the same housing conditions and rat facility throughout the experimental period (22 months). For one week, animals had free access to a semi-synthetic powdered diet prepared according to the Teklad control diet (#TD 89248) which consisted of 22% casein (vitamin free), 48.5% sucrose, 15% corn starch, 5% corn oil, 4.6% fiber (cellulose), 3.9% mineral mix and 1% vitamin mix (Teklad Test Diets, Madison, WI, USA). After this acclimatization period, rats were randomly assigned to a diet containing either low (L; ~100 μg/kg diet), adequate (A; ~500 μg/kg diet) or high (H; ~1500 μg/kg diet) levels of K_1. These diets compared to the Teklad control diet (#TD 89248) except for vitamin K, where menadione was replaced by K_1 (Sigma Chemicals, St-Louis, MO, USA). The powder diets were prepared in our laboratory and K_1 concentrations evaluated by HPLC analysis were: Mean ± SEM, $n = 8$; 104 ± 9 μg/kg diet, 433 ± 13 μg/kg diet, and 1668 ± 9 μg/kg diet, respectively. These dietary concentrations of K_1 were chosen to provide rats with a range of intakes around the minimal amount required for normal coagulation activity namely 500 μg K_1/kg diet [34]. Rats had free access to water and food. Food intake and body weights were recorded every 2 weeks, and the health of the rats was monitored regularly by a veterinarian throughout the experimental period. Distinct groups of male and female rats from each dietary group were killed at 3, 12 and 22 months of age ($n = 5$–7/sex/age/diet), after having been food deprived overnight prior to the day of the experiment.

Study 2. A total of 48 rats were used for this study. 4-week-old male and female Sprague–Dawley rats were obtained from Charles Rivers Canada, Inc. (St Constant, QC, Canada). Animals were individually housed in wire-bottom cages under constant temperature of 22 °C and a 12 h light/12 h dark cycle. After one week of acclimatization, rats were given free access to the Teklad control diet (#TD 89248) (described above) where menadione was replaced by K_1 (Sigma Chemicals, St-Louis, MO, USA) at a concentration of ~500 μg/kg diet (Mean ± SEM, $n = 8$; 479 ± 13 μg K_1/kg diet by analysis). At 8 months of age, 16 male and 16 female rats were randomized in two dietary groups: one group was given free access to food (*ad libitum* (*AL*)) while the second group was subjected to a 20% reduction in daily caloric intake for two weeks, and 40% (CR) thereafter based on the mean intake of *AL* rats. A gradual approach to CR was adopted to minimize stress on the animals. Diet fed the CR rats was adjusted for vitamins (including K_1) and minerals, so that intakes of micronutrients were identical to those of *AL* animals: 22% casein (vitamin free), 48.5% sucrose, 15% corn starch, 5% corn oil, 4.6% fiber (cellulose), 5.85% mineral mix, 1.67% vitamin mix (Teklad Test Diets, Madison, WI, USA), and 835 μg K_1/kg diet. Eight males and eight females aged three months and fed *AL* since weaning, served as the "young" control group. All animals had free access to water. Food intake and body weights were assessed weekly and every two weeks respectively, and health of the rats was monitored regularly by a veterinarian throughout the study. Distinct groups of male and female rats were killed at 3 and 20 (*AL* and CR) months of age ($n = 6$–8/group, after having been food deprived overnight prior to the day of the experiment.

2.2. Sacrifice Procedure (Applies to Both Studies)

On the day of sacrifice, rats were anesthetized with sodium pentobarbital (45 mg/Kg body weight, ip), blood was withdrawn from the abdominal aorta and collected in a vacutainer containing 9:1, v/v trisodium citrate (Becton Dickinson Co, Rutherford, NJ, USA), and plasma was immediately separated by a 10-min centrifugation (500× g at 4 °C). The liver, heart, kidneys, spleen, brain, ovaries or testis were harvested, washed in 0.9% saline solution, weighed and stored at −80 °C until analysis.

2.3. Analytical Procedure (Applies to Both Studies)

Phylloquinone and MK-4 were quantified by HPLC as previously described [35]. Briefly, tissue samples were pulverized in anhydrous Na_2SO_4 (10 times tissue weight) and extracted for 1 h in 10 mL of acetone containing an internal standard (2 ng/50 μL 2-Methyl-3-(3,7,11,15,19-pentamethyl-2-eicosenyl)-1,4-naphthalenedione—also referred to as (K_1(25)) (GL Synthesis Inc., Worcester, MA, USA). Extracts were centrifuged (500× g at 4 °C for 10 min), dried under nitrogen at 45 °C and the solid residue was reextracted with 6 mL of hexane and 2 mL of water for 3 min. After centrifugation, the top hexane layer was dried under nitrogen and redissolved in 2 mL of hexane for solid phase extraction on 3 mL silica gel columns (JT Baker Inc., Phillipsburg, NJ, USA). The K_1 and MK-4 fraction was eluted with 8 mL of hexane:diethyl ether (97:3, v/v), evaporated under nitrogen and the residue dissolved in 0.02 mL of dimethyl chloride and 0.180 mL methanol containing aqueous phase (10 mmol/L zinc chloride, 10 mmol/L acetic acid and 5 mmol/L sodium acetate; 5 mL aqueous phase was added to 1 L methanol). Quantitative analysis of the vitamers was performed by reverse-phase HPLC using a C-18 reverse phase column and fluorescence detection. The calibration standard consisted of a mixture of K_1, MK-4 and $K_1(25)$ at 2 ng/50 µL. The percent recovery for the samples was calculated from the internal standard and found to be 85%–90%. Tissue concentrations are expressed relative to wet weight. Plasma K_1 and MK-4 concentrations were quantified using the same HPLC technique as previously described [36,37].

Prothrombin times (PT) and activated partial thromboplastin times (APTT) were performed on an AC/100 Automated Clot Timer (Fisher Scientific Ltd, Montreal, QC, Canada) using thromboplastin and cephalin reagents (Sigma Chemical, St-Louis, MO, USA).

2.4. Statistical Analysis

All data are expressed as the mean $\pm$ SEM. Study 1. Body weight, food intake, K_1 intake, PT, APTT, plasma and tissue K_1 and MK-4 were analysed with respect to diet, sex and age, by three-way ANOVA (main effects) followed by pairwise multiple comparisons (Holm–Sidak method). Homogeneity of variance for ANOVA was assessed using the Shapiro–Wilk test and variables that were not normally distributed were log-transformed prior to the analysis. The effect of diet was further tested within each sex and age group by conducting distinct one-way ANOVA's followed by Tukey's *post hoc* tests. Tissue K_1 and MK-4 concentration differences were tested in 12-month-old male and female rats fed the adequate diet (as reference groups), using one-way ANOVA's followed by Tukey's *post hoc* tests. Study 2. Body weight, food intake, K_1 intake, PT, APTT, plasma and tissue K_1 and MK-4 were assessed in males and females with respect to age and diet, with distinct one-way ANOVA's followed by Tukey's post hoc tests. Homogeneity of variance for ANOVA was assessed using the Shapiro-Wilk test and variables that were not normally distributed were log-transformed prior to the analysis. Student' *t*-test was used to further assess the effect of CR at 20 months, and that of sex for given age and diet groups. Differences were considered significant at $p < 0.05$. Three-way analyses of variance were conducted using SigmaPlot version 12.0 (Systat Software, Inc., San Jose, CA, USA) whereas one-way analyses of variance and *t*-tests were conducted using GraphPad Prism6 version 6.01 (GraphPad Software, Inc., La Jolla, CA, USA).

3. Results

3.1. Study 1

3.1.1. Body Weights, Food, and K_1 Intakes

Mean body weights (BW) of male (M) and female (F) rats at 3, 12, and 22 months of age are presented in Figure 1 for the low (L), adequate (A) and high (H) dietary groups, respectively. Body weights increased with age in both males and females ($p < 0.001$). At all ages, body weights were higher in males than in females ($p < 0.001$) but were not affected by diet.

Daily food (g) and K_1 (µg) intakes expressed per 100 g·BW are presented in Table 1 for 3-, 12-, and 22-month-old male and female rats fed the L, A or H diets. Food intakes decreased with age in both males and females ($p < 0.001$) and were higher in females than in males at 3- and 12- but not at 22-months of age ($p < 0.001$). Food intakes did not vary among the dietary groups in males at any age in contrast to females where, at 3 months, food intakes were significantly higher in the H than in the L and A groups ($p < 0.05$). Phylloquinone intakes decreased with age irrespective of diet in both males and females ($p < 0.001$), and were higher in females than in males at 3 and 12 but not at 22 months of age ($p < 0.001$). As expected, K_1 intakes were significantly different between each dietary group, in both sexes ($p < 0.001$).

BODY WEIGHT

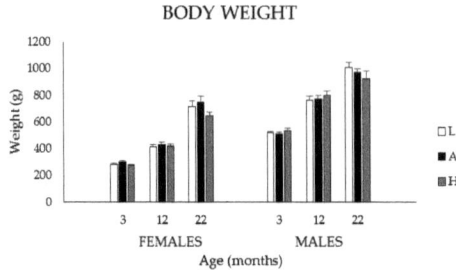

Figure 1. Mean body weights of 3-, 12-, and 22-month-old male (M) and female (F) Sprague–Dawley rats fed the L, A or H diets throughout their lives. Based on the 3-way ANOVA analysis, body weights increased with age in both M and F ($p < 0.001$). At all ages, body weights were higher in M than in F ($p < 0.001$) but were not affected by diet ($p = 0.258$), a finding confirmed by the individual one-way ANOVAs conducted at the group level. Values are expressed as mean $\pm$ SEM. (3 months F: $n = 16$/diet gp (group); M: $n = 16$/diet gp; 12 months F: $n = 15$–16/diet gp; M: $n = 16$/diet gp; 22 months F: $n = 6$–7/diet gp; M: $n = 7$–9/diet gp).

Table 1. Daily food (g/100 g body weight (BW)) and K_1 (μg/100 g·BW) intakes of 3-, 12-, and 22-month-old male (M) and female (F) Sprague–Dawley rats fed the low (L), adequate (A) or high (H) diets throughout their lives.

Age (Months)	Diet	Food Intake (g/100 BW/Day)		K_1 Intake (μg/100 g· BW/Day)	
		F	M	F	M
	L	5.7 ± 0.2	4.5 ± 0.1	562.6 ± 15.9	444.6 ± 9.4
3	A	5.6 ± 0.2	4.5 ± 0.1	2780.4 ± 83.0 [c]	2204.8 ± 56.2 [c]
	H	6.3 ± 0.1 [a,b]	4.7 ± 0.2	9433.2 ± 164.3 [a,b]	7022.3 ± 217.7 [a,b]
	L	4.2 ± 0.2	3.0 ± 0.1	414.9 ± 15.3	297.2 ± 11.6
12	A	4.2 ± 0.2	3.2 ± 0.1	2063.6 ± 101.2 [c]	1574.8 ± 51.4 [c]
	H	3.8 ± 0.2	3.0 ± 0.1	5987.3 ± 174.2 [a,b]	4386.0 ± 165.9 [a,b]
	L	2.6 ± 0.2	2.7 ± 0.1	253.6 ± 14.4	268.9 ± 9.9
22	A	2.5 ± 0.2	2.6 ± 0.1	1231.5 ± 85.6 [c]	1281.9 ± 43.5 [c]
	H	2.8 ± 0.2	2.7 ± 0.2	4141.4 ± 245.1 [a,b]	3954.1 ± 229.3 [a,b]

Based on the 3-way ANOVA analysis, food intakes decreased with age in both sexes ($p < 0.001$) and were higher in F than in M at 3 and 12 but not at 22 months of age ($p < 0.001$). Food intakes did not vary according to diet in M in contrast to F where, at 3 months, food intakes were significantly higher in the H than L and A groups ($p < 0.05$). Phylloquinone intakes decreased with age irrespective of diet in both sexes ($p < 0.001$) and were higher in F than in M at 3 and 12 but not at 22 months of age ($p < 0.001$). Phylloquinone intakes were significantly different between each dietary group, in both sexes ($p < 0.001$). The effect of diet was further tested within each sex and age group by one-way ANOVA's followed by Tukey's *post hoc* tests; [a]: $p < 0.05$ between H and L group same age and sex; [b]: $p < 0.05$ between H and A group same age and sex; [c]: $p < 0.05$ between A and L group same age and sex. Values are expressed as mean $\pm$ SEM; n for each group are as in Figure 1.

3.1.2. Plasma and Tissue K_1, MK-4, and Total VK (K_1 + MK-4) Concentrations, and MK-4/Total VK Ratios

Plasma and tissue (the liver, heart, kidneys, spleen, brain, ovaries and testes) K_1, MK-4 and total VK (K_1 + MK-4) concentrations are presented in Table 2. In plasma, there were no main sex or age effects but in most groups, K_1 concentrations increased with dietary K_1 (F:H *vs.* A and L in all age groups; M:H *vs.* A and L at 12 months, H *vs.* L at 3 and 22 months ($p < 0.05$). No MK-4 could be detected in plasma hence group differences for total VK values are as those for K_1.

Table 2. Plasma and tissue (liver, heart, kidneys, spleen, brain, ovaries and testes) K_1, MK-4 and total (K_1 + MK-4) vitamin K (VK) concentrations of 3-, 12-, and 22-month-old M and F Sprague–Dawley rats fed the L, A or H diets throughout their lives.

Organ (Months)	VK Diet (µg)	K1		MK-4		K1 + MK4	
		F	M	F	M	F	M
				pmol/g or L Plasma			
Plasma							
3	L	0.14 ± 0.11	0.04 ± 0.09	nd	nd	0.14 ± 0.11	0.04 ± 0.09
	A	0.21 ± 0.08	0.27 ± 0.17	nd	nd	0.21 ± 0.08	0.27 ± 0.17
	H	0.67 ± 0.35 [a,b]	0.41 ± 0.30 [a]	nd	nd	0.67 ± 0.35 [a,b]	0.41 ± 0.30 [a]
12	L	0.36 ± 0.29	0.21 ± 0.08	nd	nd	0.36 ± 0.29	0.21 ± 0.08
	A	0.44 ± 0.08	0.15 ± 0.08	nd	nd	0.44 ± 0.08	0.15 ± 0.08
	H	1.83 ± 0.53 [a,b]	0.76 ± 0.43 [a,b]	nd	nd	1.83 ± 0.53 [a,b]	0.76 ± 0.43 [a,b]
22	L	0.96 ± 0.35	0.84 ± 0.97	nd	nd	0.96 ± 0.35	0.84 ± 0.97
	A	1.83 ± 0.58	1.19 ± 0.42	nd	nd	1.83 ± 0.58	1.19 ± 0.42
	H	4.60 ± 1.63 [a,b]	2.29 ± 1.08 [a]	nd	nd	4.60 ± 1.63 [a,b]	2.29 ± 1.08 [a]
Liver							
3	L	46.4 ± 4.9	43.0 ± 13.9	26.7 ± 2.6	16.4 ± 3.5	73.1 ± 6.3	59.5 ± 16.4
	A	49.8 ± 7.7	68.6 ± 25.7	37.4 ± 7.2	10.2 ± 3.2	87.2 ± 12.5	78.8 ± 27.3
	H	199.6 ± 30.0 [a,b]	73.3 ± 19.5	135.5 ± 14.6 [a,b]	14.5 ± 2.9	335.1 ± 32.7 [a,b]	87.8 ± 17.7
12	L	71.5 ± 14.3	33.7 ± 7.8	35.8 ± 7.4	23.6 ± 7.7	107.3 ± 20.7	57.4 ± 11.3
	A	171.9 ± 43.8 [c]	44.3 ± 6.8	68.4 ± 10.9	31.9 ± 7.6	240.3 ± 41.5 [c]	76.2 ± 12.7
	H	410.3 ± 13.9 [a,b]	122.5 ± 37.6 [a]	142.7 ± 10.9 [a]	38.9 ± 11.8	553.0 ± 22.4 [a]	161.5 ± 43.4 [a]
22	L	34.7 ± 2.9	25.6 ± 5.4	65.0 ± 9.3	57.5 ± 8.8	99.7 ± 8.1	83.1 ± 13.7
	A	69.2 ± 12.6 [c]	52.6 ± 8.5	81.0 ± 17.9	58.8 ± 7.8	150.2 ± 21.7	111.4 ± 8.3
	H	191.1 ± 14.3 [a,b]	79.1 ± 19.1 [a]	104.4 ± 18.0	61.7 ± 16.0	295.4 ± 29.9 [a]	140.8 ± 25.8
Heart							
3	L	13.2 ± 1.7	9.5 ± 0.3	19.5 ± 2.2	9.7 ± 1.6	32.7 ± 3.2	19.2 ± 1.7
	A	32.1 ± 2.1 [c]	31.2 ± 1.9 [c]	25.0 ± 2.4	26.6 ± 5.2 [c]	57.1 ± 2.9 [c]	57.7 ± 5.6 [c]
	H	300.4 ± 74.4 [a,b]	188.1 ± 42.1 [a,b]	265.9 ± 60.2 [a,b]	59.9 ± 11.5 [a,b]	566.2 ± 134.4 [a,b]	248.0 ± 52.6 [a,b]
12	L	16.3 ± 0.7	15.6 ± 5.3	17.7 ± 2.7	34.7 ± 20.9	34.0 ± 3.4	50.2 ± 26.0
	A	41.5 ± 6.4 [c]	32.1 ± 4.0 [c]	27.7 ± 4.3	15.7 ± 3.6	69.2 ± 10.4 [c]	47.7 ± 7.4
	H	225.6 ± 32.0 [a,b]	213.9 ± 42.6 [a,b]	165.9 ± 24.6 [a,b]	79.6 ± 11.4 [a,b]	391.5 ± 51.9 [a,b]	293.4 ± 52.9 [a,b]
22	L	30.8 ± 4.7	30.1 ± 2.8	56.9 ± 3.5	43.5 ± 3.8	87.6 ± 5.1	73.6 ± 3.1
	A	54.9 ± 7.3 [c]	47.1 ± 7.7	62.5 ± 7.7	42.0 ± 8.1	117.4 ± 12.1	89.1 ± 15.4
	H	106.3 ± 14.4 [a,b]	100.9 ± 39.0 [a]	104.0 ± 24.1	89.7 ± 25.8	210.2 ± 37.1 [a,b]	190.6 ± 56.1

Table 2. *Cont.*

Organ (Months)	VK Diet (µg)	K1		MK-4		K1 + MK4	
		F	M	F	M	F	M
				pmol/g or L Plasma			
Kidneys							
3	L	2.8 ± 0.5	4.7 ± 0.6	17.6 ± 3.2	11.9 ± 3.5	20.4 ± 3.6	16.6 ± 3.2
	A	9.3 ± 4.3	6.5 ± 1.4	29.9 ± 2.9	14.7 ± 3.7	39.2 ± 4.9	21.1 ± 3.1
	H	18.7 ± 4.7	10.2 ± 2.2	176.7 ± 24.6 [a]	34.9 ± 9.2	195.4 ± 28.1 [a,b]	45.1 ± 10.9 [a]
12	L	4.3 ± 1.1	3.7 ± 0.8	28.5 ± 8.8	12.1 ± 3.8	32.8 ± 9.5	15.8 ± 4.4
	A	6.0 ± 1.2	6.6 ± 1.1	32.6 ± 8.4	22.1 ± 5.8	38.6 ± 9.6	28.8 ± 6.8
	H	32.0 ± 4.6 [a,b]	6.4 ± 1.8	154.1 ± 34.8 [a,b]	32.2 ± 8.5 [a]	186.1 ± 30.3 [a,b]	38.6 ± 8.9 [a]
22	L	7.7 ± 0.9	3.6 ± 0.5	30.8 ± 4.5	26.3 ± 3.0	38.5 ± 4.7	30.0 ± 3.1
	A	11.6 ± 1.1	7.8 ± 0.6 [c]	52.4 ± 7.1	38.9 ± 3.7	63.9 ± 7.6 [c]	46.7 ± 4.2
	H	30.6 ± 9.8 [a,b]	20.3 ± 5.5 [a,b]	42.3 ± 8.6	19.4 ± 8.4	72.9 ± 13.3 [a]	39.7 ± 12.8
Spleen							
3	L	16.7 ± 1.5	16.6 ± 2.3	17.2 ± 3.2	8.6 ± 1.9	33.9 ± 4.0	25.1 ± 3.3
	A	24.9 ± 4.4	28.0 ± 3.4 [c]	23.6 ± 6.8	17.1 ± 3.9	48.5 ± 9.6	45.1 ± 4.7
	H	80.1 ± 17.8 [a,b]	49.4 ± 6.0 [a,b]	73.1 ± 15.3 [a,b]	37.6 ± 4.2 [a,b]	153.2 ± 28.7 [a,b]	86.9 ± 5.1 [a]
12	L	15.5 ± 1.8	15.5 ± 6.8	17.5 ± 3.5	11.4 ± 4.4	33.0 ± 5.2	26.8 ± 10.6
	A	30.4 ± 4.5 [c]	31.8 ± 10.4	50.9 ± 11.9	47.2 ± 17.1	81.3 ± 15.2	79.0 ± 26.6
	H	110.9 ± 17.7 [a,b]	38.2 ± 7.0	66.8 ± 8.7	35.7 ± 12.5	177.6 ± 22.8 [a]	73.8 ± 18.2 [a]
22	L	18.8 ± 3.9	22.7 ± 6.0	43.1 ± 10.6	56.3 ± 14.4	61.8 ± 10.8	79.0 ± 19.4
	A	28.4 ± 4.7	26.1 ± 3.8	67.1 ± 8.9	48.3 ± 7.8	95.5 ± 13.2	74.3 ± 11.1
	H	91.9 ± 14.9 [a,b]	126.7 ± 17.2 [a,b]	101.5 ± 21.1 [a]	120.6 ± 22.1	193.4 ± 31.1 [a,b]	247.2 ± 35.9 [a,b]
Brain							
3	L	2.0 ± 0.7	2.3 ± 0.4	54.2 ± 7.1	21.1 ± 1.6	56.2 ± 7.3	23.4 ± 1.3
	A	4.3 ± 0.8	3.7 ± 0.6	64.5 ± 4.8	47.2 ± 5.6 [c]	68.8 ± 5.1	51.0 ± 5.7 [c]
	H	8.0 ± 0.7 [a,b]	8.4 ± 0.9 [a,b]	197.5 ± 7.6 [a,b]	144.3 ± 12.0 [a,b]	205.4 ± 8.0 [a,b]	152.6 ± 12.7 [a,b]
12	L	1.6 ± 0.3	2.6 ± 1.2	47.1 ± 4.1	46.9 ± 18.9	48.7 ± 4.0	49.5 ± 20.1
	A	4.2 ± 0.4 [c]	3.3 ± 0.5	71.9 ± 7.1 [c]	40.6 ± 3.9	76.1 ± 7.3 [c]	43.9 ± 4.4
	H	7.4 ± 1.2 [a,b]	9.1 ± 2.3 [a]	187.2 ± 20.8 [a,b]	157.6 ± 10.5 [a,b]	194.6 ± 20.7 [a,b]	166.7 ± 12.4 [a,b]
22	L	2.2 ± 0.3	3.9 ± 0.2	53.5 ± 5.9	56.8 ± 11.9	55.7 ± 6.0	60.6 ± 11.8
	A	3.2 ± 0.2	3.4 ± 0.4	66.7 ± 7.9	85.5 ± 4.1	70.0 ± 8.0	88.9 ± 4.2
	H	4.4 ± 0.8 [a]	5.4 ± 1.7	70.0 ± 8.5	63.3 ± 20.5	74.4 ± 9.0	68.7 ± 21.9

Table 2. *Cont.*

Organ (Months)	VK Diet (μg)	K1		MK-4		K1 + MK4	
		F	M	F	M	F	M
		pmol/g or L Plasma					
Ovaries							
3	L	89.1 ± 35.9		190.6 ± 39.1		279.7 ± 34.4	
	A	133.3 ± 19.2		296.1 ± 100.0		429.5 ± 98.5	
	H	267.6 ± 42.4 [a]		616.4 ± 48.2 [a]		884.0 ± 89.7 [a,b]	
12	L	60.0 ± 22.1		187.1 ± 39.9		247.1 ± 54.7	
	A	218.2 ± 9.2 [c]		517.2 ± 93.4 [c]		735.4 ± 99.8 [c]	
	H	424.4 ± 46.6 [a]		762.1 ± 67.3 [a]		1186.5 ± 111.2 [a]	
22	L	183.9 ± 32.3		516.2 ± 72.2		700.1 ± 99.4	
	A	307.8 ± 50.2		706.6 ± 90.7		1014.4 ± 138.4	
	H	416.6 ± 46.7		656.7 ± 49.6		1073.3 ± 51.8	
Testes							
3	L		13.4 ± 4.5		63.8 ± 7.2		77.3 ± 6.6
	A		7.2 ± 1.4		134.5 ± 15.8 [c]		141.6 ± 16.3 [c]
	H		11.8 ± 3.6		292.4 ± 30.0 [a,b]		304.1 ± 28.6 [a,b]
12	L		9.9 ± 4.8		83.4 ± 28.3		93.3 ± 29.4
	A		20.9 ± 12.8		258.7 ± 43.6 [c]		279.7 ± 51.4 [c]
	H		22.0 ± 11.8		299.1 ± 52.3 [a]		321.1 ± 45.0 [a]
22	L		4.5 ± 0.6		64.3 ± 8.1		68.8 ± 8.2
	A		6.8 ± 0.6		96.3 ± 8.3 [c]		103.1 ± 8.7 [c]
	H		13.3 ± 1.9 [a,b]		81.4 ± 9.5		94.7 ± 9.7

Main sex, diet and age effects were assessed by conducting 3-way ANOVAs followed by pairwise multiple comparisons; results for these analyses are presented in the text (Section 3.1.2). The effect of diet on plasma and tissue K1, MK-4 and total VK concentrations were further tested within each sex and age group by one-way ANOVA's followed by Tukey's *post hoc* tests; [a]: $p < 0.05$ between H and L groups same age and sex, [b]: $p < 0.05$ between H and A groups same age and sex, [c]: $p < 0.05$ between A and L groups same age and sex. Values are expressed as mean ± SEM; $n = 5$–7/sex/age/diet groups. MK-4: menaquinone-4. nd: non-detectable.

Tissue K_1 concentrations were highest in ovaries and liver and lowest in the brain and kidneys, other tissues presenting intermediate levels ($p < 0.001$). A main sex effect was seen for the liver, kidneys, and heart, females showing higher K_1 concentrations than males ($p < 0.001$). The 3-way ANOVA also revealed a main diet effect for most organs ($p < 0.001$), differences being more frequently observed between the L and H, and the A and H groups ($p < 0.05$); dietary group differences (one-way ANOVA) are detailed in Table 2. A significant main effect was observed for age in the liver, heart, kidneys, and ovaries but differences varied according to organs and dietary groups ($p < 0.001$). Specifically, in the liver, K_1 concentrations increased between 3 and 12 months and were decreased at 22 months ($p < 0.05$). In the heart and kidneys, K_1 concentrations at 3 and 12 months were generally similar and were increased at 22 months, the extent of the change varying according to sex and dietary groups ($p < 0.05$). Finally, in ovaries, concentrations were observed to increase throughout life in all dietary groups ($p < 0.05$).

Tissue MK-4 concentrations were highest in ovaries and testes followed by the brain, the lowest amounts being seen in the heart and kidneys ($p < 0.001$). A main sex effect was observed for the liver, heart, kidneys, and the brain with females showing higher concentrations than males ($p < 0.001$). In most cases, the sex effect was observed at all ages and tended to be more pronounced in the H group ($p < 0.05$).

As for K_1, MK-4 tissue concentrations varied as a function of diet, differences being mainly observed between the L and H, and the A and H groups ($p < 0.05$); dietary group differences (one-way ANOVA) are detailed in Table 2. The 3-way ANOVA also revealed a main age effect in all organs, differences varying according to organs, sex (when applicable), and dietary groups ($p < 0.001$). In liver and ovary, concentrations increased throughout life in all dietary groups ($p < 0.05$) whereas in the heart, kidneys, spleen, and the brain, the extent of age-associated increases varied according to sex and dietary groups. In testes, concentrations were comparable at 3 and 12 months (for a given dietary group), and were significantly decreased at 22 months, mainly due to the lower concentrations of rats fed the A and H diets ($p < 0.05$).

Tissue total VK (K_1 + MK-4) concentrations were highest in ovaries followed by testes and liver, concentrations in other organs being statistically similar ($p < 0.001$). Except for the spleen, a main sex effect was observed in all organs, females showing higher total VK concentrations than males ($p < 0.001$). In the liver, the sex effect was observed at all ages and in most dietary groups while in the heart, kidneys and the brain, sex effect was more pronounced at 3 and 12 months in the H diet ($p < 0.05$). A main diet effect was also seen in most organs ($p < 0.001$), differences being mainly observed between the L and H, and the A and H groups ($p < 0.05$); dietary group differences (one-way ANOVA) are detailed in Table 2. The 3-way ANOVA also revealed a significant main effect for age in all organs, differences varying according to organs, sex (when applicable), and dietary groups ($p < 0.001$).

Specifically, in the liver, total VK concentrations increased between 3 and 12 months and decreased in the second year of life, the age effect being more pronounced in females fed the A and H diets ($p < 0.05$). In spleen, total VK concentrations were increased at 22 months compared to 3 and 12 months, the effect being particularly marked in males fed the H diet ($p < 0.05$). In brain, in both sexes, concentrations were comparable at 3 and 12 months (for a given dietary group) and were decreased at 22 months, largely due to the lower concentrations of rats fed the H diet ($p < 0.05$). In ovaries, total VK contents increased throughout life, the extent and time of change depending on the dietary groups ($p < 0.05$). Finally, in testes, total VK concentrations were comparable at 3 and 12 months (for a given dietary group), and were significantly decreased at 22 months, mainly due to the lower concentrations of rats fed the A and H diets ($p < 0.05$).

In light of the growing importance of MK-4 in various physiological functions, tissue MK-4 relative to total VK was computed for each organ in all animals as the ratio MK-4/total VK (Figure 2) (In plasma, MK-4 could not be detected hence no ratios were computed for this variable). In contrast to what is observed for K_1, MK-4, and total VK, the MK-4/total VK ratios were much less affected by sex, diet, and age. Furthermore, MK-4 represents the main K vitamer in a number of organs. This is notably the case for the brain where the MK-4/total VK ratios are close to one irrespective of sex, diet and age. Menaquinone-4 is also the preferred K vitamer in testes and kidneys while ovaries, spleen, heart, and liver present more of a mixture of the two vitamers ($p < 0.001$). The 3-way ANOVA revealed a main sex effect in the heart, kidneys, and brain ($p < 0.001$), females showing higher ratios than males, ($p < 0.05$). The main diet effects were seen in all organs except for spleen ($p < 0.001$), ratios tending to be higher in the L diet groups ($p < 0.05$); dietary group differences (one-way ANOVA) are detailed in Figure 2. Finally, the 3-way ANOVA also revealed an age effect in liver, heart and spleen ($p < 0.001$). Specifically, in liver and spleen, ratios were increased at 22 months (*vs.* 3 and 12 months) notably in rats fed the L and A diets ($p < 0.05$). In the heart, ratios were increased at 22 months (*vs.* 3 and 12 months) especially in rats fed the A and H diets ($p < 0.05$).

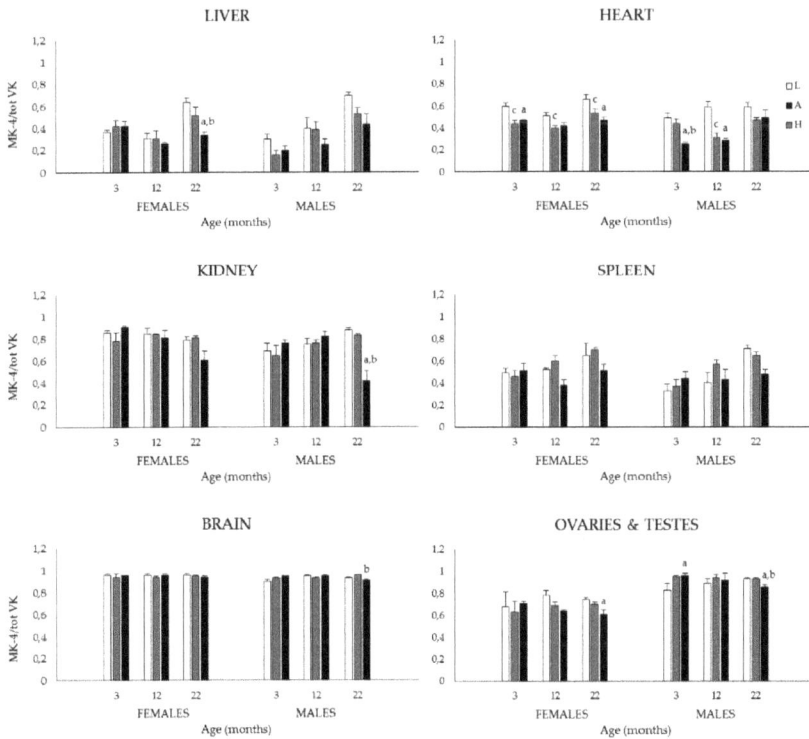

Figure 2. Tissue MK-4/total VK ratios of 3-, 12-, and 22-month-old M and F Sprague–Dawley rats fed the L, A or H diets throughout their lives. No ratios were computed for plasma as MK-4 could not be detected. Main sex, diet and age effects were assessed by conducting 3-way ANOVAs followed by pairwise multiple comparisons; results for these analyses are presented in the text (Section 3.1.2). The effect of diet on tissue MK-4/total VK ratios were further tested within each sex and age group by one-way ANOVA's followed by Tukey's *post hoc* tests; [a]: $p < 0.05$ between H and L group same age and sex; [b]: $p < 0.05$ between H and A group same age and sex; [c]: $p < 0.05$ between A and L group same age and sex. Values are expressed as mean $\pm$ SEM; $n = 5$–7/sex/age/diet groups.

3.1.3. Prothrombin and Activated Partial Thromboplastin Times

Results for prothrombin (PT) and activated partial thromboplastin (APTT) times are presented in Figure 3. The 3-way ANOVA revealed no main sex and age effects for either variable. However, dietary K_1 intakes significantly affected the coagulation times of male rats fed the L diet. Specifically, the low

K_1 containing diet was associated with increased PT in 3-month-old (*vs.* H diet), and increased APTT in 3- (*vs.* A and H diets) and 12-month-old (*vs.* H diet) male rats ($p < 0.05$).

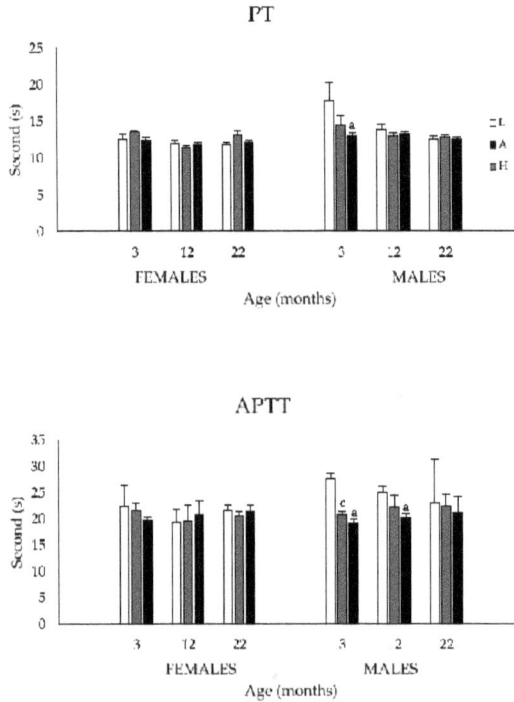

Figure 3. Prothrombin (PT) and activated partial thromboplastin (APTT) times of 3-, 12-, and 22-month-old M and F Sprague–Dawley rats fed the L, A or H diets throughout their lives. The 3-way ANOVA revealed no main sex and age effects for either variables. In contrast, a diet effect was observed in M rats fed the L diet. Specifically, this diet was associated with increased PT at 3 months and increased APTT at 3 and 12 months; [a]: $p < 0.05$ between H and L group same age and sex; [c]: $p < 0.05$ between A and L group same age and sex (one-way ANOVA). Values are expressed as mean ± SEM; $n = 4$–7/sex/age/diet groups.

3.2. Study 2

3.2.1. Body Weights, Food, and K_1 Intakes

Body weights, daily food (g/day and g/100 g· BW/day), and K_1 (µg/day and µg/100 g· BW) intakes of 3- and 20-month-old male and female Sprague–Dawley rats fed an *ad libitum* (AL) or calorie restricted (CR) diet are presented in Table 3. In all age and diet groups, body weights were significantly higher in male than female rats ($p < 0.05$). In animals of both sexes fed the AL diet, body weights were significantly increased at 20 months compared to 3 months and as expected, were signifiantly lower in the 20 CR than 20 AL group ($p < 0.05$).

Table 3. Body weights, daily food (g/day and g/100 g· BW/day), and K$_1$ (µg/day and µg/100 g· BW) intakes of 3- and 20-month-old M and F Sprague–Dawley rats fed an *ad libitum* (AL) or calorie restricted (CR) diet.

Age (Months)	Diet	Body Weight (g)		Food Intake (g/Day)		K$_1$ Intake (µg/Day)		Food Intake (g/100 g· BW/Day)		K$_1$ Intake (µg/100 g· BW/Day)	
		F	M	F	M	F	M	F	M	F	M
3	AL	277 ± 35 ^{z}	523 ± 73	16.5 ± 1.7 ^{z}	22.5 ± 1.3	8.3 ± 0.8 ^{z}	11.2 ± 0.6	6.0 ± 0.5 ^{z}	4.3 ± 0.4	3.0 ± 0.2 ^{z}	2.2 ± 0.2
20	AL	647 ± 171 ^{y,z}	939 ± 132 ^{y}	18.0 ± 3.5 ^{z}	27.1 ± 3.8 ^{y}	9.0 ± 1.8	13.6 ± 9.3	2.9 ± 0.5 ^{y}	2.9 ± 0.4 ^{y}	1.4 ± 0.2 ^{y}	1.4 ± 0.2 ^{y}
	CR	281 ± 29 ^{z,*}	484 ± 37 *	11.0 ^{x,z,*}	16.0 ^{x,*}	9.2 *	13.3	4.6 ^{x,z,*}	3.9 *	3.8 ^{x,z,*}	3.3 ^{x,*}

In all age and diet groups, body weights were higher in M than F ($p < 0.05$). In both sexes fed the AL diet, body weights were significantly increased at 20 months (*vs.* 3 months) and significantly decreased in 20 CR rats (*vs.* 20 AL) ($p < 0.05$). Food intakes expressed as g/day were significantly higher in M than F in all age and diet groups, and were higher in 20 AL *vs.* 3 groups ($p < 0.05$). As expected, food intakes were lower in the 20 CR than in 20 AL groups (both sexes; $p < 0.05$). Phylloquinone intakes µg/day were significantly higher in M than F (3 and 20 CR) but were similar among age and diet groups ($p < 0.05$). When expressed per 100 g· BW, food and K$_1$ intakes (µg/100 g· BW/day) were higher in F than M (3 and 20 CR groups), were lower in older animals fed the AL diet (*vs.* 3 months), and were higher in the 20 CR *vs.* 20 AL groups ($p < 0.05$); ^{x}: $p < 0.05$ between 20 CR and 3-month group, same sex; ^{y}: $p < 0.05$ between 20 AL and 3-month group, same sex; ^{z}: $p < 0.05$ between M and F, same age and diet; *: $p < 0.05$ between 20 AL and 20 CR, same sex. Values are expressed as mean ± SEM; $n = 6$–8/sex/age/diet groups.

Food intakes expressed as g/day were significantly higher in males than in females in all age and diet groups, and were higher in 20 *AL vs.* 3-month-old groups ($p < 0.05$). In both sexes and, as expected, food intakes of 20 CR rats were lower than those of the 20 *AL* group and also of the 3-month-old groups ($p < 0.05$). Phylloquinone (K_1) intakes expressed as µg/day were significantly higher in males than in females (3 and 20 CR groups; ($p < 0.05$) but did not differ among age and diet groups.

Given the impact of the CR model on body weights, food (g) and K_1 (µg) intakes are also reported per 100 g· BW. When expressed in this manner, food intakes were significantly higher in females than in males in the 3-month and 20 CR groups ($p < 0.05$), and were significantly lower in older animals (F: 20 *AL vs.* 3 months, 20 CR *vs.* 3 months; M: 20 *AL vs.* 3 months, $p < 0.05$). In addition, and in both sexeses, were lower in the 20 *AL vs.* 3-month-old group ($p < 0.05$).

Finally, when expressed as µg/100 g· BW/day, K_1 intakes were significantly higher in females than in males in the 3-month and 20 CR groups ($p < 0.05$), and in both sexes, were lower in the 20 *AL vs.* 3-month-old group ($p < 0.05$). As mentioned previously, the diet fed the CR rats was adjusted to contain similar amounts of vitamins (including K_1) and minerals as that fed the *AL* group. However, due to their lower body weights at 20 months, in both sexeses, K_1 intakes (µg/100 g· BW/day) of CR rats were significantly higher than those fed the *AL* diet ($p < 0.05$).

3.2.2. Plasma and Tissue K_1, MK-4, and Total VK (K_1 + MK-4) Concentrations, and MK-4/Total VK Ratios

Plasma and tissue (the liver, heart, kidneys, spleen, brain, ovaries and testes) K_1, MK-4 and total VK (K_1 + MK-4) concentrations of 3- and 20-month-old male and female Sprague–Dawley rats fed an *AL* or CR diet are presented in Table 4. In both sexes, plasma K_1 concentrations were significantly increased at 20 (*AL* and CR) compared to 3 months, and were significantly higher in females than males ($p < 0.05$). A diet effect was also observed in both sexeses at 20 months, rats fed the CR diet showing decreased K_1 concentrations compared to those of the respective *AL* groups ($p < 0.05$). Menaquinone-4 was undetectable in plasma, hence group differences for total VK values are as those for K_1.

Table 4. Plasma and tissue (the liver, heart, kidneys, spleen, brain, ovaries and testes) K_1, MK-4 and total VK (K_1 + MK-4) concentrations of 3- and 20-month-old M and F Sprague–Dawley rats fed an *AL* or CR diet.

Diet		K1		MK-4		K1 + MK4	
		F	M	F	M	F	M
		pmol/g or L Plasma		pmol/g or L Plasma		pmol/g or L Plasma	
				Plasma			
3	AL	0.21 ± 0.03	0.25 ± 0.08	nd	nd	0.21 ± 0.03	0.25 ± 0.08
20	AL	1.73 ± 0.15 [y,z]	1.12 ± 0.11 [y]	nd	nd	1.73 ± 0.15 [y,z]	1.12 ± 0.11 [y]
	CR	1.35 ± 0.10 [x,z,*]	0.85 ± 0.07 [x,*]	nd	nd	1.35 ± 0.10 [x,*]	0.85 ± 0.07 [x,*]
				Liver			
3	AL	54.2 ± 8.1	48.4 ± 17.9	43.4 ± 3.6 [z]	18.5 ± 2.1	97.6 ± 7.7	56.9 ± 20.0
20	AL	71.2 ± 7.9	50.7 ± 6.1	66.6 ± 12.0	54.5 ± 6.1 [y]	137.8 ± 17.9	105.2 ± 7.2 [y]
	CR	49.0 ± 5.7 *	50.6 ± 6.6	61.6 ± 8.2	48.6 ± 5.6 [x]	110.6 ± 10.5	99.2 ± 7.3 [x]
				Heart			
3	AL	32.1 ± 2.1	31.2 ± 1.9	24.7 ± 2.4	26.2 ± 5.1	56.7 ± 2.9	57.4 ± 5.5
20	AL	47.2 ± 6.4	46.9 ± 5.1	55.5 ± 5.6 [y]	43.3 ± 5.6	102.8 ± 10.2 [y]	90.2 ± 9.6 [y]
	CR	32.7 ± 6.8	41.5 ± 5.8	53.6 ± 4.8 [x,z]	38.7 ± 4.6	86.3 ± 9.0	80.2 ± 7.4
				Kidney			
3	AL	9.3 ± 4.3	5.6 ± 1.4	29.5 ± 2.8 [z]	12.0 ± 3.3	38.7 ± 4.9 [z]	17.6 ± 3.5
20	AL	11.8 ± 1.1 [z]	7.6 ± 0.4	54.5 ± 4.7 [y,z]	35.0 ± 3.9 [y]	66.3 ± 5.1 [y,z]	42.6 ± 4.3 [y]
	CR	10.1 ± 1.0 [z]	6.2 ± 0.4 *	45.3 ± 4.7 [z]	33.2 ± 1.6 [x]	55.4 ± 5.0 [z]	39.4 ± 1.5 [x]

Table 4. *Cont.*

Diet		K1		MK-4		K1 + MK4	
		F	M	F	M	F	M
		pmol/g or L Plasma		pmol/g or L Plasma		pmol/g or L Plasma	
		Spleen					
3	AL	23.6 ± 5.1	25.1 ± 2.3	17.0 ± 3.0	19.7 ± 3.7	40.6 ± 7.0	44.8 ± 5.3
20	AL	26.9 ± 3.2	23.5 ± 2.2	64.0 ± 7.2 [y,z]	41.1 ± 4.4 [y]	90.9 ± 8.9 [y,z]	64.6 ± 6.3
	CR	24.2 ± 3.0	23.0 ± 3.0	53.7 ± 6.0 [x]	42.8 ± 5.7 [x]	77.9 ± 7.8 [x]	65.7 ± 7.2
		Brain					
3	AL	4.3 ± 0.8	3.7 ± 0.6	63.6 ± 4.7 [z]	46.6 ± 5.5	67.9 ± 5.0 [z]	50.3 ± 5.6
20	AL	3.5 ± 0.4	3.6 ± 0.4	69.9 ± 5.6	66.3 ± 7.3	73.4 ± 5.8	70.0 ± 7.3
	CR	4.6 ± 0.4	3.9 ± 0.4	52.9 ± 5.8 *	54.8 ± 7.2	57.4 ± 5.9	58.7 ± 7.4
		Ovaries					
3	AL	133.7 ± 19.6		426.5 ± 114.9		560.2 ± 133.1	
20	AL	278.5 ± 27.4 [y]		636.3 ± 58.5		914.8 ± 76.7 [y]	
	CR	240.5 ± 28.0 [x]		453.4 ± 42.1 *		693.9 ± 65.0 *	
		Testes					
3	AL		6.1 ± 1.0		131.8 ± 19.0		137.9 ± 19.6
20	AL		6.1 ± 0.6		110.4 ± 7.8		116.5 ± 7.8
	CR		4.6 ± 0.3		123.6 ± 8.9		128.2 ± 8.7

Age and diet effects were determined in M and F by conducting distinct one-way ANOVA's followed by Tukey's *post hoc* tests. Student' *t*-test was used to further assess the effect of CR at 20 months, and that of sex *i.e.*, given age and diet group. [x]: $p < 0.05$ between 20 CR and 3-months, same sex; [y]: $p < 0.05$ between 20 AL and 3 months, same sex; [z]: $p < 0.05$ between M and F, same age and diet; *: $p < 0.05$ between 20 AL and 20 CR, same sex. Values are expressed as mean $\pm$ SEM; $n = 6$–8/sex/age/diet groups.

Tissue K_1, MK-4, and total VK content profiles were similar to those reported in Study 1. Ovaries contained the highest amounts of total VK with high levels of both K vitamers ($p < 0.001$). Similarly, organs differed in their relative K_1 and MK-4 contents (Table 4) with much higher MK-4/total VK ratios in organs such as the brain, testes, and kidneys (*i.e.*, 0.8–0.95) than in the liver and heart (*i.e.*, ~0.5).

Regarging K_1, there was a general trend for concentrations to be higher in females than in males, this difference reaching statistical significance in kidneys ($p < 0.05$). In both sexes and for most organs, K_1 concentrations were similar at 3 and 20 months except for ovaries where concentrations were significantly increased at 20 compared to 3 months ($p < 0.05$). Finally, and although differences reached statistical significance only in the liver (F) and kidneys (M) ($p < 0.05$), K_1 concentrations at 20 months tended to be lower in the CR than in the AL groups (Table 4).

In contrast to K_1, MK-4 concentrations were much more affected by sex with females showing higher concentrations than males in the liver (3 months), heart (20 CR), kidneys (all groups), spleen (20 AL), and the brain (3 months) ($p < 0.05$). In a number of organs, MK-4 concentrations also increased as a function of age, the effect being particularly marked in the liver (M: 20 AL, 20 CR), heart (F: 20 AL, 20 CR), kidneys (M: 20 AL, 20 CR; F: 20 AL), and spleen (M and F: 20 AL, 20 CR), ($p < 0.05$). Finally, as observed for K_1, MK-4 concentrations tended to be lower in rats fed the CR regimen, differences reaching statistical significance in brain (F) and ovaries ($p < 0.05$) (Table 4).

As for the individual K vitamers, females generally presented higher tissue total VK concentrations than males, differences reaching statistical significance in kidney (all groups), spleen (20 AL), and brain (3 months) ($p < 0.05$). Similarly, total VK was generally increased at 20 months when compared to tissue concentrations at 3 months, the effect being more often observed in old rats fed the AL regimen liver (M: 20 AL, 20 CR), heart (M and F: 20 AL), kidney (M: 20 AL, 20 CR; F: 20 AL), spleen (F: 20 AL, 20 CR), and ovaries (20 AL). Finally, as oberved for individual K vitamers, the CR regimen was associated, at 20 months, with lower total VK concentrations, differences reaching statistical significance in ovaries ($p < 0.05$) (Table 4).

Finally, MK-4/total VK ratios were little affected by sex although they were significantly higher in females than males in liver (3 months) and heart (20 CR) ($p < 0.05$) (Figure 4). As observed in study 1, ratios were increased at 20 months in the liver (M: 20 AL, 20 CR), heart (F: 20 CR), kidneys (M: 20 AL, 20 CR), and spleen (M and F: 20 AL, 20 CR) ($p < 0.05$). Finally, MK-4/total VK ratios at 20 months were largely unaffected by the CR regimen with only the ratio for brain (F) being statistically decreased in CR compared to that in the AL group ($p < 0.05$).

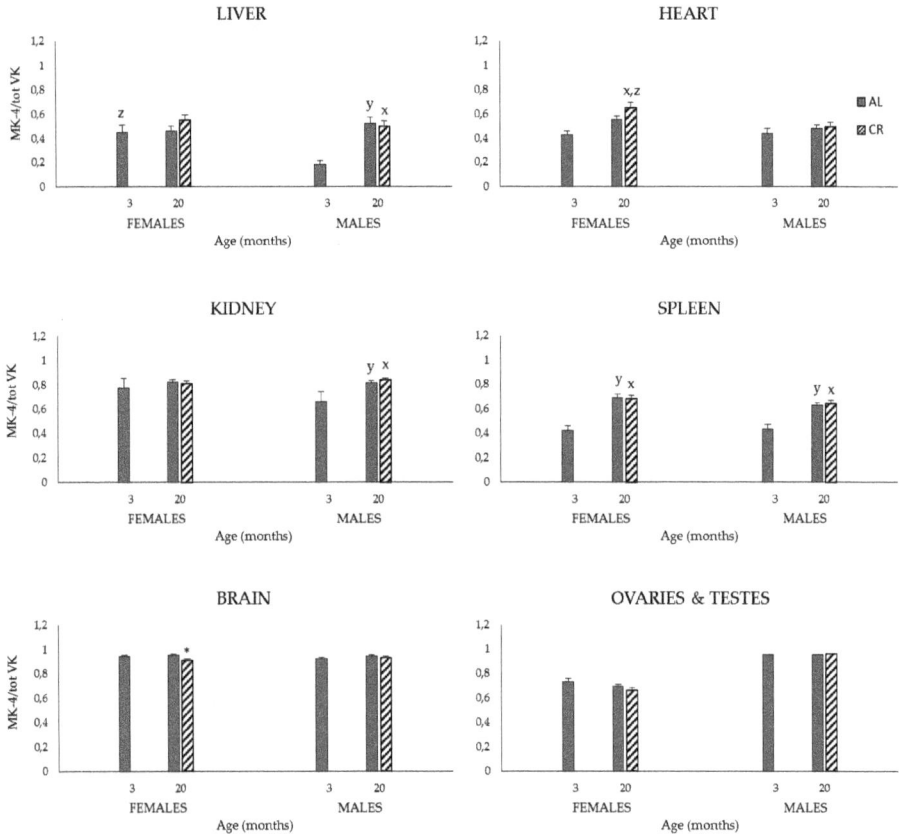

Figure 4. Tissue MK-4/total VK ratios of 3- and 20-month-old M and F Sprague–Dawley rats fed an AL or CR diet. Age and diet effects were determined in M and F by conducting distinct one-way ANOVA's followed by Tukey's *post hoc* tests. Student' *t*-test was used to further assess the effect of CR at 20 months, and that of sex i.e., given age and diet group. [x]: $p < 0.05$ between 20 CR and 3 months, same sex; [y]: $p < 0.05$ between 20 AL and 3 months, same sex; [z]: $p < 0.05$ between M and F, same age and diet; [*]: $p < 0.05$ between 20 AL and 20 CR, same sex. Values are expressed as mean $\pm$ SEM; $n = 6$–8/sex/age/diet groups.

3.2.3. Prothrombin and Activated Partial Thromboplastin Times

Results for prothrombin (PT) and activated partial thromboplastin (APTT) times are presented in Table 5. At 20 months of age, a diet effect was observed in male rats, the mean PT value of CR rats being statistically increased compared to that of AL animals ($p < 0.05$), and comparable to that of rats aged 3 months. A sex effect was also observed for PT in 20-month-old rats fed the CR diet, males showing a statistically higher mean value than females ($p < 0.05$).

Table 5. Prothrombin (PT) and activated partial thromboplastin (APTT) times of 3- and 20-month-old M and F Sprague–Dawley rats fed an *AL* or CR diet.

Age (Months)	Diet	PT		APTT	
		(s)			
		M	**F**	**M**	**F**
3	AL	14.5 ± 1.2	13.5 ± 0.3	20.8 ± 1.2	21.6 ± 1.3
20	AL	12.8 ± 0.2	12.8 ± 0.3	21.7 ± 1.4	20.0 ± 1.6
	CR	$14.0 \pm 0.4^{z,*}$	12.9 ± 0.2	23.3 ± 1.6	20.3 ± 1.1

At 20 months, the mean PT value of M fed the CR diet was statistically higher than that of the 20 *AL* group ($p < 0.05$), and comparable to that of male rats aged 3 months. A sex effect was observed in 20-month-old rats fed the CR diet, M showing a statistically higher mean value than F ($p < 0.05$). ^{x}: $p < 0.05$ between 20 CR and 3-months, same sex; ^{y}: $p < 0.05$ between 20 *AL* and 3 months, same sex; ^{z}: $p < 0.05$ between M and F, same age and diet; *: $p < 0.05$ between 20 *AL* and 20 CR, same sex. Values are expressed as mean $\pm$ SEM; $n = 6$–8/sex/age/diet groups.

4. Discussion

All K vitamers classically serve as cofactors in a carboxylation reaction that results in the conversion of specific glutamic acid residues to gamma-carboxyglutamic acid in precursor proteins *i.e.*, VKDPs. In addition, there is increasing evidence that K_1 and MK-4 have additional actions outside their role as enzymatic cofactor, e.g., inflammation, oxidative stress. In recent years, VK has been associated with a number of age-related conditions such as osteoporosis [1], the calcification process [3], insulin resistance [4,38], cancer [39], and cognitive decline [11]. This report aimed to investigate the influence of lifetime dietary VK exposure on the tissue content and distribution of the K_1 and MK-4 vitamers at different life stages in male and female rats fed different diets since weaning, or subjected to caloric restriction, a life-prolonging model.

4.1. Study 1

In the first study, conducted in 3-, 12- and 22-month-old male and female rats fed different K_1 diets since weaning, body weights were found to increase with age in both sexes but were not significantly affected by lifetime K_1 intakes. Body weights have been shown to increase during aging in rodents and our results concur with previous studies [40,41]. The lack of effect of K_1 intakes on body weights is of interest given the recently proposed role of VK in energy metabolism. In a series of studies using murine models, a specific form of the VKDP osteocalcin has been shown to modulate glucose and insulin metabolism, energy expenditure, and fat mass [4]. Although the endocrine role of osteocalcin remains an intense subject of debate, other studies conducted in rats [42] and humans [38,43] point to potential beneficial effects of increased VK intakes on metabolic profile and body weights. The trend towards lower body weights observed at 22 months in both males and females fed the H diet goes along those lines.

Plasma K_1 increased as a function of diet in both sexes, however, no MK-4 could be detected under our experimental conditions. The presence of MK-4 in the circulation in response to K_1 intake has been variable, some studies reporting low [6,27,28] or undetectable [8] values. Tissue contents and distribution of the K vitamers were found to differ, with K_1 as the predominant vitamer in some organs *i.e.*, the liver, heart, and MK-4 in others *i.e.*, testes and brain. Such differential distributions of the K vitamers were observed in previous short-term studies [6,8,26,29]. One notable finding of the present study, however, is the large amount of total VK observed in ovaries, this organ being rich in both K_1 and MK-4 vitamers. High levels of VK have been reported in a previous study [29], although levels were significantly lower than those reported here. Differences in strain (Brown–Norway *vs.* Sprague–Dawley) and VK content of the diets could explain the differences between the two studies. However, the high VK content of ovaries is intriguing as this organ is not known to be particularly rich in either of the known VKDPs. Whether the K vitamers possess actions in the ovary beyond their role in the carboxylation reaction remains to be determined; however, in a series of older studies, VK was shown to possess estrogenic activity. Specifically, treatment of castrate mice with either K_1 and menadione resulted in increases in uterine weights and cornification of the vaginal epithelium [44].

Increasing K_1 intake generally resulted in higher tissue K_1 and MK-4, differences being mainly observed between the L and H, and the A and H groups suggesting that intakes >500 µg K_1/kg diet are needed for tissue accumulation. These results are in line with those of previous studies conducted in normal [26] and germ-free [45] rats. In the great majority of organs, total VK tissue contents were higher in females than in males, the effect being mainly seen at 3 and 12 months of age. This finding has been observed by others [29,30] and is likely explained by the facilitatory action of estrogens on the intestinal absorption of K_1 [46]. As discussed below, this estrogenic effect on VK absorption could contribute to the greater resistance of female rats to VK deficiency. Concentrations of the K vitamers and total VK were also affected by age in a number of organs (*i.e.*, the liver, spleen, brain, ovaries and testes), differences varying according to organs, sex (when applicable), and dietary groups. Except for ovaries for which VK contents increased throughout life, total VK concentrations either increased between 3 and 12 months or were comparable, and decreased in the second year of life. In 3-, 12- and 24-months old Brown–Norway rats which had been fed a nonpurified diet (NIH 31 M), liver K_1 was found to be increased and MK-4 to be decreased in the heart, kidneys, lung, and cerebellum of old animals [29]. In a more recent study conducted in Fisher 344 male rats aged two, 12, and 24 months, a 28-day administration of a low K_1 containing diet (~200 µg K_1/kg diet) was associated with higher MK-4 concentrations in the liver, spleen, kidneys, heart, and cortex (myelin) in 24- compared to two-month-old rats; the opposite effect was observed for testes [28]. Divergent results among studies could be explained by differences in experimental design *i.e.*, VK contents of the diets, duration of exposure, *etc.*, and strain of animals.

In light of the growing importance of MK-4 in various physiological functions and given that the aging process can affect enzymatic activities [32,47] which could include those involved in the K_1 to MK-4 conversion, we assessed the relative MK-4 to total VK tissue content (MK-4/total VK) in all organs. In contrast to what was observed for K_1, MK-4, and total VK, the MK-4/total VK ratios were much less affected by sex, diet, and age. Regarding the latter, an interesting trend was observed. In high MK-4 containing organs such as the brain, testes, kidneys and ovaries, the high MK-4/total VK ratios were maintained in old age, this finding being observed for both sexes and in most dietary groups. In organs with lower MK-4 contents *i.e.*, liver, heart and spleen, MK-4/total VK ratios tended to increase with age in both sexes and dietary groups. Hence, irrespective of an organ's usual MK-4 content, the proportion of this vitamer relative to total VK appears to increase with age. Whether this trend reflects an increased physiological demand for MK-4 in handling age-related conditions such as inflammation and oxidative stress remains to be established, but such hypothesis should be pursued in future studies.

Male rats have long been shown to be less resistant to VK deficiency compared to females [30,48,49]. The increased PT and APTT observed in young male rats fed the L diet corroborate these observations and confirm earlier findings that diets containing <500 µg K_1/kg diet are insufficient to maintain normal coagulation [34]. It should be mentioned that, despite their increased coagulation times, no rat presented signs of bleeding or died due to hemorrhage.

4.2. Study 2

By virtue of its nature, the CR dietary regimen resulted in significantly lower body weights in old CR compared to *AL* groups. As a corollary to this and because the diet fed the CR rats was adjusted to contain equimolar amounts of vitamins and minerals as that fed the *AL* group, K_1 intakes of CR rats were significantly higher than those fed the *AL* diet when expressed per unit body weight (Table 3). As shown in Table 4, the dietary regimen had no impact on the K vitamer profile in plasma and tissues, organs rich in K_1 (*i.e.*, liver, heart) and MK-4 (*i.e.*, brain, testes) being those observed in study 1. Likewise, ovaries were found to contain high quantities of both K vitamers and the highest

VK content of all organs. The general trend for higher VK tissue concentrations in females than in males was also observed, the effect being particularly marked for the MK-4 vitamer. Age had little effect on K_1 tissue contents in contrast to MK-4, which were generally increased at 20 months compared to 3 months. Interestingly, despite the fact that rats fed the CR regimen consumed more K_1 per unit body weight than their *AL* counterparts since adulthood, their tissue K_1 and MK-4 contents at 20 months tended to be decreased when compared to those of the *AL* group. Lower tissue MK-4 content could be the result of lower synthesis from K_1 or greater tissue utilization. Although assessing the activity of the UBIAD1 enzyme would have provided useful information regarding tissues' synthetic capacities, this hypothesis is unlikely given that the MK-4/total VK ratios at 20 months were largely unaffected by CR. The second hypothesis probably represents a more plausible explanation as the aging process is characterized by molecular and cellular events that leads to impaired function and increased vulnerability to death [47,50]. In fact, a study conducted in 4-, 19- and 28-month-old rats aiming at assessing the impact of CR on α-tocopherol tissue distribution point in this direction. Compared to tissues of 19-month-old *AL* rats, α-tocopherol concentrations in CR rats were found to be lower by 48% in plasma, 30% in kidneys, 60% in the liver, and 44% in the heart homogenate. These results were interpreted as reflecting a greater utilization of tissue α-tocopherol in limiting the age-induced oxidative damage to membranes [51].

Finally, in this study, coagulation times were increased in old male rats fed the *AL* diet (PT, $p < 0.05$; trend for APTT). The fact that animals subjected to CR were able to maintain a more youthful coagulation profile *i.e.*, similar to that of 3-month-old animals, supports the notion that this dietary regimen is associated with a greater utilization of the K vitamers.

5. Conclusions

Dietary K_1 intakes around the minimal amount required for normal blood coagulation had no significant influence on body weights of both male and female rats at different life stages. Tissue contents of the K vitamers differed according to organs, were generally higher in females than in males, and increased with K_1 intake. The MK-4/total VK ratios tended to increase with age, possibly reflecting an increased physiological demand for MK-4 during aging. Our study also confirmed the greater susceptibility of male rats to VK insufficiency, notably at a younger age.

Despite lifelong higher K_1 intakes per unit body weight, tissue K_1 and MK-4 contents at 20 months were generally lower in CR rats compared to their *AL* counterparts. Whether the lower tissue MK-4 content is the result of lower synthesis from K_1 or greater tissue utilization remains to be determined. However, the more youthful coagulation profile observed in old CR rats (*vs.* *AL* rats) tends to support the notion that CR is associated with greater utilization of the K vitamers to sustain physiological functions.

Acknowledgments: This work was supported by the Natural Sciences and Engineering Research Council of Canada (NSERC). The authors wish to thank Mses Sylvie Roy, Bouchra Ouliass, and Elisabeth Bélanger for their valuable assistance in the preparation of this manuscript.

Author Contributions: Guylaine Ferland designed the studies. Isabelle Doucet and Dominique Mainville conducted the experimental work and analyses. All 3 authors contributed to interpretation of the data and writing of the manuscript. All authors reviewed the final manuscript.

Conflicts of Interest: The authors declare no conflict of interest.

References

1. Booth, S.L. Roles for vitamin K beyond coagulation. *Annu. Rev. Nutr.* **2009**, *29*, 89–110. [CrossRef] [PubMed]
2. Ferland, G. The discovery of vitamin K and its clinical applications. *Ann. Nutr. Metab.* **2012**, *61*, 213–218. [CrossRef] [PubMed]
3. Beulens, J.W.; Booth, S.L.; van den Heuvel, E.G.; Stoecklin, E.; Baka, A.; Vermeer, C. The role of menaquinones (vitamin K_2) in human health. *Br. J. Nutr.* **2013**, *110*, 1357–1368. [CrossRef] [PubMed]

4. Ferron, M.; Lacombe, J. Regulation of energy metabolism by the skeleton: Osteocalcin and beyond. *Arch. Biochem. Biophys.* **2014**, *561*, 137–146. [CrossRef] [PubMed]
5. Shearer, M.J.; Newman, P. Recent trends in the metabolism and cell biology of vitamin K with special reference to vitamin K cycling and mk-4 biosynthesis. *J. Lipid Res.* **2014**, *55*, 345–362. [CrossRef] [PubMed]
6. Thijssen, H.H.; Drittij-Reijnders, M.J. Vitamin K distribution in rat tissues: Dietary phylloquinone is a source of tissue menaquinone-4. *Br. J. Nutr.* **1994**, *72*, 415–425. [CrossRef] [PubMed]
7. Thijssen, H.H.; Drittij-Reijnders, M.J.; Fischer, M.A. Phylloquinone and menaquinone-4 distribution in rats: Synthesis rather than uptake determines menaquinone-4 organ concentrations. *J. Nutr.* **1996**, *126*, 537–543. [PubMed]
8. Al Rajabi, A.; Booth, S.L.; Peterson, J.W.; Choi, S.W.; Suttie, J.W.; Shea, M.K.; Miao, B.; Grusak, M.A.; Fu, X. Deuterium-labeled phylloquinone has tissue-specific conversion to menaquinone-4 among fischer 344 male rats. *J. Nutr.* **2012**, *142*, 841–845. [CrossRef] [PubMed]
9. Hirota, Y.; Tsugawa, N.; Nakagawa, K.; Suhara, Y.; Tanaka, K.; Uchino, Y.; Takeuchi, A.; Sawada, N.; Kamao, M.; Wada, A.; *et al.* Menadione (vitamin K_3) is a catabolic product of oral phylloquinone (vitamin K_1) in the intestine and a circulating precursor of tissue menaquinone-4 (vitamin K_2) in rats. *J. Biol. Chem.* **2013**, *288*, 33071–33080. [CrossRef] [PubMed]
10. Nakagawa, K.; Sawada, N.; Hirota, Y.; Uchino, Y.; Suhara, Y.; Hasegawa, T.; Amizuka, N.; Okamoto, T.; Tsugawa, N.; Kamao, M.; *et al.* Vitamin K2 biosynthetic enzyme, UBIAD1 is essential for embryonic development of mice. *PLoS ONE* **2014**, *9*, e104078. [CrossRef] [PubMed]
11. Ferland, G. Vitamin K, an emerging nutrient in brain function. *Biofactors* **2012**, *38*, 151–157. [CrossRef] [PubMed]
12. Reddi, K.; Henderson, B.; Meghji, S.; Wilson, M.; Poole, S.; Hopper, C.; Harris, M.; Hodges, S.J. Interleukin 6 production by lipopolysaccharide-stimulated human fibroblasts is potently inhibited by naphthoquinone (vitamin K) compounds. *Cytokine* **1995**, *7*, 287–290. [CrossRef] [PubMed]
13. Ohsaki, Y.; Shirakawa, H.; Hiwatashi, K.; Furukawa, Y.; Mizutani, T.; Komai, M. Vitamin K suppresses lipopolysaccharide-induced inflammation in the rat. *Biosci. Biotechnol. Biochem.* **2006**, *70*, 926–932. [CrossRef] [PubMed]
14. Ohsaki, Y.; Shirakawa, H.; Miura, A.; Giriwono, P.E.; Sato, S.; Ohashi, A.; Iribe, M.; Goto, T.; Komai, M. Vitamin K suppresses the lipopolysaccharide-induced expression of inflammatory cytokines in cultured macrophage-like cells via the inhibition of the activation of nuclear factor κB through the repression of IKKalpha/beta phosphorylation. *J. Nutr. Biochem.* **2010**, *21*, 1120–1126. [CrossRef] [PubMed]
15. Moriya, M.; Nakatsuji, Y.; Okuno, T.; Hamasaki, T.; Sawada, M.; Sakoda, S. Vitamin K_2 ameliorates experimental autoimmune encephalomyelitis in lewis rats. *J. Neuroimmunol.* **2005**, *170*, 11–20. [CrossRef] [PubMed]
16. Li, J.; Lin, J.C.; Wang, H.; Peterson, J.W.; Furie, B.C.; Furie, B.; Booth, S.L.; Volpe, J.J.; Rosenberg, P.A. Novel role of vitamin K in preventing oxidative injury to developing oligodendrocytes and neurons. *J. Neurosci.* **2003**, *23*, 5816–5826. [PubMed]
17. Li, J.; Wang, H.; Rosenberg, P.A. Vitamin K prevents oxidative cell death by inhibiting activation of 12-lipoxygenase in developing oligodendrocytes. *J. Neurosci. Res.* **2009**, *87*, 1997–2005. [CrossRef] [PubMed]
18. Shibayama-Imazu, T.; Aiuchi, T.; Nakaya, K. Vitamin K_2-mediated apoptosis in cancer cells: Role of mitochondrial transmembrane potential. *Vitam. Horm.* **2008**, *78*, 211–226. [PubMed]
19. Ozaki, I.; Zhang, H.; Mizuta, T.; Ide, Y.; Eguchi, Y.; Yasutake, T.; Sakamaki, T.; Pestell, R.G.; Yamamoto, K. Menatetrenone, a vitamin K_2 analogue, inhibits hepatocellular carcinoma cell growth by suppressing cyclin D1 expression through inhibition of nuclear factor κB activation. *Clin. Cancer Res.* **2007**, *13*, 2236–2245. [CrossRef] [PubMed]
20. Tabb, M.M.; Sun, A.; Zhou, C.; Grun, F.; Errandi, J.; Romero, K.; Pham, H.; Inoue, S.; Mallick, S.; Lin, M.; *et al.* Vitamin K_2 regulation of bone homeostasis is mediated by the steroid and xenobiotic receptor SXR. *J. Biol. Chem.* **2003**, *278*, 43919–43927. [CrossRef] [PubMed]
21. Ichikawa, T.; Horie-Inoue, K.; Ikeda, K.; Blumberg, B.; Inoue, S. Steroid and xenobiotic receptor SXR mediates vitamin K_2-activated transcription of extracellular matrix-related genes and collagen accumulation in osteoblastic cells. *J. Biol. Chem.* **2006**, *281*, 16927–16934. [CrossRef] [PubMed]

22. Tsang, C.K.; Kamei, Y. Novel effect of vitamin K$_1$ (phylloquinone) and vitamin K$_2$ (menaquinone) on promoting nerve growth factor-mediated neurite outgrowth from PC12D cells. *Neurosci. Lett.* **2002**, *323*, 9–12. [CrossRef]

23. Otsuka, M.; Kato, N.; Shao, R.X.; Hoshida, Y.; Ijichi, H.; Koike, Y.; Taniguchi, H.; Moriyama, M.; Shiratori, Y.; Kawabe, T.; *et al.* Vitamin K$_2$ inhibits the growth and invasiveness of hepatocellular carcinoma cells via protein kinase A activation. *Hepatology* **2004**, *40*, 243–251. [CrossRef] [PubMed]

24. Ichikawa, T.; Horie-Inoue, K.; Ikeda, K.; Blumberg, B.; Inoue, S. Vitamin K$_2$ induces phosphorylation of protein kinase A and expression of novel target genes in osteoblastic cells. *J. Mol. Endocrinol.* **2007**, *39*, 239–247. [CrossRef] [PubMed]

25. Ito, A.; Shirakawa, H.; Takumi, N.; Minegishi, Y.; Ohashi, A.; Howlader, Z.H.; Ohsaki, Y.; Sato, T.; Goto, T.; Komai, M. Menaquinone-4 enhances testosterone production in rats and testis-derived tumor cells. *Lipids Health Dis.* **2011**, *10*, 158. [CrossRef] [PubMed]

26. Ronden, J.E.; Thijssen, H.H.; Vermeer, C. Tissue distribution of K-vitamers under different nutritional regimens in the rat. *Biochim. Biophys. Acta* **1998**, *1379*, 16–22. [CrossRef]

27. Sato, T.; Ozaki, R.; Kamo, S.; Hara, Y.; Konishi, S.; Isobe, Y.; Saitoh, S.; Harada, H. The biological activity and tissue distribution of 2′,3′-dihydrophylloquinone in rats. *Biochim. Biophys. Acta* **2003**, *1622*, 145–150. [CrossRef]

28. Booth, S.L.; Peterson, J.W.; Smith, D.; Shea, M.K.; Chamberland, J.; Crivello, N. Age and dietary form of vitamin K affect menaquinone-4 concentrations in male fischer 344 rats. *J. Nutr.* **2008**, *138*, 492–496. [PubMed]

29. Huber, A.M.; Davidson, K.W.; O'Brien-Morse, M.E.; Sadowski, J.A. Tissue phylloquinone and menaquinones in rats are affected by age and gender. *J. Nutr.* **1999**, *129*, 1039–1044. [PubMed]

30. Huber, A.M.; Davidson, K.W.; O'Brien-Morse, M.E.; Sadowski, J.A. Gender differences in hepatic phylloquinone and menaquinones in the vitamin K-deficient and -supplemented rat. *Biochim. Biophys. Acta* **1999**, *1426*, 43–52. [CrossRef]

31. Anton, B.; Vitetta, L.; Cortizo, F.; Sali, A. Can we delay aging? The biology and science of aging. *Ann. N. Y. Acad. Sci.* **2005**, *1057*, 525–535. [CrossRef] [PubMed]

32. Speakman, J.R.; Mitchell, S.E. Caloric restriction. *Mol. Asp. Med.* **2011**, *32*, 159–221. [CrossRef] [PubMed]

33. Fontana, L.; Partridge, L. Promoting health and longevity through diet: From model organisms to humans. *Cell* **2015**, *161*, 106–118. [CrossRef] [PubMed]

34. Kindberg, C.G.; Suttie, J.W. Effect of various intakes of phylloquinone on signs of vitamin K deficiency and serum and liver phylloquinone concentrations in the rat. *J. Nutr.* **1989**, *119*, 175–180. [PubMed]

35. Carrie, I.; Portoukalian, J.; Vicaretti, R.; Rochford, J.; Potvin, S.; Ferland, G. Menaquinone-4 concentration is correlated with sphingolipid concentrations in rat brain. *J. Nutr.* **2004**, *134*, 167–172. [PubMed]

36. Davidson, K.W.; Sadowski, J.A. Determination of vitamin K compounds in plasma or serum by high-performance liquid chromatography using postcolumn chemical reduction and fluorimetric detection. *Methods Enzymol.* **1997**, *282*, 408–421. [PubMed]

37. Wang, L.Y.; Bates, C.J.; Yan, L.; Harrington, D.J.; Shearer, M.J.; Prentice, A. Determination of phylloquinone (vitamin K$_1$) in plasma and serum by HPLC with fluorescence detection. *Clin. Chim. Acta* **2004**, *347*, 199–207. [CrossRef] [PubMed]

38. Booth, S.L.; Centi, A.J.; Gundberg, C. Bone as an endocrine organ relevant to diabetes. *Curr. Diab. Rep.* **2014**, *14*, 556. [CrossRef] [PubMed]

39. Tokita, H.; Tsuchida, A.; Miyazawa, K.; Ohyashiki, K.; Katayanagi, S.; Sudo, H.; Enomoto, M.; Takagi, Y.; Aoki, T. Vitamin K$_2$-induced antitumor effects via cell-cycle arrest and apoptosis in gastric cancer cell lines. *Int. J. Mol. Med.* **2006**, *17*, 235–243. [CrossRef] [PubMed]

40. Menard, C.; Quirion, R.; Bouchard, S.; Ferland, G.; Gaudreau, P. Glutamatergic signaling and low prodynorphin expression are associated with intact memory and reduced anxiety in rat models of healthy aging. *Front. Aging Neurosci.* **2014**, *6*, 81. [PubMed]

41. Moyse, E.; Bedard, K.; Segura, S.; Mahaut, S.; Tardivel, C.; Ferland, G.; Lebrun, B.; Gaudreau, P. Effects of aging and caloric restriction on brainstem satiety center signals in rats. *Mech. Ageing Dev.* **2012**, *133*, 83–91. [CrossRef] [PubMed]

42. Sogabe, N.; Maruyama, R.; Baba, O.; Hosoi, T.; Goseki-Sone, M. Effects of long-term vitamin K$_1$ (phylloquinone) or vitamin K$_2$ (menaquinone-4) supplementation on body composition and serum parameters in rats. *Bone* **2011**, *48*, 1036–1042. [CrossRef] [PubMed]

43. Knapen, M.H.; Schurgers, L.J.; Shearer, M.J.; Newman, P.; Theuwissen, E.; Vermeer, C. Association of vitamin K status with adiponectin and body composition in healthy subjects: Uncarboxylated osteocalcin is not associated with fat mass and body weight. *Br. J. Nutr.* **2012**, *108*, 1017–1024. [CrossRef] [PubMed]
44. Mellette, S.J. Interrelationships between vitamin K and estrogenic hormones. *Am. J. Clin. Nutr.* **1961**, *9*, 108–116. [PubMed]
45. Ronden, J.E.; Drittij-Reijnders, M.J.; Vermeer, C.; Thijssen, H.H. Intestinal flora is not an intermediate in the phylloquinone-menaquinone-4 conversion in the rat. *Biochim. Biophys. Acta* **1998**, *1379*, 69–75. [CrossRef]
46. Jolly, D.W.; Craig, C.; Nelson, T.E., Jr. Estrogen and prothrombin synthesis: Effect of estrogen on absorption of vitamin K1. *Am. J. Physiol.* **1977**, *232*, H12–H17. [PubMed]
47. Lopez-Otin, C.; Blasco, M.A.; Partridge, L.; Serrano, M.; Kroemer, G. The hallmarks of aging. *Cell* **2013**, *153*, 1194–1217. [CrossRef] [PubMed]
48. Metta, V.A.; Mameesh, M.S.; Johnson, B.C. Vitamin K deficiency in rats induced by the feeding of irradiated beef. *J. Nutr.* **1959**, *69*, 18–22. [PubMed]
49. Gustafsson, B.E.; Daft, F.S.; Mc, D.E.; Smith, J.C.; Fitzgerald, R.J. Effects of vitamin K-active compounds and intestinal microorganisms in vitamin K-deficient germfree rats. *J. Nutr.* **1962**, *78*, 461–468. [PubMed]
50. Kenessary, A.; Zhumadilov, Z.; Nurgozhin, T.; Kipling, D.; Yeoman, M.; Cox, L.; Ostler, E.; Faragher, R. Biomarkers, interventions and healthy ageing. *New Biotechnol.* **2013**, *30*, 373–377. [CrossRef] [PubMed]
51. Kamzalov, S.; Sohal, R.S. Effect of age and caloric restriction on coenzyme q and alpha-tocopherol levels in the rat. *Exp. Gerontol.* **2004**, *39*, 1199–1205. [CrossRef] [PubMed]

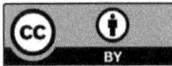

MDPI AG

St. Alban-Anlage 66

4052 Basel, Switzerland

Tel. +41 61 683 77 34

Fax +41 61 302 89 18

http://www.mdpi.com

Nutrients Editorial Office

E-mail: nutrients @mdpi.com

http://www.mdpi.com/journal/nutrients